Essential Vascular Surgery

For WB Saunders

Commissioning Editor Margaret Macdonald
Project Manager Mark Sanderson
Copy Editor Lucy Gardner
Indexer John Sampson

Essential Vascular Surgery

Edited by

Alun H Davies MA DM FRCS
Senior Lecturer and Honorary Consultant
in General and Vascular Surgery
Division of Surgery, Anaesthetics and Intensive Care
Imperial College School of Medicine
Charing Cross Hospital
London, UK

Jonathan D Beard FRCS ChM
Consultant Vascular Surgeon
Sheffield Vascular Institute
Northern General Hospital NHS Trust
Sheffield, UK

Michael G Wyatt MD MSc FRCS
Consultant Vascular Surgeon
Northern Vascular Centre
Freeman Hospital
Newcastle upon Tyne, UK

WB Saunders Company Limited
London   Philadelphia   Toronto   Sydney   Tokyo

WB Saunders Company Limited
An imprint of Harcourt Brace and Company Limited

© Harcourt Brace and Company Limited 1999

Ⓦ is a registered trademark of Harcourt Brace and Company Limited

First published 1999

ISBN 0-7020-2326-4

British Library Cataloguing in Publication Data
A catalogue record for this book is available from the British Library

Library of Congress Cataloging in Publication Data
A catalog record for this book is available from the Library of Congress

Note
Medical knowledge is constantly changing. As new information becomes
available, changes in treatment, procedures, equipment and the use of drugs
become necessary. The editors, contributors and the publishers have, as far as
it is possible, taken care to ensure that the information given in this text is
accurate and up to date. However, readers are strongly advised to confirm that
the information, especially with regard to drug usage, complies with the latest
legislation and standards of practice.

The
Publisher's
policy is to use
**paper manufactured
from sustainable forests**
||

Typeset by Expo Holdings Sdn. Bhd, Malaysia
Printed in China

Contents

Contributors

Petter Aadahl MD PhD
Department of Anaesthesiology
University Hospital of Trondheim
Trondheim, Norway

Jonathan D Beard FRCS ChM
Consultant Vascular Surgeon
Sheffield Vascular Institute
Northern General Hospital NHS Trust
Sheffield, UK

Andrew JM Boulton MD FRCP
Professor, Department of Medicine
Manchester Royal Infirmary
Manchester, UK

Kevin G Burnand MS FRCS
Chairman of GKT Department of
Surgery
St Thomas' Hospital
London, UK

S Byford BSc MSc
Centre for Health Economics
University of York
York, UK

Bruce Campbell MS FRCP FRCS
Consultant in Vascular and General
Surgery
Royal Devon and Exeter Hospital
Exeter, UK

John Chamberlain FRCS (Ed) FRCS
(Eng)
Consultant Vascular Surgeon
Northern Vascular Unit
Freeman Hospital
Newcastle upon Tyne, UK

Trevor Cleveland FRCS FRCR
Senior Lecturer in Vascular Radiology
Sheffield Vascular Institute
Northern General Hospital NHS Trust
Sheffield, UK

Alun H Davies MA DM FRCS
Senior Lecturer and Honorary
Consultant in General and Vascular
Surgery
Division of Surgery, Anaesthetics and
Intensive Care
Imperial College School of Medicine
Charing Cross Hospital
London, UK

FGR Fowkes PhD FRCP FFPHM
Professor, Wolfson Unit for Prevention
of Peripheral Vascular Diseases
Public Health Sciences
University of Edinburgh
Edinburgh, UK

Neil CM Fyfe MChir FRCS FRCP
Department of Rehabilitation
Medicine
Freeman Hospital
Newcastle upon Tyne, UK

Peter A Gaines MRCP FRCR
Sheffield Vascular Unit
Northern General Hospital NHS
Trust
Sheffield, UK

AM Garratt PhD
National Centre for Health Outcomes
Unit of Health-Care Epidemiology
Department of Public Health
University of Oxford
Oxford, UK

Roger M Greenhalgh MA MD MChir
FRCS
Professor of Surgery
Imperial College School of Medicine
Charing Cross Hospital
London, UK

George Hamilton MB ChB FRCS
Consultant Vascular Surgeon
Royal Free Hampstead NHS Trust
Royal Free and University College
School of Medicine
London, UK

Michelle Hayes MD FRCA
Consultant Anaesthetist
Magill Department of Anaesthesia
Chelsea and Westminster Hospital
London, UK

Edward Housley FRCP (Edin) FRCP
(Lond)
Consultant Physician
Peripheral Vascular Clinic
Royal Infirmary
Edinburgh, UK

James Jackson MRCP FRCR
Senior Lecturer and Consultant
Radiologist
Imperial College School of Medicine
Hammersmith Hospital
London, UK

Nick JM London MRCP FRCS MD
Professor of Surgery
Department of Surgery
Leicester University
Leicester, UK

Jan Lundbom MD
Department of Surgery
University Hospital of Trondheim
Trondheim, Norway

Shane TR MacSweeney MA MChir
FRCS
Consultant Vascular Surgeon
Department of Vascular and
Endovascular Surgery
University Hospital
Nottingham, UK

Derek Manas BSc MBBCh FCS(SA)
Consultant Surgeon in Transplant
Surgery
Freeman Hospital
Honorary Clinical Lecturer in
Transplant Surgery
University of Newcastle
Newcastle upon Tyne, UK

Catharine L McGuinness FRCS
Surgical Unit
St Thomas' Hospital
London, UK

Hans O Myhre MD PhD
Professor and Chairman
Department of Surgery
University Hospital of Trondheim
Trondheim, Norway

A Ross Naylor MD FRCS
Consultant Vascular Surgeon and
Honorary Senior Lecturer in Surgery
Department of Surgery
Leicester Royal Infirmary
Leicester, UK

Mark Palazzo MD FRCA FRCP
Department of Anaesthetics
Charing Cross Hospital
London, UK

JF Price BSc MBChB
Clinical Lecturer
Wolfson Unit for Prevention of
Peripheral Vascular Disease
Public Health Sciences
University of Edinburgh
Edinburgh, UK

Jonathan E Shaw MRCP
Research Fellow
Department of Medicine
Manchester Royal Infirmary
Manchester, UK

Clifford P Shearman BSc MS FRCS
Department of Vascular Surgery
Southampton University Hospital
Southampton, UK

JF Thompson MS FRCS
Consultant Vascular and General
Surgeon
Exeter Vascular Service
Royal Devon & Exeter Hospitals
Exeter, UK

DJ Torgerson PhD
Centre for Health Economics
University of York
York, UK

Alasdair J Walker FRCS
Consultant Vascular and General
Surgeon
Vascular Unit
Derriford Hospital
Plymouth, UK

Ian M Williams MD FRCS
Department of Vascular Surgery
St Mary's Hospital
London, UK

John HN Wolfe MS FRCS
Department of Vascular Surgery
St Mary's Hospital
London, UK

Michael G Wyatt MD MSc FRCS
Consultant Vascular Surgeon
Northern Vascular Centre
Freeman Hospital
Newcastle upon Tyne, UK

Preface

Essential Vascular Surgery is an easy-to-use text, covering the basic principles of vascular disease and its management. It has been written in a straightforward format and each chapter uses a similar style to lead the reader through the various aspects of arterial and venous disease in a didactic and problem-orientated way. At the end of each chapter, there is a summary list and areas of controversy are highlighted. Instead of producing a referenced text, each chapter contains a list of key references which will enable the reader to acquire further information if necessary.

The text is aimed at surgical trainees and residents but it will also provide an invaluable guide for all health care professionals interested in vascular disorders.

Acknowledgement

The editors would like to thank all the contributors for their hard work in the preparation of this text and would also like to thank the editorial staff at the publishers for their help in producing this text.

Alun H Davies
Jonathan D Beard
Michael G Wyatt

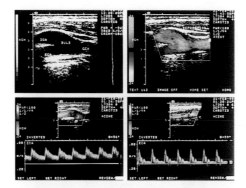

Plate 1. Duplex scanning couples real-time B-mode ultrasound imaging of vessels: in this case, the carotid bifurcation (top left) with pulsed Doppler which can sample the blood flow waveform from any point within the lumen (bottom left and right). Colour Doppler represents the duration and velocity of flow by colour (red to blue) and saturation (colour to white), respectively (top right). (See p. 50.)

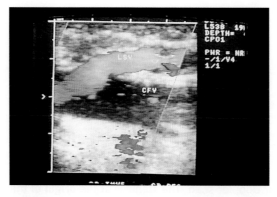

Plate 2. Colour Doppler scan of an incompetent saphenofemoral junction (represented in monochrome). There is reflux down the long saphenous vein (LSV) on release of calf compression, whereas the valves in the common femoral vein (CFV) are competent (no flow). (See p. 57.)

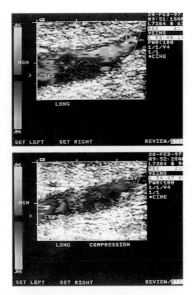

Plate 3. Colour Doppler scan of superficial femoral vein containing non-occlusive thrombus (represented in monochrome). The thrombus is more echogenic than non-flowing blood and is black compared with flowing blood (coloured). The vein can only be partly compressed (bottom scan). (See p. 60.)

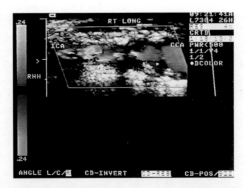

Plate 4. Colour Doppler scan. The stenosis at the origin of the internal carotid artery can be estimated from the proportion of the lumen occupied by plaque (black) and by the increased blood velocity (represented by a shift towards white). The most accurate parameter is the peak systolic velocity of the pulsed Doppler waveform (not shown). (See p. 124.)

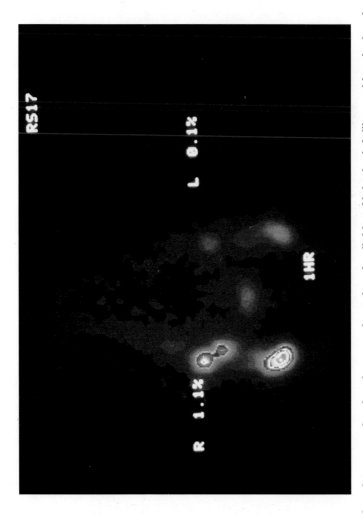

Plate 5. Lymphoscintogram showing decreased uptake of colloid at 1h in the left iliac and inguinal nodes, confirming left-sided lymphatic obstruction. (See p. 284.)

1
Aetiology of Vascular Disease

Michael G Wyatt

Introduction

Vascular disease is common in modern society and primarily involves the arterial and venous components of the peripheral circulation. In the middle-aged and elderly population, at any one time between 5% and 7% will be suffering symptoms attributable to either coronary or peripheral atherosclerosis and 20% will suffer from various degrees of venous insufficiency.

The aetiology of both peripheral atherosclerosis and chronic venous insufficiency is complex and as yet the causation of each condition is not fully understood. To help understand the mechanisms resulting in these conditions, the basic anatomy and physiology of the arterial and venous systems are described at the beginning of each section below.

Arterial system

Anatomy

The arterial system is a complex and highly organized structured organ that must withstand the stress of pulsatile arterial blood flow.

Large and medium sized arteries consist of three distinct layers, each of which must remain intact for normal function:

- intima;
- media;
- adventitia.

The *intima* is the innermost layer. It consists of a monolayer of flat endothelial cells with a thin underlying matrix of collagen and elastic fibres. The *internal elastic membrane* separates the intima from the media.

The *media* is a relatively thick middle layer which contains varying amounts of collagen, smooth muscle and elastic fibres. The content of elastic fibres decreases with increasing distance of the artery from the heart. The innermost portion of the media is nourished by the circulating blood and the outermost by small vessels which penetrate its outer wall (vasa vasorum). These vessels may be affected by the athero-sclerotic process leading to a decrease in wall strength. An *external elastic membrane* separates the media from the adventitia.

The outer layer of the artery is the *adventitia*. Although it may appear thin and weak, its high elastic and collagen content make it a key element in the overall strength of the artery.

Pathophysiology

The basic principles of fluid dynamics can help to explain the physio-logic consequences of arterial occlusive and aneurysmal disease.

Occlusive disease

As blood flow to an extremity or organ is reduced by the formation of atherosclerotic plaques, symptoms will eventually become apparent. This occurs when a critical arterial stenosis is reached (75% of cross-sectional area, 50% of vessel diameter). At this degree of vessel stenosis, both blood flow and pressure begin to fall (Fig. 1.1). Other factors which influence the degree of critical stenosis to a lesser extent include:

- length of stenosis;
- blood viscosity;
- peripheral resistance.

The longer the stenosis, the earlier is the critical stenosis reached. In addition, flow and pressure across a stenosis diminish more quickly if the

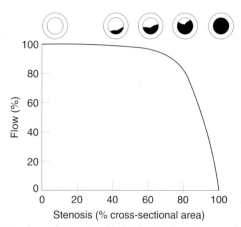

Fig. 1.1. Blood flow in relation to degree of arterial stenosis. Note that blood flow remains relatively normal until the cross-sectional area of the vessel is reduced to 25%. (Adapted from May AG *et al.* Critical arterial stenosis. *Surgery* 1963; **54**:250.)

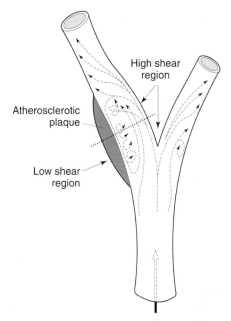

Fig. 1.2. **Relationship between low and high shear stress at the carotid bifurcation. Atherosclerotic plaques tend to develop on the outer wall of the internal carotid artery at areas of boundary layer separation and low shear stress.** (Adapted from Zarins CK *et al.* Atherosclerotic plaque distribution and flow velocity profiles in the carotid bifurcation. In: Bergan JJ, Yao JST (eds) *Cerebrovascular Insufficiency.* New York: Grune and Stratton, 1983.)

blood is more viscous. In patients with a low peripheral resistance, flow is increased but turbulence around the stenosis is worsened and pressure across the lesion may drop.

Turbulence is the most important cause of blood flow and pressure drop across a vascular stenosis. Indeed, it has been shown that atherosclerotic plaques tend to form at areas of blood separation and low shear stress. At these arterial bifurcations, although flow in the centre of the vessel is rapid and laminar, the flow in the boundary area adjacent to this fast flow is often slowed and may even be reversed, especially in the presence of an atherosclerotic plaque (Fig. 1.2).

Aneurysmal disease

The pathophysiological mechanisms that result in aneurysm formation are multifactorial (Fig. 1.3). Aneurysms form as a result of degeneration and weakening of the components of their arterial wall. Rupture occurs if the intraluminal pressure exceeds the tensile strength of the wall.

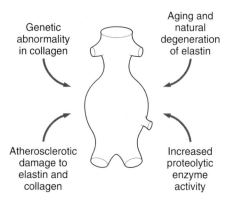

Fig. 1.3. Factors which may contribute to the development of arterial aneurysms.

The aetiology of arterial wall degeneration is not fully understood; nevertheless, certain haemodynamic principles may assist the understanding of aneurysm formation. These include:

- reflective pressure waves at iliac bifurcation;
- paucity of vasa vasorum in abdominal aorta;
- collagen and elastic defects associated with certain connective tissue disorders, e.g. Marfan's syndrome.

When arterial flow reaches a bifurcation (e.g. aortic flow into iliacs), some of the flow is reflected against the arterial wall just proximal to this bifurcation. When the ratio of the cross-sectional areas of the outflow arteries (e.g. iliacs) to the inflow artery (e.g. aorta) is approximately 1.0, this reflective pressure wave is minimal. With advancing age, this ratio decreases and the pressure of the reflective blood flow increases. This may result in dilatation of the vessel at this point (aortic aneurysm).

In addition, with the development of atherosclerosis in the abdominal aorta, the aortic vasa vasorum is obliterated. This may result in necrosis of the media which causes weakening and aneurysmal dilatation of the aorta.

Finally, in certain connective tissue diseases such as Marfan's syndrome, defects in the structural integrity of the vessel collagen and elastin content are found. Again, this may predispose to aneurysm formation.

Atherosclerosis

The aetiology of most arterial disease in the modern world is atherosclerosis. Atherosclerosis describes a combination of changes in the intima and media of an artery. These changes include:

Table 1.1. **Major risk factors for atherosclerosis.**

Positive	Men >45 years
	Women >55 years or premature menopause (no HRT)
	Family history of premature atherosclerosis
	Smoking
	Hypertension
	HDL <35 mg/dl
	Diabetes mellitus
Negative	HDL cholesterol >60 mg/dl

- focal accumulation of lipids;
- haemorrhage;
- fibrous tissue;
- calcium deposits.

The causes of atherosclerosis are multifactorial and involve a combination of hereditary factors, hypertension, raised cholesterol, diabetes, diet, lack of exercise and smoking. Not all of these are essential to the development of atherosclerosis, but all have a role to play and are involved in the progression of this common disorder of the peripheral arterial system. The major risk factors for the development of atherosclerosis are listed in Table 1.1.

Cigarette smoking

Cigarette smokers are at high risk of developing symptoms of peripheral artherosclerosis. With continuation of the habit, the condition progresses and can result in amputation, myocardial infarction and increased failure rates in vascular grafts.

Smokers have up to a 4-fold chance of developing peripheral atherosclerosis compared with those who have never smoked and cigarette smoking appears to be the single most important risk factor in the development of peripheral vascular disease. Current smoking is estimated to cause 14–53% of disease and if ex-smokers are included, this figure rises. Recent studies have suggested that 80% of cases of intermittent claudication can be attributed to smoking.

Exact mechanisms for the causation of atherosclerosis by smoking are unknown. Intermittent carbon monoxidaemia probably predisposes to arterial wall injury by producing increased plasma flux and increased entry of Low-density lipoproteins (LDLs) and other proteins. Cigarette smoking also causes increased platelet reactivity, promotes peripheral vasoconstriction and is associated with reduced high-density lipoprotein (HDL) levels.

In addition, smokers have lower intakes of antioxidants such as β-carotene and vitamin C. This antioxidant deficiency may in itself be

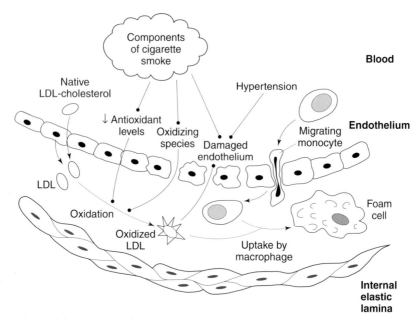

Fig. 1.4. Interactions between smoking, hypertension, LDL-cholesterol and antioxidants in the formation of foam cells. (Reproduced from Leng FC, Fowkes FGR. Epidemiology and risk factors for peripheral vascular disease. In: Beard D, Gaines PA (eds) *Vascular and Endovascular Surgery*. Philadelphia: WB Saunders, 1998 with permission.)

responsible for some of the peripheral atherosclerosis associated with smoking. The very act of smoking a cigarette will also have a deleterious effect on antioxidant status due to the many reactive oxidizing species found in the gas and tar phase of tobacco smoke. Therefore, the combination of an enhanced free radical load and a low antioxidant intake in smokers will result in increased oxidation of fatty acids and atherogenicity of LDL cholesterol (Fig. 1.4).

Lipid abnormalities

Cholesterol

Arterial disease was first induced in rabbits over 80 years ago by feeding them cholesterol. Evidence of a causal role for fats in human arterial disease is steadily increasing. These include epidemiological (see Chapter 2) and metabolic studies and are supported by several intervention trials involving both cholesterol-lowering drugs and diet.

The first clear evidence of a link between raised blood cholesterol and the subsequent development of atherosclerosis came from the

Framingham study. There is now a strong case to support the relationship between fats and the development of atherosclerosis.

Biochemical measures which predict the risk of atherosclerotic disease include:

- total serum cholesterol;
- LDL-cholesterol;
- HDL-cholesterol.

Lipoproteins

Lipoproteins are large complexes containing cholesterol, cholesteryl esters, triglyceride, phospholipid and protein in varying quantities. LDLs are the main carriers of cholesterol from the liver to the peripheral tissues. High levels of LDL-cholesterol promote atherosclerosis. By contrast, HDLs transfer cholesterol from the peripheral tissues back to the liver. High levels of HDL-cholesterol are a negative risk factor for the development of atherosclerosis. There is also some evidence that HDL-cholesterol levels may be related to cigarette smoking and reduced physical activity.

Nevertheless, at all ages, serum cholesterol tends to mirror LDL-cholesterol levels and measurement of serum cholesterol remains the most important indicator of risk. Measurement of LDLs and HDLs provides refined risk estimates for the development of peripheral atherosclerosis. Favourable levels in middle-aged men are:

- total cholesterol <185 mg/dl;
- LDL <140 mg/dl;
- HDL >45 mg/dl.

Apolipoproteins

Another factor which may be important in the development of atherosclerosis is the presence of apolipoproteins A and B. These are moieties of the protein constituent of the lipoprotein molecule and are found in chylomicrons. They have an important role in the absorption and transport of cholesterol and triglycerides. The measurement of apolipoprotein levels in the peripheral circulation may discriminate between patients with atherosclerosis and normal controls with more accuracy than lipid or lipoprotein levels alone.

Apolipoprotein B is associated with LDL-cholesterol and a tendency for this lipoprotein to enter the arterial wall. This is genetically linked to obesity and a tendency to develop coronary artery disease. Genetic hyperlipidaemia, such as familial hypercholesterolaemia Type II, is due to a lack of LDL receptors, mainly in the hepatocytes. This causes an inability to incorporate and metabolize LDLs within the liver. Exceedingly high LDL levels and premature death from atherosclerosis inevitably result.

Apolipoprotein A is the main constituent of HDL-cholesterols and is a 'helper protein'. High HDL levels are markers of relative immunity from coronary artery disease and are associated with fewer and less severe atherosclerotic lesions. High HDL levels are found in people who take regular exercise and those who stop smoking.

Antioxidant status

Antioxidants protect polyunsaturated fatty acids from peroxidation and occur naturally as vitamins A, C, E and the provitamin β-carotene. It is known that the production of lipid peroxides following fatty-acid peroxidation is related to the severity of aortic atherosclerosis. In addition, plasma lipid peroxide levels are higher in patients with peripheral vascular disease than controls. Although a lower dietary intake of vitamins C, A and D has been found in patients with peripheral vascular disease, the causal relationship remains to be proven.

The oxidation of LDL-cholesterol that occurs in the absence of antioxidants is thought to encourage their subsequent uptake by macrophages, forming the cholesterol-laden foam cell (Fig. 1.4). Conclusive evidence of the role of antioxidants in the prevention of atherosclerosis is awaited.

Hypertension

Hypertension is a major cardiovascular risk factor and has been associated with the presence of peripheral vascular disease in many studies. Patients with intermittent claudication generally have higher mean blood pressures than normal controls and the control of hypertension can prolong life by reducing the risk of myocardial infarction.

Atherosclerosis due to hyperlipidaemia is accelerated by chronic hypertension in experimental animals. This effect has not been proven in humans; nevertheless, the cause of accelerated atheroma in hypertensive patients appears to relate to continued haemodynamic injury. This accelerates plaque growth and promotes plaque complications. It appears to exacerbate the effect of smoking by increasing nicotine movement across the endothelial cell membrane.

Diabetes mellitus

Types I and II diabetes mellitus are major risk factors for the development and progression of atherosclerosis. Diabetics have more severe atherosclerosis at an earlier age than non-diabetics, and in the absence of other risk factors this atherosclerosis tends to involve the infragenicular arteries, sparing the more proximal arterial tree.

The mechanism by which diabetes accelerates the development of peripheral atherosclerosis is unknown. Insulin therapy can control the hyperlipidaemia associated with diabetes and decrease total cholesterol synthesis, but the role of glucose intolerance in the aetiology of peripheral vascular disease is not fully understood.

Rheological factors

Other factors thought to influence the development and progression of atherosclerosis include fibrinogen and haemostatic factors. Increased fibrinogen is a significant risk factor for myocardial infarction and is found in elevated concentrations in patients with intermittent claudication. Blood viscosity is also higher in patients with intermittent claudication and some studies have also shown a raised haematocrit. There is also a raised fibrinogen lysis time, decreased fibrinolytic activity and raised levels of factor VIII, XIII, plasminogen and antiplasmin in these subjects. In addition, platelet function is altered with low counts, increased aggregatability and decreased platelet survival times. The levels of von Willebrand factor, β-thromboglobulin, plasminogen activator inhibitor and fibrin-degradation products are raised in patients with peripheral arterial disease, although these may be related more to smoking.

These results indicate that patients with peripheral vascular disease have an increased thrombogenic tendency, although why this contributes to chronic vessel wall damage is unclear. It would, however, appear that these rheological factors are important in producing superimposed plaque thrombosis and arterial occlusion in the presence of established atherosclerosis.

Other risk factors

These include:

- lack of exercise;
- obesity;
- psychological factors.

Physically active men have less chance of developing ischaemic heart disease than sedentary men. Obesity is controversial. It is known that life-expectancy increases with weight reduction, but this reduction may be related to other risk factors. Finally, psychological studies have shown an increased risk of coronary artery, cerebrovascular and peripheral vascular disease in Type IA personalities. These people are competitive, ambitious and stressed.

The atheromatous plaque

The degree of severity of atheromatous plaques is dependent upon plaque type and its stage of development. They commonly contain three components (Table 1.2).

Table 1.2. **Main components of atherosclerotic plaques.**

Cholesterol	Mainly cholesteryl esters
Cells	Mainly smooth muscle, macrophages and others
Fibrous proteins	Mainly collagen, elastin and glycosaminoglycan

The development of atherosclerosis is a complex biochemical and cellular process. The gross appearance and development of an atherosclerotic plaque can be divided into three major stages.

- early lesions;
- fibrous plaques;
- complicated lesions.

Early lesions

Early lesions usually appear as fatty streaks in young adult life. They are minimally raised, yellow lesions often found in infants and children. They consist of lipid deposits within macrophages and in smooth muscle cells. These lipids are similar to plasma lipids and may have entered the arterial wall from the blood stream.

Fibrous plaques

These are more advanced atheromatous lesion. They are composed of large numbers of smooth muscle cells and connective tissue, which form a fibrous cap over an inner yellow core containing mainly cholesterol esters (Fig. 1.5).

Fibrous plaques appear chronologically after fatty streaks, often in the same anatomical locations. They can also arise following conversion of mural thrombus into atheroma. These fibrous plaques gradually encroach into the arterial lumen until flow is compromised and obstructed, resulting in arterial occlusion.

Arteries containing fibrous plaques often exhibit periarterial inflammation, fibrosis and lymphocytic infiltration which relates linearly to disease severity. Neovascularization from the adventitia characterizes intermediate and fibrous plaque lesions.

Complicated lesions

Fibrous plaques complicated by calcification, ulceration, haemorrhage or extensive necrosis compromise end-stage atherosclerosis. These represent late developments in fibrous plaques and are associated with the clinical complications of stroke, gangrene and myocardial infarction.

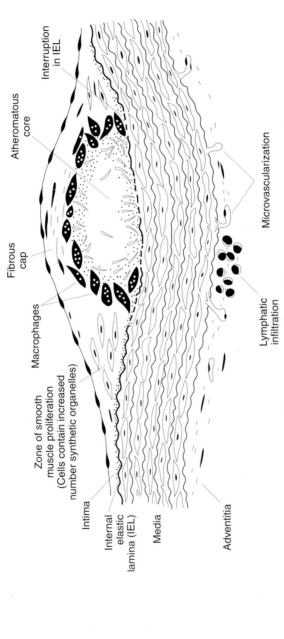

Fig. 1.5. **Fibrous atheromatous plaque.** (Reproduced from DePalma RG. The pathology of atheromas. In: Bell PRF, Jamieson CW, Ruckley CV (eds) *Surgical Management of Vascular Disease.* London: WB Saunders, 1992, with permission.)

Labels in figure:

Interruption in IEL

Atheromatous core

Fibrous cap

Macrophages

Zone of smooth muscle proliferation (Cells contain increased number synthetic organelles)

Intima

Internal elastic lamina (IEL)

Media

Adventitia

Microvascularization

Lymphatic infiltration

Aneurysms are also manifestations of advanced atherosclerosis and represent a unique atherosclerotic response which may be genetically conditioned.

Mechanisms of atherosclerosis

The mechanisms for the development of atherosclerosis remain controversial, but may involve mechanical injury, i.e. hypertension. A suggested series of events is as follows:

- Platelets adhere to any defect in the endothelial lining and discharge their granules.
- The release of serotonin, platelet factor 4 and catecholamines encourages the accumulation of more platelets.
- Fibrin appears and a thrombus is formed whose size and colour depends on flow velocity.
- Smooth muscle cells in the media are stimulated to proliferate by platelet-derived growth factor (PDGF).
- Smooth muscle cells break through internal elastic lamina to produce the earliest lesions of occlusive arterial disease.
- LDL receptors in these cells take up cholesterol from circulating lipoproteins. Cholesterol also accumulates independently and the lesion grows.
- Degeneration eventually occurs producing the large extravascular atheromatous deposits known as atheroma.

The effect of individual risk factors on the development of atherosclerosis remains unknown and is the subject of continuing research.

Non-atheromatous arterial disease

The pathology of non-atheromatous vascular disease is poorly understood. *Fibromuscular dysplasia* is an uncommon condition occurring in middle-aged men or younger women (see Chapter 9). It affects the medial layer of the artery and manifests as cerebrovascular insufficiency or hypertension. More often than not it presents as an incidental finding during arteriography for an unrelated condition. The renal, carotid and cerebral arteries are frequently involved and aneurysmal formation is a recognized complication of this condition.

Arteritis is a term loosely applied to a series of uncommon, poorly described conditions which tend to affect younger patients and more central arteries than atherosclerosis.

Venous system

Anatomy

Veins can be divided into the:

- superficial system;
- deep system;
- perforator system.

The *superficial system* has fairly thick-walled muscular veins, whereas the *deep veins* are thinner and accompany the arteries. *Communicating veins* perforate the muscle fascia to connect the deep and superficial systems. Normally, blood flows from the superficial to deep systems via these perforating veins. This one-way flow is assisted by one-way valves within the perforators.

Valves are found in most veins and play a central role in most venous disorders. Normal venous valves are bicuspid, opening to allow blood to flow towards the heart and closing to prevent reflux. The greatest number of valves is found in the lower leg. Valve numbers decrease as the inguinal ligament is approached. A single valve is found in the external iliac or common femoral vein and none is found in the inferior vena cava.

Venous return is assisted by the calf muscle pump. When the leg muscles (mainly soleus and gastrocnemius) contract around intra-muscular and surrounding veins, blood is pumped towards the heart. This mechanism may provide as much as 30% of the energy required to circulate the blood during strenuous exercise.

Each vein consists of three layers, but the composition and function of these differs from that of the adjacent arterial system by having:

- a relatively thin wall;
- less elastic tissue;
- a media that is mostly composed of smooth muscle (venules lack a media and smooth muscle);
- an adventitia composed of collagen and elastin which forms the major portion of large veins;
- vasa vasorum do not completely penetrate vein wall. Most nourishment comes from the contained blood flow.

Pathophysiology

The pathophysiology of venous disease relates to two mechanisms:

- valve insufficiency;
- venous obstruction.

In the normal situation, a standing individual has a venous pressure at the ankle equal to a column of blood rising to the right heart. This pressure approximates to arterial pressure. With exercise, the calf muscle pump moves blood from the superficial system, through the communicating veins to the deep system and on to the heart. Pressure in the foot vein will drop by approximately 70%.

When patients with *varicose veins* exercise, their foot pressures drop by only 30–40%. Although blood may flow normally into the deep system, as much as 25% of all femoral flow may reflux back into the superficial system and a circular motion ensues.

In patients with *chronic venous insufficiency*, the problem of venous obstruction is often added to that of valve insufficiency. These patients have usually suffered deep venous thrombosis (DVT), resulting in deep venous occlusion and damage/insufficiency of their deep venous valves. The venous obstruction tends to be of less importance and this usually decreases with time as recanalization occurs. The major pathology is incompetence of the deep venous valves which is permanent. This results in a minimal drop in venous pressure with exercise due to poor calf muscle pump function in the presence of deep venous incompetence. High ankle and foot venous pressures result in chronic oedema and heavy (40 mmHg) support stockings are often required to assist venous emptying.

Varicose veins

Varicose veins affect approximately 20% of the adult population and are either primary or secondary (following DVT, etc.).

Primary varicose veins are due to valvular failure, the cause of which is usually unclear. Theories include:

- primary valve failure secondary to degenerative changes in the valve annulus and leaflets;
- secondary valve failure due to a developmental weakness in the vein wall. This leads to secondary widening of the valve commissures and incompetence.

In each case, reverse flow and incompetence turbulence lead to incompetence, lengthening and tortuosity of subjacent vein.

In the usual situation, venous return against gravity relies on muscle pumps within the foot, calf and thigh. With muscle contraction, blood is squeezed into the deep veins and back towards the right ventricle. Perforating veins ensure that the direction of blood flow is from the superficial to the deep veins. On relaxation, reflux is prevented by valves within the superficial, deep and perforator systems. In the presence of muscle pump or valve failure or venous obstruction, this mechanism fails and venous hypertension ensues. This may promote the formation of varicose veins but may also contribute to the development of lipodermatosclerosis and venous ulceration.

Chronic venous insufficiency

Chronic venous insufficiency describes disease of the lower limbs where venous return is impaired by reflux, obstruction or muscle pump failure. This results in sustained venous hypertension which may manifest as swelling, eczema, lipodermatosclerosis and ulceration of the leg.

The causes of venous hypertension are:

- superficial venous reflux (long or short saphenous vein);
- deep venous reflux (primary or secondary to DVT);
- perforating vein reflux;
- deep venous occlusion;
- inadequate muscle pump (neurological/musculoskeletal).

The aetiology of chronic venous insufficiency involves several mechanisms, mostly involving venous reflux. Initially, most venous ulcers were thought to be secondary to previous DVT. With the advent of duplex scanning, it is now apparent that there is a group of patients with primary deep venous reflux. In addition, the superficial systems are more important than at first thought. The iliofemoral, long saphenous and popliteal veins have the greatest effect on haemodynamics and skin changes. The superficial femoral, profunda femoris and short saphenous veins have a lesser effect. By contrast, isolated perforator incompetence alone appears to have little significance in the aetiology of venous ulceration; there is almost always underlying superficial or deep reflux.

Despite this knowledge, the pathophysiological pathway from venous hypertension, through lipodermatosclerosis to venous ulceration is not fully understood. The two most popular theories for this evolution are:

- fibrin cuff theory;
- white cell trapping theory.

Fibrin cuff theory

It has been shown that a rise in venous pressure is directly transmitted to the capillary bed. This results in capillary elongation and 'opening' of the pores between the capillary cells. Larger molecules, such as fibrinogen, can now leave the capillaries and enter the pericapillary tissue space. A polymerizing reaction occurs to form fibrin which deposits itself around the capillary in a 'cuff'. This fibrin cuff then acts as a barrier to oxygen, resulting in local tissue ischaemia and cell death and eventually producing ulceration.

White cell trapping theory

This theory proposes that white cells can get 'stuck' within the capillary bed due to their large size. This is more likely to occur in the presence of a reduced perfusion pressure across the capillary bed secondary to an increase in venous pressure. Red cells gradually build up behind this obstruction to flow and these move the white cells along to the postcapillary venule. Here they are forced to marginate and adhere to the endothelial wall. The 'trapped' white cells subsequently become activated, releasing proteolytic enzymes and oxygen free radicals. These produce endothelial damage and tissue destruction. In turn, this results in endothelium permeability and fibrin deposition. In addition, perfusion is reduced by the trapped white cells and local ischaemia is produced.

Other mechanisms

Other mechanisms which may be important include:

● arteriovenous communications;
● trap hypothesis;
● tissue pressure;
● cutaneous iron overload.

It has been shown that blood draining from a limb with varicose veins or venous ulceration has a higher oxygen content than blood draining from a normal limb. The reason for this is unknown, but it has been proposed that there are direct communications between small arteries and veins in the legs of patients with venous disease. These *arteriovenous communications* may divert blood away from the skin and have a role in the development of venous ulceration.

Wound fluid from venous ulcers fails to stimulate *in vitro* proliferation of some cell types responsible for wound healing. This may be due to the trapping of growth factors and other stimulatory substances by macromolecules such as fibrinogen and α_2-macroglobulin which leak into the dermis in the presence of venous hypertension. Although not all growth factors are '*trapped*' in this way, there may be sufficient disturbance at a local level to upset the balance of tissue viability.

Both tissue and intravascular hydrostatic pressure are raised in a limb with chronic venous insufficiency. In the upper calf these changes may result in an increase in limb volume. This is not possible around the gaiter due to the tightness of the skin and the increased ratio of bone: tissue in this area. In the absence of such volume increase, a rise in *tissue pressure* in this area may lead to venous ulceration.

With the rise in hydrostatic pressure, which accompanies venous hypertension, capillary permeability increases and red cells are extravasated within the pericapillary tissues. As they degenerate, iron is released from the haemoglobin and deposited within the dermis. When excess iron is deposited, the local ferritin-binding capacity of the tissues is exceeded and iron becomes available in its bivalent form. This results in the production of oxygen free radicals and lipid peroxides which in turn can lead to tissue destruction.

Summary

- Vascular disease is common in modern society and affects both the arterial and venous systems.
- The aetiology of both artherosclerosis and chronic venous insufficiency is multifactorial and complex.
- The major risk factor for the development of atherosclerosis is smoking.
- There is clear evidence of a link between serum cholesterol and atherosclerosis.
- Primary varicose veins develop due to valve failure, the cause of which is usually unclear.
- The aetiology of chronic venous sufficiency is not fully understood.

Areas of controversy

- Relative role of the various risk factors in the development of atherosclerosis.
- Mechanisms for the development of atherosclerosis.
- Pathophysiological pathway from venous hypertension to varicose ulceration.

Further reading

- DePalma RG. The pathology of atheromas: theories of aetiology and evolution of atheromatous plaques. In: Bell PRF, Jamieson CW, Ruckley CV (eds) *Surgical Management of Vascular Disease*. London: WB Saunders, 1992, pp 21–34.
- Eastcott HHG, Rose GA. Causes and mechanisms of arterial disease. In: Eastcott HHG (ed) *Arterial Surgery*. Edinburgh: Churchill Livingstone, 1992, pp 1–30.
- Leng GC, Fowkes FGR. Epidemiology and risk factors for peripheral arterial disease. In: Beard JD, Gaines PA (eds) *Vascular and Endovascular Surgery*. Philadelphia: WB Saunders, 1998, pp 1–24.
- Lees TA, Redwood NFW. Chronic venous insufficiency and lymphoedema. In: Beard JD, Gaines PA (eds) *Vascular and Endovascular Surgery*. Philadelphia: WB Saunders, 1998, pp 397–432.
- Bradbury AW, Ruckley CV. Varicose veins. In: Beard JD, Gaines PA (eds) *Vascular and Endovascular Surgery*. Philadelphia: WB Saunders, 1998, pp 433–460.

2

Epidemiology of Peripheral Vascular Disease

JF Price and FGR Fowkes

Introduction

Epidemiological research into peripheral vascular diseases has increased in recent years, and there is now a substantial amount of data available on incidence, prevalence, risk factors and prognosis. A knowledge of the epidemiology of peripheral vascular diseases is important in predicting health-care use and evaluating treatment, and for a basic understanding of the disease processes themselves.

Arterial disease of the lower limbs

Arterial disease of the lower limbs includes conditions such as inflammatory arteritis, vasospastic disorders and medial calcification. However, by far the commonest cause of peripheral arterial disease is atherosclerosis, consisting of a slow accumulation of lipids and fibrosis in the arterial intima (see Chapter 1).

Atherosclerotic disease of the lower limbs ranges from mild asymptomatic disease to severe limb-threatening ischaemia. Asymptomatic disease can be measured by clinical tests such as the ankle brachial pressure index, the ratio of systolic blood pressure in the ankle to that in the arm (see Chapter 3). This is important in identifying people who are at risk of developing intermittent claudication and is also indicative of more widespread atherosclerosis, such as ischaemic heart disease and cerebrovascular disease. However, the conditions presenting most commonly to vascular surgeons are intermittent claudication and critical limb ischaemia.

Intermittent claudication

Intermittent claudication is the prime symptom of arterial disease of the lower limb. It is characterized by pain in the muscles of the leg when walking which is relieved by rest.

Incidence and prevalence

The prevalence of intermittent claudication in the general population ranges from 1% to 7% in middle-aged men and from 0.5% to 4.5% in middle-aged women, depending on the population examined. For example, in Scotland, intermittent claudication affects 4.5% of the population aged between 55 and 74 years. In the USA, the biennial incidence of intermittent claudication (the development of new cases over 2 years in a population initially free of disease) has been estimated at 7.1 per 1000 men and 3.6 per 1000 women. Intermittent claudication increases with age and is 1.5–2-fold more common in men than in women.

Risk factors

Risk factors for intermittent claudication reflect those for atherosclerosis in general: cigarette smoking, hyperlipidaemia and hypertension (Table 2.1).

Table 2.1. **Suggested risk factors for atherosclerotic lower limb disease.**

Personal	Age
	Male sex
Lifestyle	Smoking
	Dietary deficiency
	Antioxidant vitamins
	Vitamin C
	α-Tocopherol
	β-Carotene
	Essential fatty acids
	Alcohol
	Lack of exercise
Physiological/biological	Diabetes/glucose intolerance
	Blood pressure
	Systolic
	Diastolic
	Body mass index
	Serum lipids
	Total cholesterol
	LDL cholesterol
	Reduced HDL-cholesterol
	Triglycerides
	Haemostatic factors
	Plasma fibrinogen
	Tissue plasminogen activator
	Rheological factors
	Blood viscosity
	Plasma viscosity
	Haematocrit

Cigarette smoking is the single most powerful risk factor for peripheral arterial disease and can increase the risk of developing disease by >10-fold. Three-quarters of cases of intermittent claudication may be attributable to smoking, which is a more important risk factor for the development of peripheral arterial disease than it is for ischaemic heart disease.

Systolic blood pressure, and possibly diastolic blood pressure, is raised in people with peripheral arterial disease. Elevated blood pressure may precede the development of disease but it may also be secondary to atherosclerotic changes in blood vessels.

Various lipids and lipid fractions have been implicated in the pathogenesis of peripheral arterial disease, and it seems fairly certain that raised serum cholesterol increases the risk of disease. In recent years, interest has concentrated on the lipoprotein subfractions of cholesterol. Low-density lipoprotein (LDL)-cholesterol is the main carrier of cholesterol from the liver to peripheral tissues and tends to reflect the role of total cholesterol as an atherosclerotic risk factor. High-density lipoprotein (HDL)-cholesterol picks up cholesterol from peripheral tissues and returns it to the liver, thus acting in opposition to LDL. HDL-cholesterol levels are low in people with peripheral arterial disease, and reduced concentrations are associated with an increased severity of disease. Serum triglyceride levels are also raised in subjects with peripheral arterial disease, but whether these are important in the development of disease in their own right is uncertain; they may simply contribute to the composition of various lipoprotein fractions.

Peripheral arterial disease is a well-known complication of diabetes mellitus. The age-adjusted prevalence of intermittent claudication is 3–4-fold higher in diabetic men and 5–6-fold higher in diabetic women than in their non-diabetic counterparts. The mechanism by which diabetes increases the risk of peripheral arterial disease is uncertain, but raised plasma glucose levels and elevated plasma insulin, which is a risk factor for coronary artery disease, may be important.

Other risk factors implicated in the pathogenesis of atherosclerosis include:

- haemostatic and rheological factors,
- deficiency of certain dietary factors, including essential fatty acids and antioxidant vitamins;
- lack of exercise;
- alcohol;
- an aggressive personality (see Chapter 1).

However, much of the evidence surrounding these factors comes from the study of coronary artery disease and their role in peripheral arterial disease is less well established.

Prognosis

Peripheral arterial disease stabilizes soon after onset in approximately 75% of patients and only 25% of claudicants deteriorate to rest pain or gangrene. A subjective improvement in symptoms does not necessarily indicate regression of atherosclerosis, but may simply represent psychological and physiological adaptation to the ischaemia, such as the development of a collateral circulation. Only 3–22% of claudicants presenting to a doctor ever require reconstructive arterial surgery, and only 1% undergo amputation.

In addition to local symptoms, claudicants have an increased prevalence of coronary artery and cerebrovascular disease; coronary disease is the commonest cause of death in subjects with peripheral arterial disease.

Critical limb ischaemia

Critical limb ischaemia has been defined as:

● persistently recurring rest pain requiring regular analgesia for >2 weeks; or
● ulceration; or
● gangrene of the foot;

plus an ankle systolic pressure <50 mmHg or absent peripheral pulses in diabetics.

Incidence and prevalence

The annual incidence of critical limb ischaemia is between 500 and 1000 per million population and up to one-quarter of these undergo major amputations. The prevalence of critical ischaemia increases with age and is higher in men than in women.

Over the past few decades, there has been a large increase in the total number of operations performed for critical limb ischaemia in Western countries. This cannot be explained solely by an increase in the elderly population or improved survival rates for diabetics. However, there is also no firm evidence that the prevalence of peripheral arterial disease has changed, and the increase may represent an increase in the number of procedures performed on each patient. Technical advances in reconstructive surgery have also led to surgery being performed earlier on those for whom amputation would not previously have been considered appropriate.

Risk factors

The risk factors which predispose to progression from the early stages of peripheral arterial disease to critical limb ischaemia are similar to those for the development of intermittent claudication, with advancing age, diabetes and cigarette smoking accounting for the majority of disease. Only 12% of patients with critical ischaemia have none of these factors.

Amputation is more common among claudicants who smoke heavily and who continue to smoke. Stopping smoking halts vascular changes and reduces the likelihood of symptomatic progression but does not reduce the risk of amputation over the subsequent 2–3 years. Diabetes is also more common among amputees than in the general population: 45% of lower limb amputees are diabetic and 56% of these are insulin dependent. Age-adjusted amputation rates are 15-fold higher in diabetics than in non-diabetics. Overall, lower limb ulceration and gangrene occur in 10% of all elderly diabetics. This propensity to critical ischaemia in diabetics is attributable not only to the development of large vessel peripheral arterial disease, but also to microangiopathy, neuropathy and infections associated with diabetes.

The role of other risk factors in the progression of peripheral arterial disease to critical ischaemia, including blood pressure, lipid levels and haemostatic factors, has not been established.

Prognosis

More than 90% of patients with critical limb ischaemia undergo major amputation, arterial reconstruction or angioplasty over the 12 months following presentation. Amputation leads to loss of mobility and independence, psychological morbidity and reduced life expectancy. Critical limb ischaemia is often fatal if left untreated, but, even after arterial reconstruction or amputation, 40–75% of patients will die within 5 years of presentation. However, peripheral arterial disease is rarely a direct cause of death and high mortality rates predominantly reflect co-existent coronary artery and cerebrovascular disease.

Abdominal aortic aneurysm

An abdominal aortic aneurysm (AAA) can be defined as a local enlargement of the lumen of the abdominal aorta (see also Chapter 11).

Incidence and prevalence

The prevalence of AAA, defined as an aortic diameter >4 cm, is about 2% in men in their late 60s and early 70s in the UK. Many of these aneurysms, detected in the general population by diagnostic ultrasound, are asymptomatic and would not normally present to a vascular surgeon. However, there is increasing interest in the prevalence of small aneurysms in the general population due to the possibility that early intervention in these cases will improve prognosis.

The number of patients with AAA presenting to vascular surgeons has increased in recent years. For example, in Scotland, admissions of patients over 50 years of age with an AAA increased from 14.5 per 100 000 in 1974 to 48.6 per 100 000 in 1984 to 156.1 per 100 000 in 1994. This is thought to be due not only to better case ascertainment but also a true increase in the incidence of AAAs.

AAAs occur more commonly in males than in females and increase quite markedly with age in both sexes. A higher prevalence is also found in whites than in blacks, which reflects the situation found in atherosclerosis. There also appears to be some geographical variation in the prevalence of AAAs, such as a 6-fold higher occurrence of disease in England and Wales compared with the US.

Risk factors

The pathogenesis of AAA involves weakening of the aortic wall due to the destruction of elastin and probably secondary failure of collagen. Atherosclerosis is the major pathology preceding the formation of aneurysms, especially in older patients. It has been suggested that atherosclerotic plaque may weaken the aortic wall either directly or through reduction in the amount of nutrient reaching the aortic media via diffusion from the aortic lumen. Alternatively, inflammatory mediators produced in response to the atherosclerotic process may destroy and weaken the aortic media. Why atherosclerosis, which generally results in narrowing of the arterial lumen, should in some instances cause dilatation is unknown. Many of the risk factors which have been shown to increase the risk of stenosing atherosclerosis have not been shown to affect aortic aneurysm formation, suggesting that different genetic or biochemical pathways may be involved. In particular, patients with aneurysmal disease have a lower incidence of diabetes and a different lipoprotein profile compared with subjects with stenosing lesions.

People who have a first-degree relative affected by AAA are at an increased risk of developing the condition themselves. This may reflect inherited defects in elastin and collagen or a genetic factor responsible for increased enzymatic destruction of these components of the aortic wall. However, although several candidate genes have been investigated, including those of elastin and collagen themselves, the precise genetic basis of aneurysm formation remains unresolved.

The strong association between cigarette smoking and AAA has been recognized for several years and the increased prevalence of aneurysms has paralleled the increased consumption of cigarettes with a lag of 40 years. Death from ruptured aneurysm is 4-fold commoner in smokers than in non-smokers. However, the toxic components of tobacco combustion associated with aneurysm formation remain to be identified.

Hypertension is also considered a risk factor for AAA. It is associated with both an increased prevalence and an increased risk of rupture. However, it is uncertain whether hypertension is involved in the pathogenesis of aneurysm or merely acts to exacerbate the effects of pre-existing weakness in the aortic wall.

Prognosis

Approximately 6% of AAAs rupture annually and 12% of those presenting clinically have ruptured. Overall, mortality from ruptured aortic aneurysm is >80%, although advances in surgery have led to recent reductions in operative mortalities in specialist centres. Many individuals with AAA die from other causes, especially co-existent cardiac and cerebrovascular disease.

Venous disease

Venous disease in the legs can range from minor asymptomatic incompetence of venous valves to disabling chronic leg ulceration. The clinical section (C) of a recently accepted classification of venous disease, the CEAP-Classification, is described in Table 2.2. Additional sections of the CEAP-Classification system take into account aetiology (E), anatomic distribution (A) and pathophysiologic dysfunction (P).

The venous conditions most commonly encountered by vascular surgeons are varicose veins, venous insufficiency and varicose ulcers.

Varicose veins

Clinically, varicose veins have been defined in several ways:

- '… any dilated, elongated or tortuous veins, irrespective of size';
- 'A varicose vein is one which has permanently lost its valvular efficiency. … As a result of continuous dilation under pressure in the course of time a varicose vein becomes elongated, tortuous, pouched and thickened'.

Table 2.2. **Clinical section of the CEAP-Classification of venous disease.**

Class 0	No visible or palpable signs of venous disease
Class 1	Telangiectases or reticular veins
Class 2	Varicose veins
Class 3	Oedema
Class 4	Skin changes ascribed to venous disease, e.g. pigmentation, venous eczema, lipodermatosclerosis
Class 5	Skin changes as defined above with healed ulceration
Class 6	Skin changes as defined above with active ulceration

Prevalence and incidence

The prevalence of all categories of varicose veins in adult Western populations is around 25–33% for women and 10–20% for men, depending on disease definitions and the population examined. Varicose veins are commoner in females than in males, with a ratio of approximately 2:1.

The prevalence of varicose veins increases with age. In men, it increases from around 3% in subjects in their 30s to nearly 40% in those over 70 years. For women in their 30s, a prevalence in the region of 20% rises to >50% in those over 70 years. Discrete reticular varices can be found in schoolchildren as young as 10–12 years of age.

The prevalence of varicose veins may also vary geographically and by race. For example, a lower prevalence has been reported in developing countries than in the West and in men born in North Africa compared with those born in Europe and America.

The annual incidence of varicose veins appears to be around 2.6% in women and 1.9% in men. Interestingly, the incidence rate, at least from age 40 years, does not increase with age. Thus, it would appear that the increasing prevalence with age is due to the relatively constant development of new cases as people grow older.

Risk factors

Numerous genetic, life-style and physiological characteristics have been suggested as possible risk factors for the development of varicose veins (Table 2.3). Many of these, e.g. a low-fibre diet and lack of exercise, are associated with 'Westernization' and may help to explain the apparent geographical variation in varicose veins. However, the evidence linking

Table 2.3. **Suggested risk factors for varicose veins.**

Pregnancy

Obesity

Genetic predisposition

'Westernization'
  Prolonged standing
  Prolonged sitting
  Tight undergarments
  Low-fibre diet/constipation
  Raised toilet seats

Life-style
  Lack of exercise
  Smoking
  Heavy lifting

Hormone levels in women
  Oral contraceptives
  Late menarche

Venous thrombosis

most of these factors to the development of varicose veins is extremely limited, with the exceptions being pregnancy and obesity.

In many women, varicose veins appear for the first time during pregnancy. Although pregnancy may merely be an exacerbating factor in those already predisposed, the risk of acquiring varicose veins increases with the woman's number of pregnancies. Women with two or more pregnancies, compared to those with a single pregnancy or no previous pregnancy, have a 20–30% increased risk of developing varicose veins. It is not clear how pregnancy might increase the risk of developing varicose veins. The role of the pregnant uterus in obstructing venous return from the legs has been questioned, largely because most varices appear during the first 3 months of pregnancy when the uterus is not large enough to cause mechanical obstruction. It has been suggested that an hormonal factor, or the additional burden of increased circulating volume of blood in the veins, could be important.

Obesity has been related to the occurrence of varicose veins in women, but the evidence that it is also a risk factor in men is not strong. Among women in the US, an excess risk of varicose veins of about 33% was found in those with a body mass index >27 kg/m. It is also not clear whether the risk increases above a certain cut-off point or is apparent across the range of body mass index.

The role of genetic predisposition and heredity in the development of varicose veins is uncertain but potentially important. The risk of varicose veins is raised in people with affected relatives, especially if the relative is male, but findings do not seem to fit with any single genetic model of inheritance. It has been suggested that an inherited factor responsible for the number of valves in veins may be important. However, a strong argument against a primary genetic cause of varicose veins is that immigrants from an area of supposedly low prevalence tend to acquire the high prevalence of their adopted country, as in the case of black immigrant Americans. This suggests an environmental rather than an hereditary cause.

Various life-style factors have been implicated in the aetiology of varicose vein, particularly those associated with Westernization. However, there is little hard evidence that these are important. These factors include prolonged standing, sitting in a chair, tight undergarments and reduced squatting to defecate. Constipation has also been implicated in the development of varicose veins, possibly as a consequence of increased intra-abdominal pressure during straining at stool. For example, in the South Pacific, the prevalence of varicose veins is low in primitive peoples, but high in more Westernized cultures where the diet contains more refined carbohydrate and less dietary fibre.

Many other factors have also been implicated:

- lack of exercise;
- cigarette smoking;

- heavy lifting;
- inguinal herniae in males;
- hormone levels in women.

In one study, valvular reflux occurred more commonly in individuals who had had a deep vein thrombosis (DVT), but in another, patients who had postoperative thrombosis did not later show a higher incidence of deep venous insufficiency. The evidence linking these factors to the occurrence of varicose veins is tenuous, and in many cases may be related more to confounding by other factors than a direct causal association.

Venous insufficiency

The prevalence of chronic venous insufficiency in the general population varies from 3% to 10%. A considerable proportion of subjects with varicose veins have evidence of the skin changes associated with prolonged stasis of venous blood flow. Oedema occurs in nearly 20% of subjects and up to 10% of women with varicose veins have signs of chronic venous insufficiency, skin changes or ulceration.

The prevalence and severity of various grades of chronic venous insufficiency are related to the severity of varicose veins. Among those with severe varicose veins (marked trunk varices), the prevalence of chronic venous insufficiency is 81% and among those with minor varicose veins (reticular veins and/or telangiectasia or 'scarcely visible trunk varices') the prevalence is 30%. The incidence of skin changes and ulceration among subjects with varicose veins indicates that 21% of those with mild varicose veins develop signs of chronic venous insufficiency whereas half of those with severe varicose veins do so. Twenty percent of subjects with severe varicose veins develop ulceration compared to only 0.8% of those with mild varicose veins.

Varicose ulcers

Chronic venous ulceration is the severest manifestation of lower limb venous disease. Although it is also the most extensively studied manifestation, care must be taken to differentiate venous ulcers from other forms of chronic leg ulcers, such as arterial and traumatic ulcers. Venous ulcers rarely occur in the foot, and above the foot only about three-quarters are thought to be due primarily to venous disease.

Prevalence and incidence

The prevalence of open (active) venous ulcers in adult Western populations is about 0.3%. For every patient with an open ulcer in the population, there would appear to be between 2 and 4 individuals with healed ulcers, so that the population prevalence of open and healed ulcers combined could be around 1%. The prevalence of ulcers is approximately 2–3-fold higher in females than males and increases consistently with age in both sexes, with the female predominance being maintained at all ages. Chronic leg ulceration is relatively uncommon below the age of 60 years.

Very little data are available on the annual incidence of venous ulcers, but it may be around 3.5 per 1000 in the population over 45 years of age.

Risk factors

The risk of ulceration increases with the severity of varicose veins. The severity of venous incompetence, as indicated by objective measures such as the ambulatory venous pressure of the foot, may also be related to the risk of ulceration. No ulceration occurs in limbs with an ambulatory venous pressure <30 mmHg, whereas a consistent increase in the prevalence of ulceration occurs with higher ambulatory venous pressure, ranging from 14% in limbs with a pressure between 31 and 40 mmHg to 100% in limbs with a pressure >90 mmHg.

It is widely believed clinically that DVT is a risk factor for the skin changes, oedema and ulceration associated with venous disease in the legs. Under these circumstances, the venous condition is sometimes referred to as the post-thrombotic syndrome. Up to 17% of subjects with chronic venous ulcers have a history of DVT and the annual incidence of ulceration in individuals who have had a DVT is around 1–2% per annum.

Several other factors are possible contributory factors to the development of venous ulceration:

- arterial disease in the lower limbs;
- minor trauma;
- oedema (not necessarily related to venous insufficiency);
- obesity;
- co-existing conditions such as arthritis or neuropathies.

However, the extent to which these factors are important is not well established.

Prognosis

Venous ulceration in the leg is a chronic condition in which healing is dependent on such factors as the size of the ulcer, age of the patient and mode of treatment. The prognosis of chronic ulcers is often poor, with only around half of ulcers healed within 4 months. The majority of ulcers recur at least once, with recurrence rates of between 3% and 30% per year. Of all ulcer patients, 45% have experienced episodes of ulceration for >10 years and approximately 20% for between 5 and 10 years.

Summary

■ The prevalence of intermittent claudication ranges from 0.5% to 7% in middle-aged populations, increases with age and is greater in men than in women.

■ Risk factors for peripheral arterial disease reflect those for atherosclerosis in general, and include smoking, hyperlipidaemia, hypertension and diabetes.

■ Intermittent claudication stabilizes soon after onset in the majority of subjects and only 1% will require amputation.

■ The annual incidence of critical limb ischaemia is between 500 and 1000 per million population.

■ More than 90% of patients with critical limb ischaemia require surgical intervention within 1 year of presentation.

■ The prevalence of abdominal aortic aneurysm (AAA) is about 2% in elderly men in the UK.

■ Risk factors for AAA include a positive family history, smoking and hypertension.

■ The prevalence of varicose veins in adult Western populations is 25–33% for women and 10–20% for men.

■ Genetic predisposition, a Western life-style and other factors may be risk factors for varicose veins, but epidemiological evidence is lacking.

■ The prevalence of venous ulcers is about 0.3% for open ulcers and 1% for open and healed ulcers combined.

■ The prognosis of chronic ulcers is often poor; only half heal within 4 months and the majority recur at least once.

Areas of controversy

■ Cause of the higher incidence of intermittent claudication in men than in women.

■ Risk factors underlying the higher incidence of peripheral arterial disease in diabetic than in non-diabetic subjects.

■ Role of risk factors in the progression of intermittent claudication to critical ischaemia.

■ Cause of the rising incidence of abdominal aortic aneurysms.

■ Role of atherosclerotic and other risk factors in the aetiology of abdominal aortic aneurysm.

■ True prevalence and incidence of varicose veins using standardized methods of definition and measurement.

■ Role of risk factors, particularly genetic polymorphisms, diet and occupation, in the aetiology of varicose veins.

■ Factors which predispose individuals with varicose veins to the development of complications, particularly ulceration.

Further reading

- Fowkes FGR (ed). *Epidemiology of Peripheral Vascular Disease.* Berlin: Springer-Verlag, 1991.
- MacSweeney STR, Powell JT, Greenhalgh RM. Pathogenesis of abdominal aortic aneurysm. *British Journal of Surgery* 1994;**81**:935–941.
- Evans CJ, Fowkes FGR, Hajivassiliou CA, Harper DR, Ruckley CV. Epidemiology of varicose veins: A review. *International Angiology* 1994;**13**:263–270.

3
History and Examination

John Chamberlain and Michael G Wyatt

Introduction

Peripheral vascular disease (PVD) may present with signs and symptoms involving the arterial, venous or lymphatic systems. The signs and symptoms of disease involving each of these systems are usually related and there may often be overlap which careful clinical history and examination will be able to separate. As disease of the arteries, veins or lymphatics may often be symptomatic of a generalized process it is essential that a complete general history and physical examination be performed in every patient.

Any diseases that affect the peripheral vessels may be associated with lesions distant from these vessels in other parts of the vasculature or may be associated with other primary disease. For example, a pulmonary embolus may be associated with acute lower limb venous thrombosis. Peripheral arterial disease is commonly associated with disease of the coronary vessels. In addition, other conditions such as diabetes, hypertension, peptic ulceration and bronchogenic carcinoma may often be present in patients with PVD.

The special clinical signs and symptoms which are associated with individual vascular conditions are discussed in future chapters. This chapter discusses the general principles of history taking and examination in these patients.

Initial evaluation

The initial history and clinical examination are extremely important in the assessment of the vascular patient because they can enable the clinician to:

- establish a preliminary diagnosis;
- determine the urgency of treatment;
- establish a rapport with the patient.

An accurate clinical impression of the problem of PVD can usually be obtained from a single history and clinical examination, consisting of inspection, palpation and auscultation.

Although most arterial and venous problems can be dealt with on an elective basis, some require more urgent treatment to save life or limb and the degree of urgency can be established at the initial patient evaluation.

Clinical history

In all patients with PVD a general history is vital and should include both symptoms and risk factors. Particular enquiry should be made as to whether the patient has a history of:

● hypertension;
● ischaemic heart disease;
● diabetes.

Patients often present with some degree of discomfort and pain associated with impaired function of the parts supplied or drained by the arteries, veins or lymphatics. The clinical signs and symptoms may be directly associated with the blood supply to the tissues or may occur at some distance from the lesion, e.g. emboli from a proximal aneurysm.

In addition to the presenting symptoms, it is important to ascertain details of family history, occupation and social history. Many vascular conditions have a familial aetiology or may be associated with particular occupations; e.g. Raynaud's phenomenon is associated with the use of vibrating tools and working in a cold environment may exacerbate peripheral vascular problems. Repeated trauma to the limbs may also aggravate PVD. A strong family history of arterial disease, whether it be due to stroke, ischaemic heart disease or arterial aneurysms, may indicate inherited factors or lipid abnormalities.

Drug therapy may also be related to the onset of vascular disorders. Antihypertensive therapy with β-blockers may exacerbate symptoms of claudication and vasospasm. Excessive oestrogen, particularly in the form of the contraceptive pill and, to a lesser extent, hormone replacement therapy promotes thrombosis in the venous system and also increases the risk of stroke.

The most important aetiological factor in arterial disease is *smoking*. The patient should be asked not only if he is smoking at present but also if he has ever smoked in the past, as the effects of tobacco can continue for a considerable time after the patient has stopped smoking.

Although a history of *alcohol intake* should be taken, there is no good evidence that heavy alcohol intake can exacerbate vascular disease. There is, however, some evidence that moderate alcohol intake may be protective.

In addition, a history of previous *radiation treatment*, e.g. for breast cancer and axillary artery stenosis/thrombosis, is important as this can lead to long-term damage to the vascular endothelium and this may lead to delayed thrombosis.

The commonest presentation of patients with venous disease is with symptoms of pain and swelling affecting the limb. For patients with superficial venous abnormalities, especially varicose veins, additional symptoms include unsightliness and episodes of superficial thrombophlebitis. Patients may complain of discolouration and pigmentation of the skin with eczema and eventually lipo-dermatosclerosis. At a very late stage ulceration may occur. With either deep or superficial venous disease, night cramps are common.

In addition to these specific features, a careful cardiac history should also be taken for patients with venous disease as right-sided heart failure may exacerbate the symptoms. The presence or past history of intra-abdominal disease may be a precipitating factor in lower limb venous problems, as may multiple pregnancies. For patients with suspected deep venous thrombosis, a careful history should be taken to exclude chest symptoms in view of the risk of pulmonary embolus.

Physical examination

The equipment required for the basic evaluation of the vascular patient is simple:

- stethoscope;
- blood pressure cuff;
- tape measure;
- hand-held Doppler.

The examination of patients with PVD is discussed separately for the arterial, venous and lymphatic systems.

Arterial examination

General examination

Most patients will have diffuse atherosclerosis and a full physical examination of the entire arterial tree is required irrespective of the presenting complaint. This should include:

- heart rate and rhythm;
- bilateral arm blood pressures;

- cardiac auscultation for arrhythmias, gallops and murmurs;
- auscultation for carotid, subclavian, abdominal and femoral bruits;
- abdominal palpation for an aortic aneurysm;
- palpation of all peripheral pulses;
- inspection of legs and feet for ulcers, gangrene and microemboli.

Head and neck

The commonest vascular disorder affecting the head and neck is athero-sclerosis of the carotid bifurcation, often involving the origin of the internal carotid artery. Stenotic disease at this site may present with either general or focal signs related to disease affecting the extracerebral vessels. Most patients referred for a vascular opinion have:

- asymptomatic carotid bruits;
- localized carotid pulsation (tortuous carotid arteries, carotid aneurysm or carotid body tumour);
- localizing neurological signs (ameurosis fugax, transient ischaemic attacks or stroke).

Inspection

The normal carotid pulse is not visible but may become apparent at the base of the right side of the neck in patients with hypertension. Often these patients are referred with a diagnosis of carotid aneurysm. This condition is rare and these patients usually are found to have a tortuous prominent carotid artery.

If a patient complains of amaurosis fugax (transient monocular blindness), retinal examination may reveal cholesterol emboli within the retinal arteries. These originate from ulcerated plaques within the carotid, innominate or arch arteries.

Palpation

Careful palpation of the carotid pulse should be undertaken; however, it is virtually impossible to distinguish between internal and external carotid artery pulsation in the mid neck where the common carotid artery bifurcates. No assumptions regarding individual patency can be made. Even in the presence of a totally occluded internal carotid artery, a strong neck pulsation is often found, provided the external carotid artery remains patent.

Palpation of the vessels in the root of the neck and at the angle of the jaw should also exclude any aneurysmal dilatation or the presence of any unrelated swelling.

Auscultation

Careful auscultation is also required for bruits. If a carotid bruit is heard on the appropriate side, there is a strong probability that this may be related to the patient's neurological signs. Urgent duplex scanning should be carried out to confirm the presence or absence of disease in the carotid territory.

The root of the neck must also be auscultated for bruits. This must be combined with careful palpation of the upper limb pulses to exclude subclavian disease. Subclavian steal syndrome typically presents with episodes of dizziness associated with the use of the upper limb and either a bruit in the neck with weak upper limb pulses or a reduction in the blood pressure on the side of the lesion.

Upper limb

The most frequent symptoms of arterial insufficiency encountered in the upper limb are:

- pain;
- pallor;
- muscle claudication with exercise.

These symptoms can be due to acute or chronic occlusive arterial disease, thoracic outlet syndrome or peripheral vasospasm (see Chapters 10 and 22).

Inspection

Pink finger tips with a capillary refilling time of <3 s usually indicates an adequate upper limb vascular supply. By contrast, an acutely ischaemic limb is usually pale with diminished movement. In a patient with chronic arterial insufficiency, muscle atrophy is often present. Microembolic infarction can be recognized in the finger tips in addition to peripheral vasospasm, skin ulceration or gangrene.

Palpation

The upper limb arterial pulsation should be palpable at the wrist (radial and ulnar), at the antecubital fossa (brachial) and in the groove between the biceps and triceps (distal axillary). Palpation can also detect skin temperature and larger aneurysms (axillary, subclavian) of the upper limb vessels.

Auscultation

Auscultation of the upper limb blood vessels should be accompanied by measurement of bilateral brachial blood pressures and examination of the supraclavicular fossa for subclavian bruits. When pulses are not readily palpable, a hand-held Doppler probe can be used to assess arterial signals and measure brachial pressures.

Abdomen

The major vascular abnormality found on abdominal examination is an abdominal aortic aneurysm. These aneurysms can either present as symptomless pulsatile abdominal swellings, or with back pain, thrombosis, embolization or rupture (see Chapter 11).

Examination of the abdominal aorta is essential in any patient who presents with symptoms of vascular disease. However, because of its retroperitoneal position, only limited information can be obtained by physical examination alone.

The patient should be lying thoroughly relaxed for this procedure. The abdominal wall may be relaxed by asking the patient to breathe gently in and out through his mouth, with his arms by his side (not behind his head).

Inspection

The normal aortic pulsation is usually not visible, except occasionally in thin young adults (often female). In the presence of visible pulsation, an underlying aortic aneurysm should be suspected.

Palpation

The palm and fingers of the examiner's hand should be curved over the side of the aneurysm so that both its anterior–posterior (pulsatile) and lateral (expansile) excursions can be felt. In a very obese patient it may be difficult to feel an aneurysm and ultrasound should be employed. Careful palpation of the distal pulses should also be carried out in these patients as there may be occlusive disease distally.

Auscultation

Often patients will be suffering from occlusive disease of their aortoiliac arteries. Auscultation of the abdomen will often reveal bruits related to these lesions. Other abdominal arteries which may be involved include the renals and mesenterics. Asymptomatic abdominal bruits may be found in young adults, especially thin women. In the absence of symptoms, these may be considered benign.

Lower limb

Clinical examination is extremely important in the management of a patient with lower limb ischaemia. Chronic and acute arterial ischaemia can produce changes easily recognizable by inspection, palpation and auscultation.

Symptoms

The majority of lower limb arterial problems present with:

- intermittent claudication;
- ischaemic rest pain, ulcers or gangrene; or
- acute arterial ischaemia (pain, pallor, paralysis, paraesthesia and pulselessness).

(see Chapters 14 and 15)

In patients who present with these symptoms, a clinical examination of the leg is the best method to assess the severity of the ischaemia and determine the urgency of further investigation and treatment.

Inspection

The appearance of the limbs should be noted and most of the important signs of chronic or acute arterial insufficiency will be readily identifiable.

In *early chronic arterial disease*, there may be no appreciable change in the appearance of the lower limb, but often muscle atrophy will be noted along with pallor on elevation with dependent rubor (positive Buerger's test). Peripheral arterial disease may lead to decreased nutrition of the periphery with brittle nails and loss of hair distally. Eventually, skin lesions may appear with pressure sores or ulceration and eventually gangrene of the digits.

Similarly, in *acute arterial insufficiency* the limb overall is pallid, but there may also be severe cyanosis accompanied by mottling. In addition, muscle weakness or paralysis of the foot becomes obvious and eventually the leg will become swollen and blistered. Gangrene is the final change in appearance, but may not occur for several days.

Palpation

All the peripheral arteries should be palpated. This along with a good clinical history is often sufficient to define the level of disease (Fig. 3.1).

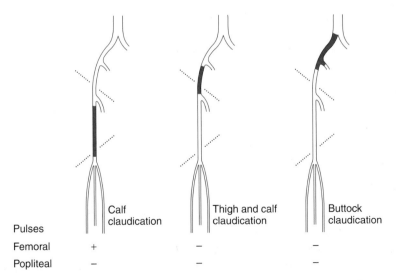

Pulses	Calf claudication	Thigh and calf claudication	Buttock claudication
Femoral	+	–	–
Popliteal	–	–	–

Fig. 3.1. Relationship of symptoms and peripheral pulses to the level of lower limb occlusive vascular disease.

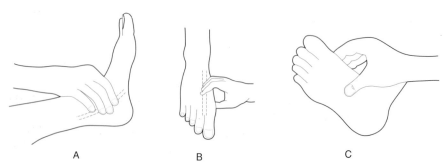

Fig. 3.2. Method of palpating the (A) posterior tibial and (B,C) dorsalis pedis pulses.

- The *posterior tibial and dorsalis pedis* pulses are usually easily found in normal individuals, although in a few patients the dorsalis pedis may be absent (Fig. 3.2).
- The *popliteal pulse* lies deeply next to the knee joint and is often most easily felt with the knee slightly flexed, the muscles relaxed and the fingers along the line of the artery in the midline (Fig. 3.3). If there is

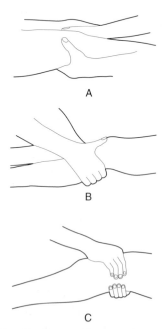

Fig. 3.3. Method of palpating the popliteal artery. (A, B) Note the thumbs are used anteriorly to steady the hands and to allow counter pressure whilst (C) the fingers are used to palpate the artery in the midline of the popliteal fossa.

doubt about this, the patient should be turned onto his face, and the knee flexed, and the examiner's fingers should palpate deeply in to the midline between the heads of gastrocnemius.

- The *femoral pulse* is found at the mid-inguinal point, just below the inguinal ligament.

One should be aware of localized disease in the distal vessels, particularly popliteal thrombosis or aneurysm, and of other conditions which may cause claudication and may temporarily occlude arteries such as popliteal entrapment syndrome. This latter condition may be detected by the disappearance of the distal pulses on hyperextending the knee.

Also, one should be aware that normal pulses at rest are possible with proximal stenotic disease. A bruit may suggest such disease and subsequent exercise testing and Doppler examination will confirm these lesions.

At all sites the rate and volume of the pulse, rigidity of the vessel and palpable calcification should be noted and whether there is dilatation of the artery suggestive of aneurysmal disease. The presence of a palpable thrill should be noted and is suggestive of a tight stenosis or an arteriovenous fistula. In addition, the temperature of the limb should also be noted, comparing one side with the other.

Palpation is also helpful in the assessment of the acutely ischaemic limb. Skin temperature can help determine the level of demarcation prior to reconstruction or amputation and muscle tenderness and tenseness are often important determinants of outcome. In addition, ischaemic sensory nerve damage can be detectable by simple pin-prick sensory examination.

Auscultation

Auscultation for bruits should be done over the peripheral arteries, particularly over the femoral artery at the groin and at the adductor hiatus. A bruit can occur in normal arteries in younger people but it may be a guide to localized stenosis. Auscultation is also important when an arteriovenous malformation is suspected. A classical 'machinery' murmur is often heard.

Further evaluation of the vessels in the limbs may be easily undertaken using Doppler techniques (see Chapter 4).

Venous examination

The venous circulation consists of a superficial subcutaneous plexus of veins and deeper muscular veins. Superficial veins have an extensive sympathetic nerve supply and a role in the reflex regulation of the circulation. Flow through the veins is produced by a combination of forces: a pressure gradient between the left ventricle and the periphery together with the assistance of muscle contraction.

Venous disease is common from the late teens onwards. It is rare in young children unless it is associated with congenital venous abnormalities. Patients with venous disease may present with asymptomatic unsightly veins only and they may request treatment for cosmetic purposes. Upper limb venous disease is less common.

Upper limbs

The main venous disorder of the upper limbs involves acute axillary or subclavian thrombosis. Patients complain of arm swelling often accompanied by a diffuse aching pain which is often worse with prolonged use or dependency. The common causes for this disorder are:

- chronic subclavian vein catheterization (parenteral nutrition, intravenous therapy);
- thoracic outlet syndrome (see Chapter 10).

Inspection

In all cases of venous disease, both limbs should be examined in a good light. In the event of subclavian vein thrombosis, the arm may appear bluish or cyanotic. Rarely, venous gangrene will develop, but these patients often have an underlying coagulopathy or malignancy. These patients will still have palpable arterial pulses and numerous venous collaterals may be present around the shoulder joint.

In general, chronic venous skin changes are not seen in the upper limb. The exception is following arteriovenous fistula formation for dialysis. These patients can develop chronically swollen upper limbs associated with hyperpigmentation and ulceration. Differentiation from chronic lymphatic obstruction is often difficult.

Palpation

Following thrombosis of the deep veins of the upper limb vessels, little useful information can be gained from attempted palpation as both the axillary and subclavian veins lie deep to the clavicle. Nevertheless, thrombosed superficial veins can present as tender 'cords' on palpation.

Auscultation

Auscultation of venous signals is not normally possible unless there is an underlying arteriovenous fistula. If deep venous signals are to be heard, a hand-held Doppler unit is required.

Lower limbs

The commonest venous problems of the legs are:

- varicose veins;
- deep venous thrombosis;
- postphlebitic syndrome.

(See Chapters 18, 19 and 20.)

For the lower limbs the patient should be examined both standing and lying with both legs completely exposed from the groin to the feet. The abnormal limb should be compared with the normal limb whenever possible.

Varicose veins

Inspection of the varicosities can provide important information as to their aetiology. Varicose veins usually involve the long saphenous system and are found on the medial side of the leg. Lesser saphenous varicosities can be seen on the posterior calf from the knee to the lateral aspect of the ankle. Likewise, varicose veins secondary to incompetent perforators may begin at or below the knee. These dilated superficial veins may be more obvious when the patient is standing and may disappear when he is lying down. Their site may give some indication as to their aetiology.

In addition, there may be superficial intradermal veins and secondary changes in the skin with eczema, ulceration and pigmentation. These skin changes may be more obvious in long-standing cases with thickening and induration of the skin and subcutaneous fat (lipodermatosclerosis). The ulceration found in the later stages is due to venous hypertension and is most commonly located on the medial side of the lower part of the leg.

Careful examination will elicit the veins involved in varicosities, particularly whether the long or short saphenous system is involved. It is to be noted, however, that veins behind the knee often connect with the long saphenous system and in order to elucidate this, careful Doppler examination may be invaluable.

In addition, veins should be palpated and a cough impulse may be elicited below non-functioning valves. This is particularly so at the saphenofemoral junction where there may be a visible swelling when the patient is standing. Care must be taken to differentiate this from other groin swellings, particularly a femoral hernia. There may be oedema in the lower part of the leg which usually is pitted. Later there may be considerable induration and within this there may be varicosities with perforating veins.

The tourniquet (Trendelenburg) test is a simple bed-side test to help determine the extent of varicosities and the site of perforating veins (Fig. 3.4). The subcutaneous veins of the patient's lower limb are excluded by a tourniquet placed around the affected limb with the patient lying down and the leg elevated. When the patient stands up, filling of the veins below the tourniquet indicates that there may be an incompetent connection between the deep superficial veins below the tourniquet. The level of this incompetent connection can be deduced from repeating the test with the tourniquet placed at different levels or by using multiple tourniquets on the leg. If multiple tourniquets are used, they should be removed from below upwards.

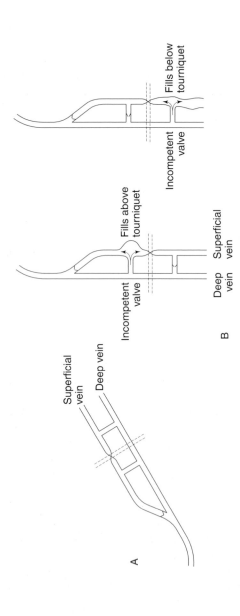

Fig. 3.4. **Principles behind the Trendelenburg test. (A) Leg elevated; (B) standing. Dotted lines represent position of the tourniquet.**

Acute venous thrombosis

Local thrombosis in the superficial veins is usually easy to diagnose from an indurated tender swelling along the line of the vein with local erythema. This can commonly occur after intravenous therapy. Inflammatory and nodular lesions of the skin, areas of fat necrosis and acute lymphangitis should be excluded.

Following an acute deep venous thrombosis, the appearance of the leg usually changes. There is swelling associated with local tenderness, pain and increased skin temperature. The calf may be tender on attempted dorsiflexion of the foot (Homan's sign), but care must be taken in eliciting this sign as it has been known for thrombi to fragment and travel proximally causing pulmonary emboli.

In the presence of deep venous thrombosis there may be muscle tenderness, but this is a variable sign and may be present in many other conditions.

An iliofemoral thrombosis presents with considerable swelling in the whole of the limb, often with superficial venous dilatation. The limb may be normal in colour or cyanotic and there may be a slight pyrexia. If the thrombus involves the inferior vena cava then both limbs will be involved. With extensive iliofemoral thrombosis (phlegmasia cerulea dolens), massive tight leg oedema, severe leg pain and cyanotic mottled skin can progress to cutaneous gangrene.

Postphlebitic syndrome

This is usually related to long-standing stasis of the venous blood flow, usually due to previous iliofemoral thrombosis, thrombophlebitis or long-standing varicose veins with subsequent venous hypertension.

The associated changes in the appearance of the lower leg are fairly specific. Because of the incompetent deep valves and associated venous hypertension, the leg becomes chronically swollen, especially around the ankle. Thickened areas of brownish pigmentation (haemosiderin) appear around the ankle and venous ulceration may develop (see Chapter 19). These ulcers are shallow, with healthy granulation tissue and they classically appear on the medial side of the ankle.

Palpation may help determine the possible cause of the leg swelling associated with chronic venous insufficiency. Occasionally, this is due to extrinsic compression by a pelvic, femoral or popliteal mass and these regions should be carefully examined

Auscultation of the lower limb veins does not provide much additional information about either superficial or deep venous flow. It can, however, be used to exclude venous abnormalities with arteriovenous fistula formation.

Doppler examination, however, is extremely helpful in the detection of both venous incompetence and thrombosis in the deep and superficial systems. In addition, duplex imaging of the lower limb venous system is a major aid to management and will help prevent recurrence after surgery (see Chapter 4).

Lymphatic examination

Chronic limb swelling may also be the result of lymphatic insufficiency. This may be due to:

- primary idiopathic lymphoedema (congenital, familial, praecox, tarda); or
- obstructive lymphoedema (malignancy, trauma, inflammatory).

(See Chapter 21.)

History

The diagnosis of a lymphatic cause of peripheral oedema is usually straightforward following the exclusion of venous or arterial disease. From the clinical history it is important to establish the presence or absence of the following features:

- limb swelling (usually distally first);
- limb heaviness;
- recurrent lymphangitis;
- skin changes: hyperkeratosis, fissuring;
- fungal infections;
- previous surgical procedure and/or radiation.

Examination

The diagnosis of lymphoedema can usually be made following the clinical examination (Fig. 3.5). It is important to look for the following clinical findings:

- limb oedema with dorsal buffalo hump of foot;
- elephantine distribution;
- lichenifiction;
- peau d'orange.

Lymphoedema of the lower limb usually involves the forefoot, sparing the metatarsal–phalangeal joint line to produce the characteristic 'buffalo-hump' when viewed laterally. With more extensive oedema, the leg develops a characteristic tree-trunk appearance. This distribution of oedema can differentiate lymphoedema form all other lower limb oedematous states.

   With more severe lymphoedema, skin changes occur. Increased vascularity may result in a pinkish tinge and there is generalized skin thickening. In advanced cases, the skin may resemble the 'skin of an orange'

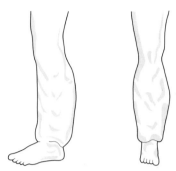

Fig. 3.5. **Lymphoedema of the lower leg. Note the chronic oedema in an elephantine distribution giving a tree-trunk appearance.**

(peau d'orange) and lichenification, hyperkeratosis and fissuring occur. In addition, the increase in lymph within the skin may encourage active fungal infection to take hold.

Summary

- Peripheral vascular disease may present with signs and symptoms involving the arterial, venous and lymphatic systems.
- A full clinical history and examination can often establish the diagnosis.
- A significant stenosis of the internal carotid artery can be suggested by history and examination, but the diagnosis can only be made following duplex scanning.
- All patients with peripheral vascular disease should have their abdomens palpated for aortic aneurysm.
- Limb swelling can be arterial, venous or lymphatic in nature.

Areas of controversy

- Should the Trendelenburg test still be used?
- Should peripheral arteries still be auscultated for bruits?
- Which varicose vein patients should be assessed with a hand-held Doppler or duplex examination?
- Do all patients with lymphoedema require a lymphangiogram?

Further reading

- Hallett JW, Brewster DC, Darling RC *Handbook of Patient Care in Vascular Surgery*. Philadelphia: Lippincott-Raven, 1995.
- Bell PRF, Jamieson CW, Ruckley CV (eds). *Surgical Management of Vascular Disease*. Philadelphia: WB Saunders, 1992.
- Eastcott HHG (ed). *Arterial Surgery*. Edinburgh: Churchill Livingstone, 1992.
- Munro JF, Ford MJ (eds). *Introduction to Clinical Examination*. Edinburgh: Churchill Livingstone, 1993.
- McLeod J (ed). *Clinical Examination*, 9th edn. Edinburgh: Churchill Livingstone, 1995.

4

Vascular Laboratory Investigation

Nick JM London

Introduction

The investigation of arterial and venous disease has undergone significant changes in recent years, largely as a result of technological advances in ultrasonography. These advances have increased the role of non-invasive imaging techniques and whereas the vascular laboratory used to be an 'optional extra', it is now an essential part of the vascular surgeon's investigational armamentarium. Whilst non-invasive imaging is by its very nature associated with minimal morbidity, perhaps a more important advantage is that it has shifted the emphasis of investigation from an anatomical towards an haemodynamic basis.

Principles of ultrasonography

In its simplest form ultrasound is transmitted as a continuous beam from a probe that contains two piezoelectric crystals. The transmitting crystal produces ultrasound at a fixed frequency (in the range 5–10 MHz for superficial vessels and 2–5 MHz for deeper vessels), whilst the receiving crystal vibrates in response to reflected waves and produces an output voltage. Conventional ultrasonography uses the reflections of ultrasound from tissue interfaces with stronger signals shown as a brighter spot on the screen (B-mode). The image produced has varying shades of grey depending on the acoustic impedance of the various tissue planes. More recently, the use of multiple transducers has allowed the production of cross-section real-time imaging.

Doppler ultrasonography makes use of the fact that the signals reflected from moving objects, such as red blood cells, will undergo a frequency shift as determined by the Doppler equation (Fig. 4.1). The output of continuous-wave Doppler ultrasound is most frequently presented as an audible signal (e.g. a hand-held pencil Doppler) or a simple tracing (Fig. 4.2). One of the problems with continuous-wave

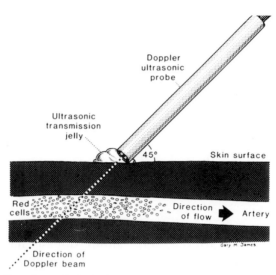

Fig. 4.1. The Doppler principle. The ultrasound reflected by the moving red cells is frequency shifted in proportion to the velocity of the blood.

ultrasonography is that there is no control over the depth of tissue which is being examined and this is solved by using pulsed ultrasound. The principle is that the depth of the tissue sample can be controlled by sending a pulse of ultrasound and closing the receiver, except when signals from a predetermined depth are returning. Thus, the centre of the artery and the areas close to the wall can be examined in turn.

The next advance in the use of ultrasonography was spectral analysis. The velocity profile provides limited information when seen as an analogue waveform; however, spectral analysis examines the complete spectrum of frequencies found in the arterial waveform during a cardiac cycle. This is most frequently carried out using real-time fast Fourier transform spectrum analysis, in which the vertical display represents the range of velocities seen at any given instant (Fig. 4.3).

Coupling the pulsed Doppler system with real-time B-mode ultrasound imaging of vessels allows the precise placement of the sample volume within the vessel lumen so that its flow patterns can be studied accurately. This combination of real-time B-mode sound imaging with pulsed Doppler ultrasound is called duplex scanning.

The final advance has been the advent of colour frequency mapping (colour Doppler). The colour assignment (red or blue) depends on the direction of blood flow, with colour saturation reflecting the magnitude of the mean Doppler frequency shift. Lower saturation (paler) indicates regions of higher blood flow, deeper colours slower flow and black the absence of flow. The particular advantage of colour Doppler is that it

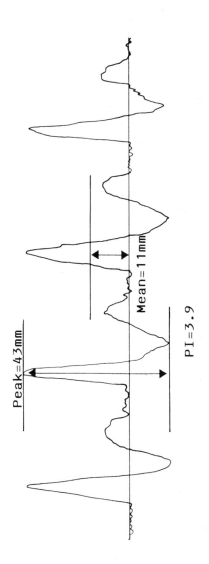
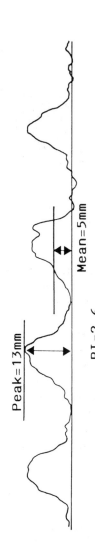

Fig. 4.2. The output of a continuous wave Doppler probe can be given as an audio signal or a simple tracing. Proximal disease causes damping of the waveform (bottom trace). The pulsality index (PI) is a method of waveform analysis (peak/mean).

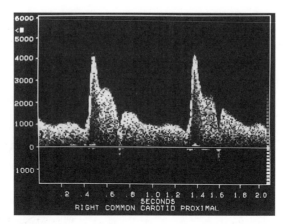

Fig. 4.3. Spectral analysis of Doppler waveform. The vertical display indicates the range of velocities present at each moment in time. In normal (laminar) blood flow, all the blood moves at the same velocity at the start of systole, i.e. there is a narrow spectrum of velocities with a dark 'window' below.

allows the rapid localization of vessels and the precise placement of pulsed Doppler sample volumes to record velocity spectra changes. In addition, spatial and temporal information of blood flow patterns can be superimposed on the B-mode grey-scale image (Plate 1).

'Power flow' Doppler is a more recent development that analyses the amplitude of the returning signal rather than its frequency and direction. The signal is sensitive to flow, has a high signal-to-noise ratio and is less dependent upon the angle of insonation than pulsed or colour flow Doppler. However, the image does not give information on the peak velocity or direction of flow and is therefore more anatomical than functional.

Cranial arteries

Colour Doppler

Although carotid angiography was the primary investigation for internal carotid artery stenosis, in many centres it has been superseded by colour Doppler scanning. Indeed, many patients now undergo carotid endarterectomy based solely on carotid colour Doppler scanning with angiography being reserved for cases that on duplex scanning have extensive disease either proximal or distal to the origin of the internal carotid artery. Extensive calcification may also impair the signal quality due to 'acoustic shadowing' The criterion most commonly used to define patients with >70% stenosis is a peak systolic velocity >180 cm/s.

The extracranial portion of the vertebral arteries can be visualized in 90% of patients using colour Doppler and its major role in this circumstance is the detection of flow and its direction. In the subclavian steal syndrome a proximal subclavian stenosis or occlusion results in diversion of blood flow into the ischaemic arm by retrograde flow down the ipsilateral vertebral artery. Using colour Doppler, this condition is identified by the detection of reversed flow in the vertebral artery compared to antegrade flow in the ipsilateral common carotid artery. The phenomenon may be spontaneous or may only appear after arm exercise.

Transcranial Doppler

The development of low-frequency pulsed-wave ultrasound has allowed insonation of the arteries comprising the circle of Willis and its principal branches. It is, however, only possible for the ultrasound beam to penetrate relatively thin areas of the skull. The most commonly used area is the temporal bone, through which most of the Circle of Willis, in particular the middle cerebral artery, can be seen. Transcranial Doppler (TCD) has the ability to 'range gate'. This enables the focusing point of the ultrasound beam to be adjusted over some distance in order to evaluate different components of the basal cerebral arteries.

The main clinical use of TCD is peri-operative monitoring in patients undergoing carotid endarterectomy. It can be used intraoperatively to monitor shunt function, indirectly assess cerebral perfusion and detect embolic events. Postoperatively, it is used to detect embolization and acute carotid thrombosis.

Upper limb arteries

A patient with symptoms of stenosis or occlusion of the arterial supply to the upper limb should have both brachial artery pressures measured and the arterial signals in the radial and ulnar arteries should be insonated using a pencil Doppler. In a patient with ischaemia of a single digit, it is useful to insonate the digital arteries because the absence of a signal suggests an embolic or thrombotic occlusion. The first line of detailed investigation should be a colour Doppler scan, starting with the subclavian artery and working peripherally. The subclavian artery should also be examined with the arm abducted and externally rotated, as in this position thoracic outlet compression syndrome (TOCS) will cause cessation of flow. Although it may be possible to make a diagnosis based solely on a colour Doppler scan, it is often necessary to perform an arteriogram if the problem lies proximally near the aortic arch.

Abdominal arteries

The first-line investigation in a patient thought to have an abdominal aortic aneurysm is B-mode ultrasonography. This is extremely accurate and has a very high sensitivity and specificity for abdominal aortic aneurysms (>99%).

In the majority of cases the vascular technologist will also be able to state whether the aneurysm is below the renal arteries and whether the iliac arteries are aneurysmal. If the ultrasonographer is confident that the aneurysm is infrarenal, then there is no indication for further imaging prior to surgery. It is important to realize that although ultrasonography may show evidence of aortic aneurysmal rupture, a normal investigation does not exclude a small rupture. Therefore, the decision to operate on painful aneurysms has to be made on clinical grounds.

To obtain adequate views of the mesenteric vessels the patient should be starved overnight both to reduce bowel gas and because a recent meal may augment mesenteric blood flow and confuse the interpretation of scans. It is possible for an experienced technician to image the origins of the coeliac, superior mesenteric and inferior mesenteric vessels. Although there are no large published series comparing colour Doppler mesenteric scanning with arteriography, it appears that colour Doppler is an ideal first-line investigation. In patients in whom the mesenteric vessels are well visualized by an experienced technician, there is no need for further investigation. However, in those in whom there is a stenosis or occlusion on duplex scanning or in whom visualization is inadequate, then arteriography with lateral views is the investigation of choice.

For the examination of the renal vessels, a low-frequency probe should be used in a fasted patient. In experienced vascular laboratories, colour Doppler can provide adequate views of the renal arteries in 85–90% of patients. As with the mesenteric vessels, if both renal arteries are clearly seen and are normal, there is no indication for angiography. If, however, the scans are abnormal or uncertain, then the next investigation of choice is arteriography.

Lower limb arteries

Ankle pressures

The first-line investigation is the measurement of ankle pressure. A standard sphygmomanometer cuff is applied to the lower third of the leg, inflated to suprasystolic levels and deflated slowly. During deflation a pencil Doppler probe is placed over the dorsalis pedis artery or the posterior tibial artery and the pressure at which blood flow is first detected in the foot is the systolic pressure. The highest pressure measured in any ankle artery is used as the numerator in the ankle-to-brachial blood pressure ratio, the ankle brachial pressure index (ABPI). The normal ABPI is >1.0 and a value of <0.9 is abnormal. Patients with claudication tend to have ABPIs in the range 0.5–0.9 whilst those with critical ischaemia usually have an index of <0.5.

Exercise test

If the diagnosis of claudication is in doubt, then the investigation of choice is an exercise test. The principle is that the limited inflow in limbs with significant arterial diseases results in a fall in pressure during exercise-induced peripheral dilatation. The test is usually performed by exercising the patient for 1 min on a treadmill at 4 km/h at a gradient of 10%. The parameters measured are the ABPI prior to and after exercise. A fall of pressure of >30 mmHg indicates the presence of significant arterial disease and the degree of fall is related to the severity of disease (Fig. 4.4). The response to treatment, e.g. exercise programmes, can be measured by walking until the onset of pain (pain-free walking distance) or the furthest distance walked (maximum walking distance).

Colour Doppler

Until recently, both the severe claudicant and all patients with critical ischaemia who were being considered for reconstruction were further

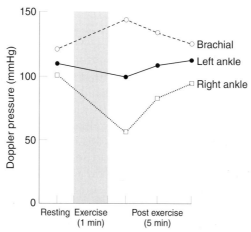

Fig. 4.4. One minute treadmill test. Resting ankle pressures are almost normal. After exercise there is a large pressure drop on the right indicating significant arterial disease.

investigated by arteriography. However, the combination of technological advances and increasingly experienced vascular technologists has meant that it is now possible to assess the lower limb vasculature in the majority of patients by colour Doppler scanning alone. The patient can be starved overnight in order to improve views of the aortoiliac segments. A complete examination of both lower limbs takes about 1.5 h.

Areas of abnormal flow are detected by colour disturbance and the peak velocity at the point of the disturbance compared with that of the artery immediately proximal. If the peak systolic velocity ratio is >2.0, then there is a significant (>50% diameter-reducing) stenosis. It is possible for lower limb angioplasty and surgery to be based solely on the result of colour Doppler scanning. It should be stressed however that this technique requires highly trained and skilled operators and is consequently very 'operator dependent'.

Papaverine test

This investigation is often considered the 'gold standard' for assessment of the aortoiliac segment. The common femoral artery is punctured by a needle or cannula connected to a pressure transducer. The brachial or radial artery is also cannulated and the femoral : brachial pressure ratio is measured. Papaverine (20 mg) is injected into the femoral artery and the percentage fall in the ratio is measured. A fall of >20% after papaverine administration indicates a significant aortoiliac stenosis (Fig. 4.5). In reality, this test is rarely required.

Demonstration of distal vessels

In critical ischaemia, arteriography may fail to demonstrate patent distal calf or pedal vessels that can be used as the outflow for femorodistal grafting. This is because these patients tend to have multiple-level disease which prevents the radiographic contrast from reaching the distal vessels.

Alternative approaches that have proved useful are pulse-generated run-off (PGR) and dependent Doppler assessment. The principle of PGR is that blood flow is generated in patent calf arteries by the application of a pulsatile pressure (250 mmHg at a rate of 50 inflations/min) to a sphygmomanometer cuff placed around the upper calf. Patent arteries can then be detected at the ankle by insonation with a 10 MHz Doppler ultrasound probe. This technique has been shown to detect up to 25% more patent vessels than angiography.

An alternative and somewhat simpler approach is that of dependent Doppler examination. This technique allows the accurate predication of calf vessels that are in continuity with the pedal arch. The leg is placed in a dependent position and a Doppler signal obtained in the first web

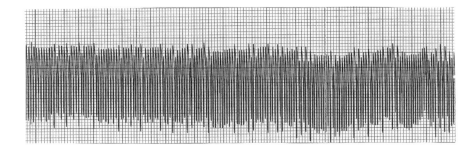

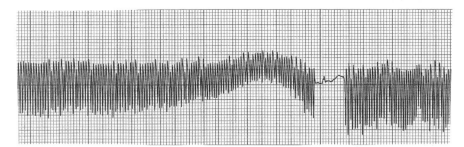

Fig. 4.5. **Papaverine test. There is a 37.5% fall in the common femoral artery pressure indicating significant aortoiliac disease.**

space over the area of the deep plantar artery. Individual calf vessels are then compressed in turn at the ankle joint. If only one calf vessel communicates with the pedal arch, then the Doppler signal is obliterated. If more than one tibial vessel is in continuity with the arch, compression results in attenuation of the pedal arch signal. The vessel that gives the greatest attenuation is defined as the major inflow vessel to the arch.

Diabetic limbs

The diabetic patient with calcified incompressible distal arteries poses a problem with respect to the measurement of ankle pressures because if the arterial wall is grossly calcified and incompressible, then falsely high ankle pressures may be obtained. One approach to this problem is the use of the pole test: a Doppler probe is placed over the patent pedal artery and the foot is elevated against a pole that is calibrated in mmHg. The point at which the pedal signal disappears is taken as the ankle pressure.

An alternative approach is the use of toe pressures as digital vessels are rarely calcified. At toe level, systolic blood pressure is usually somewhat lower than at brachial level. Toe pressure is measured by placing a pneumatic cuff around the proximal phalanx and applying a photoplethysmograph distally. The latter consists of an infrared light-emitting diode and a photosensor mounted side by side on a small probe. Because whole blood is more opaque to red and near-infrared light than the surrounding tissue, the degree to which the light is attenuated is proportional to the quantity of blood present. Normal systolic toe pressures are 80–90% of the brachial systolic pressure and range from 90–100 mmHg. Values of <30 mmHg indicate critical ischaemia.

Lower limb veins

Colour Doppler

Colour Doppler has revolutionized the investigation of the lower limb venous system in the last 5 years and has rendered lower limb venography redundant in many vascular centres. The first description of ultrasonography for the investigation of lower limb veins was in 1983 when B-mode scanning was used for the detection of deep venous thrombosis. Although it quickly became apparent that duplex scanning could demonstrate venous valve function and venous reflux, its impact was limited by the long examination time (1.5 h per limb).

The advent of colour Doppler allowed instantaneous visualization of blood flow and its direction and this technique therefore quickly became the first-line modality for investigation of the lower limb venous system. An experienced vascular technologist can perform a complete examination of a lower limb in 15 min.

The lower limb veins are examined with the legs dependent. The deep and superficial venous systems are examined with 5 MHz and 10 MHz linear-array probes, respectively. The calf muscles are manually compressed producing cephalad flow in the vein and this Doppler shift is assigned a blue colour for flow towards the heart. Sudden release of the distal compression will reveal reflux as a red colour, indicating flow away from the heart. Significant reflux is defined as reverse flow lasting >0.5 s. Using this technique, it is relatively easy to detect reflux at the saphenofemoral junction, saphenopopliteal junction and within the deep venous system, including the below-knee popliteal vein and gastrocnemius veins (Plate 2).

Pencil Doppler

Pencil Doppler has the advantage of being quick and relatively cheap. The saphenofemoral junction is examined with the patient standing and the probe placed over the common femoral vein at an angle of 45° to the horizontal. Confirmation that the probe is in the correct position is obtained by manual compression of the calf, thereby producing a marked increase in the blood velocity signal towards the heart. The patient is asked to cough or perform a Valsava manoeuvre, the calf is compressed manually and then this is suddenly released. Absence of flow during the cough or Valsava manoeuvre and on sudden release of calf compression means that there is no reflux. However, a signal lasting >0.5 s demonstrates flow away from the heart and indicates significant reflux. The reflux may also be detected in the long saphenous vein and its lateral tributary in the thigh. A tourniquet or finger placed above the probe should control the reflux.

The saphenopopliteal junction is examined with the patient standing, facing away from the examiner. The knee to be examined is slightly flexed and the Doppler probe is then positioned on the skin in the knee crease at an angle of 45° to the horizontal. Augmentation of the venous signal by compression of the calf produces an optimum venous signal. The calf is then compressed manually and venous flow in the direction of the heart is detected. Absence of flow on sudden release of the calf compression means that there is no reflux and is characteristic of a normal saphenopopliteal junction and popliteal vein. The presence of flow distally on release of compression indicates reflux in either the short saphenous or popliteal vein. In the presence of reflux, the calf compression with sudden release is repeated with the addition of finger compression of the short saphenous vein just distal to the probe. If reflux continues despite digital compression of the short saphenous vein, it is inferred that the reflux is in the popliteal vein itself.

The major limitation of pencil Doppler is that it cannot insonate an individual vessel selectively and will therefore detect velocity in any artery or vein in the path of the ultrasound beam. Thus, at the level of the groin, reflux can be detected in a tributary of the long saphenous vein, long saphenous vein itself or the common femoral vein. In the popliteal fossa, reflux may be in the short saphenous vein, popliteal vein or gastrocnemius veins. Moreover, pencil Doppler cannot demonstrate the level of the saphenopopliteal junction. It has been shown that compared to colour Doppler pencil Doppler misses 12% of saphenofemoral and 20% of saphenopopliteal junction reflux. However, when performed by an experienced clinician it is a very useful tool for the assessment of varicose veins.

Ambulatory venous pressure measurements

Ambulatory venous pressure (AVP) measurement is considered the 'gold standard' investigation for the assessment of calf muscle pump function.

The action of the calf muscle pump is to empty and reduce the pressure in the superficial veins during exercise and the measurement of the effect of exercise on superficial vein pressure is an important test of calf muscle pump function. It has been shown that superficial veins constitute a single superficial compartment so that the pressure obtained in one vein is representative of the pressure throughout the compartment.

A suitable vein on the dorsum of the foot is cannulated and the cannula connected to a pressure transducer and via an amplifier to a chart recorder. The patient holds onto a frame to support himself and the resting pressure is recorded. The patient then performs 10 heel raises at the rate of 1 per second and having finished stays still as the recovery in pressure is recorded. The parameters commonly recorded are the AVP at the end of the 10 heel raises and the time taken for the pressure to rise again to 90% of its resting value [the '90% return time' (RT90)]. The AVP measures the efficacy of the calf muscle pump whereas the RT90 measures the 'rate of reflux' in the limb. The normal AVP is 15–30 mmHg and the normal RT90 is 18–40 s (Fig. 4.6).

Photoplethysmography

The basis of any plethysmographic technique is indirectly to measure changes in the blood flow or content of an organ. In the case of photo-

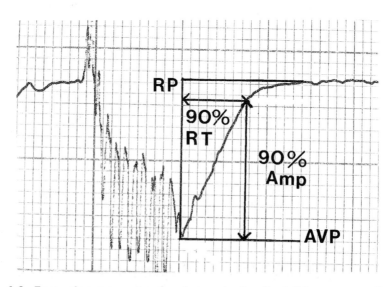

Fig. 4.6. Foot vein pressure tracing demonstrating the fall in pressure after 10 heel raises (AVP) and return to resting pressure (RP). The RT90 is the time taken for the pressure to rise to 90% of its resting value.

plethysmography (PPG) the parameter that is measured is the volume of blood in the skin capillaries, which itself correlates with the superficial venous pressure. The PPG consists of an infrared light-emitting diode and a photosensor mounted side by side on a small probe. Because whole blood is more opaque to red and near-infrared light than the surrounding tissue, the degree to which the light is attenuated is proportional to the quantity of blood present.

The probe is fixed to the skin with transparent double-sided tape and with the patient sitting, 10 heel raises are performed. The PPG trace looks very similar to an AVP recording. Most laboratories use the PPG solely for measuring RT90 because it is not possible to calibrate the PPG in terms of venous pressure. The PPG is most useful as a test for excluding venous disease and a RT90 of >18 s excludes significant venous disease. It should be noted that severe skin damage renders PPG readings difficult and/or unreliable.

Air plethysmography

Air plethysmography (APG) measures changes in the volume of a limb by measuring changes in the volume of an air-filled cuff around the limb. The APG consists of a 14-inch tubular PVC air chamber (capacity 5 litres) that surrounds the leg from knee to ankle. The chamber is inflated to 6 mmHg and connected to a pressure transducer, amplifier and recorder. A smaller bag (capacity 1 litre) placed between the air chamber and the leg is used for calibration. Initially, the patient lies supine with his legs elevated 45° to empty the veins. Calibration is performed by injecting 200 ml increments of water into the calibration bag and recording the corresponding pressure changes in the air chamber. The water is removed and the patient stands with his weight on the opposite leg, holding onto an orthopaedic frame.

An increase in leg volume occurs because of venous filling. This volume is defined as the venous volume (VV). The VV in normal limbs is 100–150 ml and in deep venous insufficiency is 70–320 ml. The time to achieve 90% venous filling is the 90% venous filling time (VFT90). The venous filling index (VFI) is defined as the ratio 90% VV/VFT90. By asking the patient to do 1 heel raise, the ejected volume (EV) and ejection fraction (EF = EV/VV × 100) as a result of the calf muscle contraction can be measured. Patients with deep venous disease have a lower EF than normals.

Finally, by asking the patient to perform 10 heel raises one can measure the residual volume (RV) and calculate the residual volume fraction (RVF = RV/VV × 100). Limbs with deep venous disease have a high RV and a high RVF. There is no evidence that this technique has any real advantage over duplex or AVPs.

Ultrasound diagnosis of deep vein thrombosis

Ultrasound scanning is increasingly used to diagnose deep vein thrombosis (DVT). In the first few days after thrombosis, the echogenicity of the thrombus is greater than that of surrounding blood. However, the echogenicity then reduces due to the breakdown of red blood cells in the thrombus and then increases again in the following weeks due to further resorption and retraction. Thus, direct visualization of thrombus is a specific but not very sensitive diagnostic test of DVT.

The usefulness of ultrasonography can be increased with compression techniques. This procedure evaluates the compressibility of the vein in transverse section during compression with the ultrasound probe. Veins containing thrombus cannot be fully compressed.

Duplex criteria to diagnose DVT include absence of spontaneous or augmented flow in occluded vein, continuous venous flow with no respiratory variation below an occluded segment and increased spontaneous flow in the main superficial veins. Colour Doppler has greatly facilitated the evaluation of pelvic and calf veins and can more easily diagnose partly occluding thrombus. The typical finding in this circumstance is a colour signal in a partly compressible segment (Plate 3). Colour Doppler scanning is now used routinely in many centres for the diagnosis of iliofemoral and femoropopliteal thrombosis and is increasingly used to image calf vein thrombosis.

Summary

- Colour Doppler is the first-line investigation for suspected carotid artery and upper limb artery disease.
- Transcranial Doppler is the commonest method of cerebral monitoring during carotid surgery.
- B-mode ultrasound is used for detecting and monitoring the growth of abdominal aortic aneurysms.
- An exercise test should be done if the diagnosis of claudication is in doubt.
- Colour Doppler should be used to investigate recurrent varicose veins or if deep venous insufficiency is suspected.
- Ambulatory venous pressure measurement is the 'gold standard' for the assessment of calf muscle pump function but is not often required.

Areas of controversy

- Will colour Doppler replace digital subtraction angiography as the investigation of choice for lower limb arterial occlusive disease?
- Can carotid surgery be safely performed on the basis of a colour Doppler scan alone?
- Is it necessary to perform a colour Doppler scan on all patients with varicose veins?

Further reading

- Gerlock AJ, Giyanani VL, Krebs CK (eds). *Applications of Non-Invasive Vascular Techniques.* Philadelphia: WB Saunders, 1988.
- Yao JST, Pearce WH (eds). *Technologies in Vascular Surgery.* Philadelphia: WB Saunders, 1992.
- Greenhalgh RM (ed). *Vascular Imaging for Surgeons.* London: WB Saunders, 1995.
- Evans DH, McDicken WN, Skidmore R, Woodcock JP (eds). *Doppler Ultrasound. Physics, Instrumentation and Clinical Applications.* Chichester: John Wiley & Sons, 1989.
- Sweibel W (ed). *Introduction to Vascular Sonography*, 3rd edn. Philadelphia: WB Saunders, 1992.
- Goldberg R, Merton DA, Deane CR (eds). *An Atlas of Ultrasound Colour Flow Imaging.* London: Martin Dunitz, 1997.

5
Radiological Investigations

Trevor Cleveland

Introduction

Radiological investigations for peripheral vascular disease must be based firmly on the principle that they should image disease which will be treatable within the context of a patient's clinical condition. In many institutions investigations are performed either in the Radiology Department or in a dedicated Vascular Laboratory. Those which may be undertaken in the latter are addressed in Chapter 4.

Diagnostic angiography

This remains the 'gold standard' investigation for the majority of manifestations of peripheral vascular disease. However, in many circumstances other non-invasive techniques have replaced arteriography.

The early enthusiasm for intravenous digital subtraction techniques (IVDSA) turned out to be unfounded and this has now largely been relegated to an imaging tool where there are no peripheral pulses. IVDSA relies on the patient's cardiac output being sufficient to produce a compact bolus by the time the blood and contrast have passed through the pulmonary circulation and into the aorta. Most patients with significant peripheral vascular disease also have coronary artery disease and as a result have reduced myocardial function. This, along with peripheral arterial occlusive disease, makes IVDSA only capable of imaging vessels as far as the femoral bifurcation with any reliability (Fig. 5.1). Consequently, most vascular radiologists electively access the arterial circulation from the left arm if femoral pulses are absent.

Pre-angiographic assessment

Despite the fact that modern angiographic techniques and equipment make angiography a low-risk procedure, it remains an invasive investigation and its safety depends upon adequate preoperative assessment. No patient should undergo arteriography unless there is a good clinical

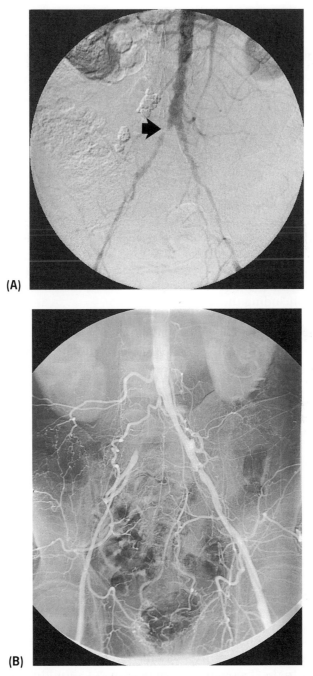

(A)

(B)

Fig. 5.1. (A) Intravenous digital subtraction angiography showing poor contrast delineation of an iliac stenosis (arrow). (B) Intra-arterial digital subtraction angiography showing much better quality images of the pelvic vessels despite a full occlusion of the common iliac artery.

indication that a treatable lesion will be found. In addition, the following specific aspects need to be addressed.

Renal function

All patients in whom arteriography is planned should have their renal function measured because iodinated contrast media are nephrotoxic. Therefore, a patient's management prior to and following angiography is dependent upon his serum creatinine. If it is 110 mmol or less, then angiography can be performed with safety. If the creatinine is between 110 and 300 mmol, then intravenous fluids should be commenced 6 h prior to arteriography to ensure a good urine output during the peri- and post-angiographic period. If cardiac function is impaired, then diuretics should be used as necessary.

A fluid balance chart should be commenced prior to arteriography and careful assessment of urine output should be made for at least 24 h following contrast injection.

If creatinine is >300 mmol, then referral to the local renal physicians is recommended so that more aggressive control of renal function can be maintained, including the use of inotropes.

Anticoagulation

Patients with peripheral vascular disease frequently have co-existing disease which requires anticoagulation, e.g. cardiac disease, prosthetic heart valves and thromboembolic disease. This group needs to be identified and anticoagulation altered appropriately. Warfarin therapy need not be interrupted for diagnostic arteriography provided that the international normalized ratio (INR) is <3. Three or four French catheter systems are used and provided no interventional procedure is contemplated at the same time, this is relatively free of haemorrhagic complications, although day-case investigation is not appropriate.

If the above is not the case, and if continuous anticoagulation is clinically indicated, then the patient must be converted to intravenous Heparin in therapeutic doses. Should continuous anticoagulation be unnecessary, then stopping warfarin 2–3 days prior to angiography, with a check INR on the day of the procedure, is usually sufficient.

Metformin

Intravascular contrast injection has been associated with an increased risk of lactic acidosis, particularly in diabetic patients with reduced renal function who are on metformin (Glucophage). The mortality of this condition is high. If possible, diabetic control should be changed to another form of oral hypoglycaemic agent, particularly if the patient has abnormal renal function.

If this is not possible or is undesirable, then metformin should be stopped 48 h prior to arteriography. The patient's renal function should be measured and managed as above for 2 days following arteriography, the renal function should again be measured and if it has not deteriorated, then metformin can safely be reintroduced. In the urgent/emergency situation when there is no time to stop metformin 48 h prior to arteriography, then it should be stopped as soon as the decision has been made to undertake angiography and the same procedures as for renal failure taken.

Hypertension

This is a relative contraindication to arteriography. In general, routine angiography should be avoided in patients with a diastolic blood pressure >100 mmHg. Blood pressure may be transiently reduced by the use of calcium channel blockers (e.g. sub-lingual nifedipine); however, this is a transitory change and long-term control of blood pressure is a part of the manipulation and control of risk factors associated with peripheral vascular disease. Therefore, long-term control of hypertension should be the aim. However, it should be remembered that many patients are understandably anxious prior to angiography and reassurance, possibly with the addition of mild sedation, will cure these 'hypertensives'.

Previous surgery

Previous vascular surgery is an important consideration in planning arteriography. Generally, percutaneous puncture sites should be chosen to avoid access through prosthetic graft material as haemostasis in these circumstances is more difficult with a consequently higher rate of haematoma formation. In addition, the potential infective consequences of direct graft puncture should be considered when planning access sites. All patients undergoing direct graft puncture should have prophylactic antibiotics.

Ability to lie flat and still

Patients need to lie flat and still for approximately 30 min for simple angiography and for up to 2–3 h for complex interventional procedures. Cardiac failure and chest infections in particular should be treated prior to catheter angiography. In general, sedation is not necessary; indeed, a degree of disinhibition may be caused by sedation and result in severe motion artefact. Good explanation and adequate analgesia are generally much more effective.

Consent

Fully informed consent should be obtained from all patients (or a relative if incapable) and should include an explanation of the specific risks associated with arteriography. Patient information sheets are a useful aid.

Post-angiographic care

Routine post-angiographic care has altered enormously as angiographic techniques have evolved from translumbar arteriography to the trans-femoral route, and catheter sizes have significantly reduced. Today most diagnostic procedures are performed through 3F or 4F catheters and are safely performed on a day-case basis, with patients confined to bed for 3–4 h only.

Routine pulse and blood pressure monitoring is important in the early stages following angiography and puncture sites should be frequently inspected for bleeding and haematoma formation. The vast majority of patients are able to rest a hand on their groin and report any such complications. The limb should be carefully observed for evidence of local or embolic complications and pulses compared with the pre-angiography status.

These precautions are all geared to the traditional approach to puncture site closure, i.e. pressure haemostasis. Recently, a number of devices have become available, at a cost, which close the arterial puncture site mechanically and allow patients in whom larger holes (up to 8F or larger) have been made, and anticoagulation given, to be managed as day cases. In general, however, these are unnecessary for simple diagnostic procedures.

Complications

Complications of angiography may be divided into those related to the contrast and those to the technique.

Contrast complications

These can be subdivided into allergic and toxic reactions.

Allergic

These are less common with modern non-ionic low osmolar contrast agents and with intra-arterial than intravenous injections. Allergic reactions to contrast include urticarial rashes, bronchospasm, laryngeal oedema and acute anaphylaxis. They are not dose related and are probably the result of mast cell degranulation.

Toxic

These reactions manifest as feelings of warmth, an unpleasant metallic taste, cardiac arrhythmias and pulmonary oedema. Unlike allergic reactions, they are dose related and are more likely to occur in dehydrated patients with extensive vascular disease.

Technique complications

These may be subdivided into those occurring locally to the puncture site and those occurring distantly.

Local

- *Haematoma/haemorrhage with subsequent false aneurysm formation.* These may be prevented by careful attention to pre-angiographic assessment of clotting disorders and anticoagulants along with adequate pressure haemostasis. Aftercare includes groin observation and gentle palpation, and should bleeding reoccur then pressure can again be applied and the vast majority of haematomata restricted to minor bruising. Compression devices are available commercially; however, for the routine diagnostic 4F angiogram an appropriately placed finger is as quick and generally better tolerated by the patient. If a false aneurysm does form, then the traditional approach is for a surgical repair; however, recently these have been successfully treated using ultrasound-controlled compression.
- *Spasm* (rare). This usually resolves spontaneously or following the administration of vasodilators (e.g. nifedipine, glyceryl trinitrate, papavarine).
- *Subintimal dissection/thrombosis.* This results in acute closure of the artery and usually requires local surgical exploration and patch repair.
- *Infection* (rare).
- *Damage to local structures,* e.g. the lateral cutaneous nerve of the thigh during femoral puncture and the brachial plexus during axillary puncture. If progressive neurological deficit occurs, then urgent decompression of the haematoma is required.
- *Arteriovenous fistula* (rare).

Distant

- *Embolic.* These usually originate from peri-catheter or guidewire thrombus which breaks away and lodges in a vessel downstream from the catheter position. Small emboli may be clinically silent and often will break up spontaneously. However, large emboli may have significant consequences, particularly if the cerebral circulation is involved. In the periphery, aspiration or surgical embolectomy may be necessary. Atheroembolism may also occur from plaque dissected by a guidewire.
- *Distant dissection.* If a guidewire or catheter is allowed to track subintimally, then a dissection flap will be raised. With retrograde punctures small dissections may not be significant, but if a flap is antegrade or contrast is injected subintimally into the flap, then these will cause significant flow limitation. Such flow-limiting dissections may now be treated with metallic stents, which reapply the intima to the media.

- *Guidewire or catheter fracture and knotting* (rare with modern equipment).

Venography

The role of contrast venography has significantly reduced in recent years as ultrasound, including Doppler and colour flow imaging, has improved (see Chapter 4). As a result, venography has been relegated to those situations where non-invasive tests have failed to give sufficient information.

Ascending venography

Ascending venography is usually performed to confirm or refute a below-knee thrombus (Fig. 5.2). A cannula is introduced into a vein on the dorsum of the foot and a tourniquet is then applied just above the ankle, thereby forcing the contrast to pass into the deep venous system. Images are therefore obtained of the deep veins and any thrombus will be identified as a filling defect within this contrast.

Varicography

A variation of ascending venography may be used to investigate recurrent varicose veins and thus is known as varicography. The varicose veins are punctured directly and contrast injected. By injecting at various levels with the patient in the semi-standing position and taking images at different obliquities, the communicating veins between the deep and varicosed systems may be identified.

A drawback with this test is that blood flow is normally from superficial to deep systems and the competence or otherwise of the perforating valves cannot be assessed. For this reason Doppler examination or colour flow imaging have largely replaced this test.

Descending venography

Evaluation of valvular damage and incompetence in the post-phlebitic limb may be performed by descending venography. This is done by accessing the appropriate femoral vein and placing the patient at approximately 60° upright tilt. Contrast is injected and the degree of reflux documented. The procedure is repeated with the patient performing a Valsalva manoeuvre. The amount of reflux can then be seen and graded if necessary. This examination has again largely been replaced by duplex imaging.

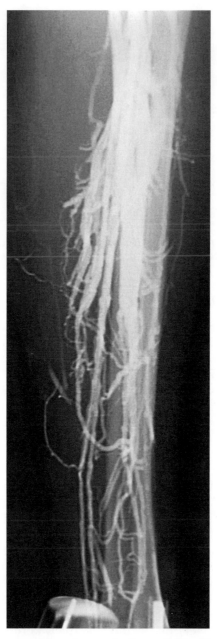

Fig. 5.2. Ascending venogram demonstrating patent calf vessels.

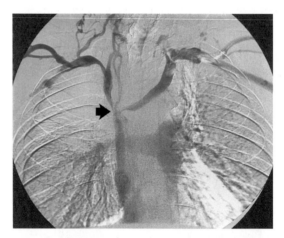

Fig. 5.3. Superior vena cavagram, following bilateral antecubital fossa injections, showing stenosis of the superior vena cava (arrow).

Upper limb venography

A subclavian vein thrombosis is also amenable to duplex assessment although the development of large collaterals may cause confusion and result in a high false negative rate. If the duplex is negative and the level of clinical suspicion is high, then a venogram may be required. In patients with the signs and symptoms of superior vena cava (SVC) obstruction, venography is needed. In these circumstances, bilateral arm vein injection on a digital subtraction unit will delineate an SVC stenosis and/or thrombosis (Fig. 5.3).

Intravascular ultrasound

Conventional ultrasound, duplex and colour Doppler are covered in Chapter 4.

Intravascular ultrasound (IVUS) is a relatively new technique in which a tiny ultrasound probe is mounted on a catheter and passed over a guidewire. As the ultrasound probe is within the lumen of the artery, very high frequency probes may be used and therefore very high resolution images obtained (Fig. 5.4.). In its infancy, IVUS catheters were large (8F, 2.5 mm in diameter) but by the late 1980s were 5F and are now as small as 2.9F (0.9 mm). Therefore, almost all arteries within the body may be imaged, including below-knee and coronary arteries.

IVUS can take very high quality 2D cross-sectional images of an artery, and with a mechanical pull-back device a 3D reconstruction of the arterial wall is possible. This technique allows evaluation of plaque morphology and

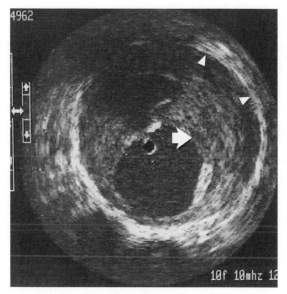

Fig. 5.4. Intravascular ultrasound of the abdominal aorta with thrombus (arrow) within an aneurysm sac (arrow heads).

composition in relation to the vessel wall and allows very precise measurements of disease bulk. The size of the true lumen diameter can be seen and these precise measurements may be extremely useful for guidance and evaluation of subsequent interventional procedures.

IVUS, however, has significant drawbacks:

- High cost. Even ignoring the cost of the imaging hardware, each single-use catheter costs in the region of £500.
- It cannot look forward and requires significant additional catheter time in already diseased vessels.
- 3D reconstruction can only be performed after the imaging has finished and cannot be utilized at the time of the procedure.

All of these problems combine to make IVUS an attractive but rather impractical proposition for most units.

Computed tomography

Conventional CT images are obtained in the axial plane and a 2D image is obtained by assigning each small piece of the image a density, and displaying these various density levels as a degree of 'grey' between black and white. To obtain images in a longitudinal plane (i.e. as required for imaging of most blood vessels) requires many slices to be stacked next to each other and then computer reconstruction in 3D. As a result these images require large radiation doses and are very susceptible to artefact from any movement of the patient (e.g. breathing) or malpositioning of the table.

More recently, spiral (helical) CT has become available. In this technique, a 'volume' of data is collected by the X-ray tube as it 'spirals' along a length of the patient. In this way large volumes of the patient may be imaged in a single breathhold. Images may then be obtained in slices appearing exactly the same as in conventional CT, but they may be chosen in any (e.g. axial, coronal, sagital) plane. In addition, if the patient is given intravenous iodinated contrast and images are taken at an appropriate time, the arteries within the 'volume' interrogated will contain a high concentration of contrast. The high-density arteries may then be identified throughout the volume and reconstructed into a CT angiogram. These may be displayed in two main ways:

- *Maximum intensity projection* (MIP) produces images rather similar to conventional angiography but with additional soft tissue information (Fig. 5.5).
- Shaded surface display (SSD) gives images which appear like arterial casts (Fig. 5.6).

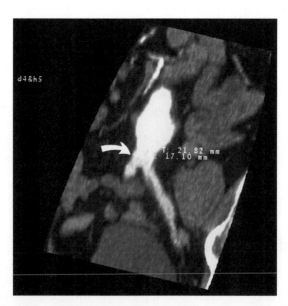

Fig. 5.5. Spiral CT (maximum intensity projection) of an aortic bifurcation (curved arrow) with an aneurysm above.

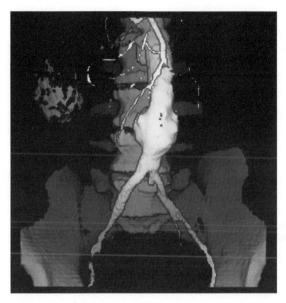

Fig. 5.6. **Same patient as in Fig. 5.5 showing the infrarenal aorta and aortic birfurcation (shaded surface display).**

CT angiography does, however, have limitations:

- A relatively high radiation dosage is required in comparison to DSA. The resolution is relatively low compared with IADSA and in large patients may result in an unacceptably low signal-to-noise ratio.
- Large contrast doses (approximately 150–200 ml) are required and may be problematic in some patients.

These problems notwithstanding, CT angiography has undoubtedly found a place in the assessment of abdominal aortic aneurysms and to a lesser extent thoracic and pelvic vascular imaging. It also has advantages over magnetic resonance angiography when assessing intracranial and cerebral disease in patients with metallic prostheses and aneurysm clips.

Magnetic resonance imaging

MRI and the various MR techniques now available are used to produce 'angiograms' (MRA). MRA cannot usually match the spatial resolution of conventional angiography; however, it is sufficient to image the aorta and its major branches. The resolution of the images of smaller vessels may be improved by the use of surface coils. MRA does not involve the use of ionizing radiation and can also be used for patients with contrast allergy and/or poor renal function. The data acquired from the MRA images may then be reconstructed into 2D or 3D images. Broadly, MRAs can be obtained in five different ways.

Black blood

In most standard MR sequences, the blood which flows in vessels is unable to produce a signal and therefore an image. As a result, it appears as an absence of signal and therefore black on images. Consequently, the vessel walls can be easily visualized as can their relationship to surrounding structures. However, if blood flow is very slow, such as in an abdominal aortic aneurysm, then some signal may remain in the scan plane and will degrade the image. In addition, a poor signal-to-noise ratio makes imaging of small vessels difficult.

Time of flight

The volume of tissue under investigation is saturated with radiofrequency pulses making all of the static tissues appear dark. Blood which flows into the region will be the only tissue able to produce signal. As a result, flowing blood will appear bright and angiographic images are produced.

Phase contrast

This technique not only allows the blood vessels to be imaged, but also gives information on the direction of blood flow and the quantity of blood flowing within the area of interest.

Cine

Images are obtained of a pulsatile blood vessel and these are correlated with each phase of the cardiac cycle via the ECG. Multiple images at the same phase are then reconstructed and again at multiple phases of the cycle. These may then be used to produce a cine loop so that, for example, an aortic dissection can be readily identified with differential flow within the two lumens.

Gadolinium-enhanced MRA

This technique produces 'bright blood' rather like conventional or CT angiography. All of the above techniques work well in normal arteries with laminar blood flow. However, in the presence of peripheral vascular disease, and therefore turbulent flow, a gadolinium-enhanced MRA improves diagnostic quality (Fig. 5.7).

It is clear from the above that the possibilities for MRA are enormous and its potential has yet to be realized. It is, however, already useful in patients who have an allergy to iodinated contrast or poor renal function. Recent reports indicate that excellent images of the smaller vessels may be obtained with gadolinium-enhanced MRI. However, at present,

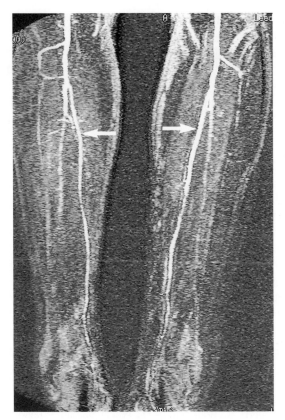

Fig. 5.7. **Magnetic resonance angiogram of the tibial vessels demonstrating bilateral patent posterior tibal arteries (arrows).**

MRA is time consuming, costly and not readily available in most UK centres. As sequences and scanners improve, MRI is likely to make a far greater impact.

Summary

- Intra-arterial digital subtraction arteriography remains the 'gold standard' for peripheral arterial imaging.
- Renal function must be checked before arteriography.
- Impaired renal function requires protection with intravenous fluids and cessation of metformin.
- Anticoagulation with warfarin can be continued during diagnostic arteriography provided the INR is <3.
- Diagnostic arteriography can be performed as a day-case procedure.

- Bleeding complications are usually due to inadequate application of pressure at the puncture site.
- Venography is no longer the investigation of choice for most venous disease.
- Spiral CT is probably the investigation of choice for elective abdominal aortic aneurysms.
- Magnetic resonance angiography cannot match the spatial resolution of arteriography at present.

Areas of controversy

- Can colour Doppler, spiral CT and MRA completely replace conventional diagnostic arteriography?
- Will interventional techniques such as angioplasty and stenting be best performed under angiographic control?
- Should intra-arterial pressure measurements always be obtained before treating stenoses?
- How should the success of surgery or angioplasty be assessed?

Further reading

- Whitehouse GH, Worthington BS (eds). *Techniques in Diagnostic Imaging.* Oxford: Blackwell, 1990.
- Fellmeth BD, Roberts AC, Bookstein JJ *et al.* Post angiographic femoral artery injuries: nonsurgical repair with US-guided compression. *Radiology* 1991;**178**:671–675.
- Edelman RR, Adamis MK, Muller M, Hochman M. MR angiography of the body. In: Edelman RR, Hesselink JR, Zlatklin Philadelphia MB (eds) *Clinical, Magnetic Resonance Imaging,* Vol II, 2nd Edn. WB Saunders, 1996, pp 1305–1329.
- Cleveland TJ, Cumberland DC, Gaines PA. Percutaneous aspiration thrombo-embolectomy to manage the embolic complications of angioplasty and as an adjunct to thrombolysis. *Clinical Radiology* 1994;**49**:549–552.
- Rubin GD, Dake MD, Semba CP. Current status of three-dimensional spiral CT scanning for imaging the vasculature. *Radiologic Clinics of North America* 1995;**33**:51–70.
- Royal College of Radiologists. Advice to members and fellows with regard to met-formin-induced lactic acidosis and X-ray contrast medium agents. *BCFR* (96) 8. London: Royal College of Radiologists, 1996.

6
Medical Management and Anticoagulation

Edward Housley

Introduction

Before the advent of effective intervention techniques, medical therapy was widely used in the treatment of intermittent claudication. Later, realization of the long-term limitations of intervention has led to a resurgence of interest in the use of medical therapy for claudication. However, the problems that bedevilled assessment of the earlier medical therapies remain:

- tendency of most patients to improve spontaneously after presentation;
- placebo effect;
- bias in reporting only positive trials in medical journals.

It is well known that after an acute arterial occlusion collateral arteries develop rapidly and 50–80% of patients will report improvement in their claudication over the next few months if they are encouraged to keep walking. Thus, great care is needed to exclude such patients from a therapeutic study.

The placebo effect is the patient's, and often the physician's, uncritical belief that the treatment will work and is particularly prevalent in claudication therapy assessments. Improvement in walking distance of 20–50% in so-called stable claudicators in the placebo arm of studies is usual and often approaches that seen in the treatment arm.

Although difficult to quantify, there is no doubt that there is a considerable degree of reporting bias of positive therapeutic studies in the medical journals, i.e. negative studies are not submitted and, even if submitted, editors are reluctant to publish them.

Finally, even where a benefit is shown in an apparently good study, this, even though statistically significant, is often clinically insignificant. For example, an increase in walking distance of 50% with a drug may seem impressive but, compared to 30% in the control group, is really only an increase of 2/13ths, i.e. 15%, which is clinically negligible.

General measures

The above criteria for proof of efficacy should apply to so-called general measures as well as drug therapy. However, as these measures are physiologically sensible, cost little or nothing and are safe, the threshold for proof of their efficacy may be lower than that for drugs.

General health

There is a high incidence of general illness, e.g. cardiac failure and anaemia, in claudicators which, if treated, may increase the walking distance considerably.

Weight reduction

This will reduce the amount of work done by the leg muscles during walking so obese patients should be strongly encouraged to lose weight.

Exercise

Exercise has been shown considerably to increase walking distance in good controlled studies. The increase is probably mainly due to collateral development but improvement in muscle metabolism, reduction of blood viscosity, increase in high-density lipoprotein cholesterol (HDL-cholesterol) and learning to walk more efficiently may also play a part.

Treadmill exercise classes have been shown to be effective but it is important to emphasize to the patient that exercise must continue after the classes have ended. Treadmill sessions of at least 1 h three times weekly, or community walking exercise of $\frac{1}{2}$–1 h a day, are necessary to show benefit. Patients will only persist with an exercise regime if it can be fitted into their lifestyle, e.g. walking to and from work, or taking the dog out twice a day.

It is important to assess the patient's ability to exercise with particular regard to co-existing angina and lower limb joint osteoarthritis before recommending an exercise programme.

Reassurance

The value of reassurance is often overlooked in a busy outpatient clinic. Many patients are there because they are afraid of gangrene. Assurance that this is unlikely, and this can be given in most cases, is of great psychological benefit and may allow the patient to accept his disability without demand for other treatment.

Foot care

In patients with severe, verging on critical, ischaemia, minor trauma such as over enthusiastic chiropody, careless trimming of toe nails or pressure on bony points, may break the skin and lead to non-healing ulcers and, eventually, gangrene. This is particularly a problem in the very elderly and poor sighted. Regular careful conservative chiropody by a chiropodist who is aware of the vascular problem is essential. Roomy soft well padded shoes or boots should be worn (see Chapter 16).

Control of risk factors

Smoking

Giving up smoking has been shown to be of benefit to claudicators. The mechanism is probably mainly by slowing the rate of development of atheroma, but possibly also by reducing hypercoagulability and the risk of thrombosis in diseased arteries and by reducing blood viscosity.

Unfortunately, the success rate for claudicators quitting is relatively low compared to patients with ischaemic heart disease (IHD), possibly because they tend to be older, and have thus smoked longer, and death is not perceived to be a consequence of continued smoking. Firm advice from the surgeon or general practitioner is the most cost-effective way of getting them to stop but anti-smoking classes or clubs may help resistant cases. Nicotine patches or chewing gum may also help.

Hyperlipidaemia

Target levels

In the last decade there has been an explosion of activity in studying the effect of lipid reduction in patients with cardiovascular disease, mostly in IHD patients but some in peripheral vascular disease patients. Recommended 'target levels' for lipids for secondary prevention have fallen drastically in this time. Current US guidelines for secondary prevention of IHD recommend reduction of the total cholesterol to <5.2 mmol/l and LDL-cholesterol to <3.1 mmol/l.

Implementation of these guidelines would result in the great majority of British claudicators being on therapy, mostly drug therapy, with enormous logistical and cost implications. In addition, the long-term side-effects of these drugs are not fully known.

Although it has been shown that reduction of the death rate from IHD continues down to these lower levels of cholesterol, the absolute benefit becomes progressively less and the problem is to decide at what level the effort outweighs the benefit. If a claudicator has IHD as well, and many do, then the target lipid levels advocated for IHD should apply. However, if the patient does not have overt IHD, and is older (where the evidence for benefit is scanty), less strict targets should be set.

It is therefore impossible to give a universal guideline level for cho-lesterol in claudicators above which treatment should be instituted. The degree of hyperlipidaemia (including the level of HDL-cholesterol, the so-called 'protective' cholesterol), ratio total : HDL-cholesterol, pres-ence of IHD and presence of other risk factors, particularly smoking, hypertension, diabetes and patient age should all be considered.

Dietary treatment

It is conventional to have a trial of diet alone, for 3–6 months, before commencing drug therapy but, in the author's experience, unless the hyperlipidaemia is very mild and due mainly to an excess intake of satu-rated fat, this is rarely successful in the long term and drug therapy will be needed. However, a trial of diet is often useful in showing the patient that diet alone will not be sufficient and that drug therapy will be needed and should be accepted. In severe hyperlipidaemia, i.e. total cholesterol >7.5 mmol/l, drug treatment should be started immediately.

Drug treatment

If drug treatment is needed for hypercholesterolaemia, and the tri-glyceride is normal, a HMG-CoA reductase inhibitor statin drug such as 10 mg simvastatin or 20 mg fluvastatin/day is the drug of choice. Lovastatin and pravastatin are alternatives. The recently introduced statin drug Atorvastatin is probably more effective and has the additional advantage of reducing triglyceride levels as well. The total cholesterol should be rechecked 6–8 weeks later and the dose progressively increased up to 40 mg simvastatin or 80 mg fluvastatin/day until the target level is reached. After the target levels of lipids have been achieved, the fre-quency of measurements can be reduced to every 6 months. An ion-exchange resin such as cholestyramine can be added in a dose of 4–8 g/day if the target level of cholesterol is not reached with the maximum dose of the statin.

Side-effects of statins and fibrates, such as liver dysfunction and myosi-tis are uncommon but serious, so regular checks of liver function and serum creatine kinase, if myositis is suspected, should be done in the first 6 months of therapy. A transient rise in liver enzyme levels up to twice normal may need only a temporary reduction in dose but higher or sus-tained elevation of enzyme levels requires withdrawal of the drug. Cholestyramine therapy can cause gastric side-effects and malabsorption of fat-soluble vitamins when used in large doses.

Drugs such as nicotinic acid derivatives have been used but side-effects, such as flushing, and their limited efficacy have made them less popular.

If hypertriglyceridaemia is a feature of the hyperlipidaemia, i.e. mixed hyperlipidaemia, and the hypercholesterolaemia is relatively mild, i.e. total cholesterol <7.5 mmol/l, a fibrate is the drug of choice as this reduces both total and LDL-cholesterol and triglyceride and raises HDL-cholesterol. Bezafibrate in a dose of 400 mg per day is usually effective. Failure of the cholesterol to reach target levels will require the addition of a statin drug as well with perhaps a slightly increased risk of myositis and liver dysfunction.

Hypertension

Sustained hypertension of >150/90 in younger patients should generally be treated but higher limits up to 160/95 may be allowed in the elderly in whom the risks of side-effects from drugs, particularly postural hypotension, are greater.

Although β-blockers do not significantly adversely affect the walking distance of claudicators, it would seem sensible to use vasodilator drugs such as ACE inhibitors to treat hypertension, rather than a β-blocker, to avoid the side-effect of reduced limb blood flow and cold extremities.

Diabetes mellitus

Good control of diabetes has been shown to retard the progress of atheroma in diabetics so tight control of blood glucose by diet, oral hypoglycaemic drugs or insulin as necessary is mandatory.

Polycythaemia

Polycythaemia is commonest in elderly men and takes two forms: relative and primary proliferative polycythaemia (polycythaemia rubra vera).

Relative polycythaemia

This type of polycythaemia, sometimes called 'stress polycythaemia', is due to reduction of plasma volume with no increase in circulating red cell mass. There is thus an increase in haemoglobin and haematocrit with normal platelet and white cell counts. This increases blood viscosity and risk of arterial thrombosis. Treatment is by repeated venesection, which is tedious and time consuming for both patient and doctor, so compliance is a problem. However, if the haematocrit is significantly raised, >0.55, it is of value. Frequent venesections of 500 ml once or twice a week are needed to lower the haematocrit to a safe level (and will make the patient mildly iron deficient), after which venesection need be done only every 1–2 months.

Primary proliferative polycythaemia

This is a myeloproliferative disorder of the bone marrow causing raised haemoglobin and white cell and platelet counts. There is a very high risk of arterial thrombosis and such patients should be referred to a haematologist for treatment with venesection and hydroxyurea.

Thrombophilia

In younger patients (<50 years) presenting with predominantly thrombotic disease and no risk factors for premature vascular disease, an inherited thrombotic disorder such as Factor V (Leiden), anticardiolipin syndrome, protein C, S or antithrombin III deficiency should be suspected. If found, referral to an haematologist for treatment with anticoagulants is advised.

Homocysteinaemia

The rare homozygous form of this genetically determined disorder has long been recognized as a cause of premature vascular disease. More recently, it has been realized that the heterozygous form, of variable degree, is also associated with premature disease. In patients presenting with vascular disease at a young age and with no obvious risk factors, the plasma homocysteine should be measured and, if raised, referral to a physician for treatment and genetic counselling is recommended.

Specific measures

Several groups of drugs have been advocated as specific treatments for intermittent claudication. These are grouped below by their alleged mode of action.

- antiplatelet drugs;
- vasodilators;
- reduction of viscosity;
- metabolic effect;
- antioxidant effect.

Antiplatelet drugs

Aspirin is used extensively in patients with claudication. It inhibits cyclo-oxygenase and thus blocks the production of the platelet aggregator thromboxane A_2. Studies have shown that it retards the rate of progression of atheroma and reduces the need for invasive intervention in claudicators. The dose is not critical but 75–150 mg/day seems to be sufficient. Treatment is recommended for patients with peripheral vascular disease and should be continued indefinitely. Aspirin is also known to have both cardiac and cerebrovascular protective effects. Contraindications are peptic ulcer or gastric irritation, with the risk of gastrointestinal bleeding, and allergy to aspirin.

Other drugs such as ticlopidine are used abroad but are associated with a small but significant risk of serious side-effects and are not licensed for use in the UK.

Vasodilators

There is no convincing evidence that any vasodilator is of benefit and none is recommended.

Viscosity-lowering drugs

Drugs such as pentoxifilline, which reduce red cell rigidity, have been extensively studied with conflicting results. The benefit, if any, is marginal and their use is not recommended.

Metabolically acting drugs

Drugs to improve the metabolic efficiency of the ischaemic leg muscle, e.g. naftidrofuryl, have been extensively studied. Their alleged benefit is not convincing. New drugs such as L-carnitine are under investigation but are still not of proven value.

Antioxidants

The role of antioxidants in the pathophysiology of atheroma and treatment of claudicators is evolving rapidly. Drugs that act as 'free radical scavengers' are being investigated but they are not yet at the stage of proven efficacy.

Anticoagulation

Prevention of arterial thrombosis, with worsening of limb ischaemia, can be achieved with aspirin or oral anticoagulants. The use of aspirin has been considered above. Use of oral anticoagulants such as warfarin is theoretically attractive but the poor risk : benefit ratio of life-long oral anticoagulation in this predominantly elderly group of patients makes this treatment inadvisable unless there is clear evidence of an underlying thrombophilia. However, acute thrombosis or embolic occlusion of a limb artery does require anticoagulation. Heparin should be given first to achieve rapid anticoagulation, followed by oral anticoagulation with warfarin to prevent extension of thrombosis or further embolization of the limb.

Heparin

Standard heparin

Heparin is a highly negatively charged conjugated polysaccharide of molecular weight varying widely between 2000 and 40 000 Da. It is known as unfractionated or standard heparin. It has to be given parenterally. The bioavailability, and thus the anticoagulant effect, of this form of heparin is variable. The half-life of the drug, given intravenously, is approximately 1 h.

An initial bolus dose of 80 unit/kg body weight should be given intravenously followed by a continuous intravenous infusion of 1200–1500 unit/h (500 unit/kg body weight/24 h). After 6 h the plasma heparin level of the initial bolus and subsequent continuous infusion should have reached and been maintained at the desired therapeutic level. The activated partial thromboplastin time (APTT) should be measured at this time to assess the level of anticoagulation. An APTT of 1.5–2.5 times the control should be aimed for. The infusion dose may need to be changed or, if the APTT is too high, the infusion may need to be held for a while. If the infusion rate is varied, the APTT should be measured after another 6 h and then at least daily thereafter.

Better control of heparin therapy can be achieved by using nomograms indicating dose adjustment, or hold, in accordance with the APTT and time. A sample nomogram is shown in Table 6.1.

If bleeding does occur, simply stopping the infusion for 1–2 h results in a subtherapeutic level of heparin and cessation of bleeding and the infusion can then be recommenced at a lower dose. In the event of serious bleeding, immediate reversal of anticoagulation can be achieved with intravenous protamine sulphate (1 mg/100 unit heparin) which carries a strong positive charge and thus combines with, and inactivates, heparin. For example, for bleeding 1 h after 5000 units of intravenous heparin administration, when approximately 2500 units would remain in the circulation the dose would be 25 mg. Side-effects such as flushing, hypotension and allergic reactions may occur. If heparin therapy has to be continued for more than a few days, significant thrombocytopenia

Table 6.1. **Heparin therapy.**

The dose of heparin should be adjusted to give an APTT 1.5–2.5 times the control. Loading dose 80 unit/kg body weight intravenously. Initial maintenance infusion 500 unit/kg body weight/24h. After 6 hours:

APTT (ratio)	Bolus	Stop (min)	Rate Change (unit/h)	Repeat APTT
<1.5	5000 units	0	+100	6 h
1.6–1.8	0	0	+100	6 h
1.9–2.7	0	0	0	Next morning
2.8–3.0	0	0	−100	Next morning
3.1–3.8	0	30	−100	6 h
>3.8	0	60	−100	6 h

may occur and regular platelet counts should be performed. Long-term heparin therapy may cause osteoporosis.

Patients on heparin should not be given aspirin or intramuscular injections.

Low-molecular-weight heparin

Low-molecular-weight heparin has a more reproducible anticoagulant effect than unfractionated heparin. It has a longer half-life and can be given as a once daily dose by subcutaneous injection. It is replacing unfractionated heparin in the treatment of venous thrombosis. However, in surgical patients, where rapid reversal of anticoagulation may be required in the event of bleeding, continuous intravenous infusion of unfractionated heparin is safer.

Warfarin

In most clinical situations heparin needs to be followed by longer term anticoagulation with warfarin. Warfarin is a competitive inhibitor of vitamin K-dependent prothrombin synthesis by the liver.

Given orally it takes 2–4 days to achieve a therapeutic effect by prolonging the prothrombin time, or international normalized ratio (INR), to 2.5–3.5 times the control. Before administration the INR and liver function tests should be measured if possible and, if normal, an initial dose of 10 mg/day prescribed. Daily INR measurements should be made and the dose reduced to 5–7 mg/day when the therapeutic range is reached. If the INR or liver function tests are abnormal before treatment, a lower dose, e.g. 5 mg, should be given and the INR checked daily before each dose is given. In patients with thrombophilic disease, such as anticardiolipin syndrome, a higher INR level of 3.0–4.5 is necessary but carries a greater risk of haemorrhage.

The main adverse effect is, of course, bleeding but in patients with the rare genetic thrombotic disorder protein C deficiency, microvascular thrombosis and cutaneous gangrene may occur as protein C is also vitamin K dependent and warfarin will worsen the condition. Bleeding in a patient with an INR in the therapeutic range is likely to be due to a pathological lesion and should be investigated.

Concomitant administration of other drugs, particularly anti-convulsants and NSAIDs, will alter the anticoagulant effect of warfarin so more frequent INR measurements should be made if these drugs are administered.

In the event of overdosage without bleeding, and an INR <7, simple withdrawal of treatment for 1–2 days will suffice to restore control. If the INR is >7, then 0.5 mg of phytomenadione (vitamin K_1) should be given intravenously as well. If bleeding is a problem, 0.5–2 mg vitamin K_1

should be given and, in severe haemorrhage, clotting factor concentrate or fresh frozen plasma should be given. Large doses of vitamin K_1, e.g. 10–20 mg, should be avoided as they make re-establishment of anti-coagulant control very difficult.

Warfarin should be avoided, if possible, in patients with a lesion that has a potential to bleed, i.e. active peptic ulcer, recent stroke, or a bleeding diathesis.

The duration of oral anticoagulation will depend on whether the indi-cation for anticoagulation persists. Embolization from a cardiac source will require permanent anticoagulation but acute thrombosis of a stenosed artery with effective surgical intervention will require treatment for only a few weeks or months.

It is most important that patients in the community on oral anti-coagulants carry an anticoagulant warning card detailing their dose and the result of their last INR test.

Summary

- Correction of risk factors is vital for the treatment of a patient with peripheral vascular disease.
- Exercise is likely to be the best first-line treatment
- Compliance with cessation of smoking, weight reduction and exercise is a major problem in the treatment of these patients.
- All patients should be on antiplatelet therapy.

Areas of controversy

- Will statin therapy improve claudication distance in addition to reducing cardiac risk?
- Is exercise better than intervention for the treatment of claudication?
- Do anticoagulants confer any benefit over antiplatelet therapy?

Further reading

- Coffman JD Intermittent claudication. In: Tooke JE, Lowe GDO (eds) *A Textbook of Vascular Medicine*. London: Edward Arnold, 1996, pp 207–220.
- Halperin JA, Creager MA. *Arterial obstructive disease of the extremities*. In: Loscalzo J, Creager MA, Dzau VJ (eds) *Vascular Medicine*. Boston: Little, Brown, 1992, pp 835–865.
- Cooke JP, Creager MA. Management of the patient with intermittent claudication. *Vascular Medicine Review* 1991;**2**:19–31.

- Rees JAE. Cholesterol lowering trials: advice for the British physician. *Journal of the Royal College of Physicians of London* 1994;**28**:70–73.
- European Atherosclerosis Society. *A Desktop Guide to the Management of Risk Factors for Coronary Heart Disease.* London: Current Medical Literature, 1992.

7

Vascular Anaesthesia

Michelle Hayes and Mark Palazzo

Introduction

Anaesthesia for patients presenting for vascular surgery is associated with a high incidence of morbidity and mortality. This is not surprising since these patients usually have extensive atherosclerotic disease due to hypertension, pre-existing renal impairment, diabetes and smoking and consequently are at risk from cardiac, renal and occasionally cerebral complications. In addition, these patients tend to be biologically elderly with poor respiratory reserve.

The risks of surgery and anaesthesia are constantly being challenged by numerous practice changes:

- no limit on age for surgery;
- less desire for conservative management by patient and surgeon;
- admission only 1–2 days before surgery.

These factors place increased demands on our care, particularly in the postoperative period.

General principles of anaesthesia

Anaesthesia can be provided by three basic techniques or a combination of techniques. These are local, regional or general anaesthesia (when paralysis is required, the patient is intubated and ventilated or when not required, the patient is allowed to breathe spontaneously). During general anaesthesia, airway protection and gaseous drug administration may be provided by a face mask, a laryngeal mask or an endotracheal tube. There are numerous drugs which may provide the necessary element of sleep, analgesia and immobility for successful anaesthesia. The basic techniques therefore will vary according to the surgery, the patient, drug characteristics and the personal preference of the anaesthetist.

Anaesthesia aims to provide:

- preoperative assessment and management that will facilitate safe operative and postoperative conditions;
- operative conditions that permit surgery;

• postoperative advice and care that provides analgesia, fluids and oxygen therapy which it is hoped will minimize complications from haemodynamic perturbations (cardiac, renal insufficiency) or poor respiratory function.

Preoperative assessment

The preoperative assessment is primarily to establish fitness for anaesthesia and surgery. Mortality attributable to anaesthesia is so low when compared to that from surgery and the patient's preoperative state that 'fitness for anaesthesia' misrepresents the purpose of preoperative assessment. Crudely put, virtually any patient admitted to hospital can be anaesthetized and woken up in the absence of surgery and recover to go home. It is the patient's physiological reserve and consequently his ability to cope with a surgical insult which determines recovery. Perfectly conducted surgery provokes a significant inflammatory response which for the majority of patients is of little consequence; however, the benefits of similar surgery in the debilitated patient may be greatly outweighed by the morbidity or mortality associated with the same inflammatory response. On the other hand, deaths directly attributable to the anaesthetic are frequently the result of error or bad management rather than the normal consequences of correctly conducted anaesthesia.

A patient's physiological reserve can be approximated from his functional status, past medical history and dependence on medication. A widely accepted assessment of preoperative physical status is the American Association of Anesthetists (ASA) classification introduced in 1941 and modified to its current form in 1961. This simple classification effectively includes functional status, past history and medication (Table 7.1)

Risk from anaesthesia alone has been debated for years and still remains poorly defined since many factors contribute to morbidity and mortality. Death directly attributable to anaesthesia has been estimated to be between 1 in 852 to 1 in 14 075. A generally accepted rate is 1 in 10 000.

Table 7.1. **ASA classification of physical status.**

Category (e: emergency)	Description
I (e)	Healthy
II (e)	Mild systemic disease — no functional limitation
III (e)	Severe systemic disease — established functional limitation
IV (e)	Severe systemic disease — constant threat to life
V (e)	Moribund — not expected to survive >24 h with or without operation

Patient characteristics

Age and sex

The overwhelming majority of patients presenting for vascular surgery are over 60 years old. Two-thirds are between 61 and 70 and the remainder except for a very small percentage are between 71 and 80. The majority of patients are male, probably reflecting the incidence of smoking in this group. However, the incidence of smoking and vascular surgery is increasing among women.

Smoking

Most patients other than those under the age of 60, whose atherosclerosis may be genetically related or as a result of diabetes, are smokers. Smoking is significantly associated with atherosclerosis and coronary artery disease. Smokers also have a high incidence of chronic pulmonary disease which almost invariably prolongs postoperative recovery due to more frequent chest infections. Smoking raises carboxyhaemoglobin which replaces oxygenated haemoglobin and shifts the position of the oxygen dissociation curve. Smoking causes marked irritability of the upper airways and promotes pulmonary secretions. These longer term effects of smoking cannot be reversed overnight but refraining from smoking overnight might help reduce carboxyhaemoglobin levels. However, if pulmonary secretions are a major problem, smoking will need to be stopped for some months before a noticeable improvement is achieved. Although associated with respiratory problems, smoking has not been independently associated with greater cardiac risk after surgery.

Co-existing disease

Atherosclerosis is a systemic disease and therefore both its causes and consequences are likely to be extremely common among vascular surgery patients. The incidence of co-existing disease is shown in Table 7.2 and risk factors associated with major vascular surgery are summarized in Table 7.3.

Table 7.2. **Co-existing disease in vascular surgery patients.**

Co-existing condition	Approximate incidence (%)
Previous myocardial infarct	50
Hypertension	50
Chronic obstructive pulmonary disease	35
Angina	15
Congestive cardiac failure	15
Renal disease	15
Diabetes	10

Table 7.3. **Risk factors associated with major vascular surgery.**

Previous myocardial infarct or angina
Congestive heart failure
Age >70 years
Significant aortic stenosis
Cardiac arrhythmias
Renal insufficiency
Pulmonary disease

Abnormal ECG at rest or exercise
Thallium redistribution on dipyridamole–thallium myocardial perfusion scan
Radionucleotide ejection fraction <0.35

Intraoperative hypotension
Intraoperative myocardial ischaemia
Intraoperative renal dysfunction

Cardiac risk assessment

The commonest cause of death in the perioperative period and early follow-up after vascular surgery is myocardial infarction (up to 50% of deaths). It is notable that the incidences of fatal and non-fatal cardio-vascular complications are similar in patients following aortic or carotid surgery but higher among those having lower limb revascularization. This might lead us to reconsider the degree of monitoring that patients having infrainguinal arterial surgery should receive in the postoperative period.

Previous myocardial infarction, particularly if recent, is associated with a high re-infarction rate and is an important reason for delaying surgery if possible. The incidence of re-infarction is greatest on the 3rd postoperative day; this is possibly associated with nocturnal hypoxaemia which is also more common on the 2nd and 3rd days.

In studies before 1980, the risk of recurrent myocardial infarction was reported to be about 30% in patients who had surgery within 3 months of an infarct and 15% in those that were between 3 and 6 months of an infarct. Beyond 6 months, the risk was estimated to be about 5% and from then on remained constant. More recent studies report reinfarction rates of between 5% and 17% for surgery within 3 months of an infarct.

Numerous studies have assessed cardiac risk in patients undergoing non-cardiac surgery. These have usually included all forms of surgery, including vascular surgery, and have tended to underestimate the risk of cardiac death in those having major vascular surgery. In the classic study by Goldman and colleagues in 1977, which assessed cardiac risk in patients undergoing non-cardiac surgery, risk of perioperative cardiac

Table 7.4. **Goldman cardiac risk index for non-cardiac surgery.**

Factor	Points
Third heart sound	11
Elevated JVP	11
Myocardial infarct within 6 months	10
Ventricular ectopics >5/min	7
Rhythm other than sinus	7
Age >70	5
Emergency operation	4
Severe aortic stenosis	3
Poor medical condition of patient.	3

Any of the following:
  PaO_2 <8 KPa (60 mmHg)
  $PaCO_2$ >6.6 KPa (50 mmHg)
  K <3.0 or HCO_3 <20 mmol/l
  Urea >50 mg/100 ml
  Creatinine >3.0 mg/100 ml
  Bedridden patient for non-cardiac reasons
  Abnormal liver function tests	

Abdominal or thoracic operation	3

complications was based on a scoring system (Table 7.4). Complications included death, myocardial infarction, pulmonary oedema and ventricular tachycardia.

The Goldman risk score does not take account of the type of surgery being undertaken and therefore, although it accurately predicts the trend of risk, it underestimates the overall risk of mortality and morbidity associated with vascular surgery. When Goldman's data are re-examined, it emerges that overall the risk of severe cardiac complications for a patient undergoing abdominal aortic surgery is 10-fold that of a patient undergoing minor surgery and 2.5-fold greater than patients undergoing other major surgery.

Evidence of heart failure prior to surgery is the most significant risk determinant of perioperative cardiac complications.

Although it would appear from studies to date that the best indicator of coronary artery disease is the history (chest pain, etc.) combined with predisposing causes such as diabetes, smoking and hypertension (sensitivity and specificity of the history range between 80% and 91%), further investigations are required to improve the detection of patients at risk of cardiac complications following major vascular surgery. It is important to point out that the possibility of cardiac complications is not excluded in a patient deemed low risk based on the Goldman risk score.

Cardiac investigations

ECG

Unfortunately, an ECG is an inadequate screen for the presence of ischaemic heart disease.

Exercise testing

Exercise testing is useful for the detection of subclinical coronary artery disease. However, many patients are unable to exercise their limbs sufficiently to generate the heart rate or systolic blood pressure required to achieve the myocardial stress necessary for satisfactory testing. Equally, their ability to exercise may be limited by pulmonary dysfunction.

Although a positive exercise test may add a further 10% to the sensitivity of a typical history of angina (85–95%), a negative test in a patient with a typical history of angina still has a 60% sensitivity for coronary artery disease. False positives and false negatives do occur and therefore exercise testing alone is insufficient to detect coronary artery disease. However, in general, poor exercise testing has been correlated with a poor postoperative prognosis in vascular surgery; consequently, in patients with an unreliable history, exercise testing may be a useful non-invasive tool in estimating risk.

Echocardiography

Two-dimensional echocardiography is the commonest method of assessing ventricular wall motion and ejection fraction. Echocardiography can also be used with pharmacological methods that induce myocardial stress (e.g. dobutamine and dipyridamole echocardiography). Dobutamine is predominantly a β-agonist inotrope which increases heart rate and contractility, whereas dipyridamole is a vasodilator which provokes a reflex tachycardia.

Radionuclide ventriculography

Radionuclide ventriculography relies on the detection of γ-radioactivity passing through the heart following an intravenous injection of, usually, a mixture of the patient's blood or albumin with technetium-99 m. Left ventricular function can be estimated by:

- *Multiple uptake gated acquisition (MUGA) scans* in which the injectate circulates for numerous cardiac cycles.

The 'images' are obtained over set periods which are timed from the R wave of the ECG. This allows identification of end diastole and end systole during which the γ-radioactivity is counted and directly related to the volumes. Background activity from the lungs is accounted for in the calculation of the ejection fraction. This method also allows estimation of ventricular wall motion abnormalities.

- The *first-pass method* relies on an intravenous injection and a rapid-response γ-camera which detects the flow over the heart in the first 15–20 s.

Both MUGA and 'first-pass' scans have been shown to be accurate assessments of left ventricular function. Although left ventricular function is an independent predictor of long-term outcome, its relationship to perioperative outcome is not clear. However, many feel intuitively that assessment of left ventricular function may help select patients who would benefit from more intensive monitoring. This information can be more conveniently obtained by echocardiography.

Exercise thallium scans

Thallium-201 is a radioactive potassium analogue. When injected, it is distributed to perfused myocardium which shows up as a generalized white area on the scan. This technique is combined with exercise and may demonstrate perfusion defects (black areas) in areas supplied by stenosed vessels. Initial filling defects on the scan may indicate ischaemia or an area of previous infarct. If the scans are repeated after a few hours, some of these defects may disappear, thus separating areas of ischaemia from those of infarct. It has been suggested that the presence of these filling defects, which later disappear and indicate ischaemia, are associated with upto a 20-fold increase in significant cardiovascular-related events in the perioperative period.

   The same limitations that apply to standard exercise testing apply to thallium scans (see above). However, it has been suggested that the thallium scan provides as much data at 85% of the maximum heart rate achieved on standard testing. Thus, at heart rates of 105–110, a thallium scan gives the same information as a more vigorous standard ECG-based exercise test. Thallium-201 exercise scanning has a sensitivity of 80% and specificity of 90% for detecting coronary artery disease compared to 60% and 80%, respectively, for standard exercise testing. Thallium scanning also provides information on left ventricular wall thickness.

Dipyridamole–thallium scintigraphy

Dipyridamole is an antiplatelet agent which also has vasodilatory properties. Infusion leads to a tachycardia and increased coronary flow. This modification of thallium scanning is particularly useful in patients who are unable to perform an exercise test. Dipyridamole–thallium scanning appears to be most helpful when used in conjunction with clinical assessment further to evaluate patients with an intermediate number of risk factors. Patients with three or more risk factors and those without any represent high- and low-risk groups, respectively, and in these two groups this imaging is probably unnecessary.

Preoperative management

Patients with cardiac risk

Clinical assessment attempts to identify patients at low, intermediate and high risk for adverse cardiac outcomes. Patients estimated to be at *high risk* of experiencing postoperative cardiac complications based on exercise testing and history of angina or previous infarcts should undergo coronary angiography and possibly corrective surgery before embarking on major vascular surgery. However, the value of prophylactic coronary artery surgery remains controversial and should be only carried out on the merits of the patient's anginal symptoms and not just to increase safety of the vascular procedure. Patients classified as *intermediate risk* benefit most from further investigations. Clearly, the emergency presentation of patients with a ruptured aneurysm or severely ischaemic limbs cannot afford the time for investigations.

In all cases, measures such as perioperative monitoring and maximizing medical treatment with antianginal therapy go without saying. There is some evidence that administration of β-blockers perioperatively reduces long-term cardiac morbidity and mortality in at-risk patients undergoing non-cardiac surgery. It has also been suggested that clonidine may be a useful agent for reducing the surgical stress response. However, as these measures have not yet been proven, they are not incorporated into routine anaesthetic practice. Long-acting β-blockers can significantly complicate haemodynamic management. The lack of tachycardia may disguise volume loss and impair the normal postoperative response to stress and infection that may be necessary for survival.

In the preparation of patients at risk of congestive heart failure, it is important that over-enthusiastic 'anti-failure' treatment does not render the patient hypovolaemic. This presents considerable risks of severe hypotension at induction, the consequences of which may be cerebral, cardiac and renal ischaemia. Since the therapy of such an event in the first instance is volume loading, there is the risk of the myocardial stress being further complicated by a sudden fluid load and precipitation of pulmonary oedema.

Hypertension

Approximately half of patients presenting for major vascular surgery have chronic hypertension. These patients develop vascular hyper-reactivity and left ventricular hypertrophy due to the increased systolic load on the left ventricle. Since the hypertrophied left ventricle requires higher filling pressures, the cardiac output and blood pressure are sensitive to hypovolaemia.

Current recommendations are that all hypertensive patients should receive their medication prior to surgery. Ideally, diastolic blood pressure should be below 100 mmHg and systolic below 180 mmHg. Every day practice suggests that untreated hypertensives have very labile blood pressure under anaesthesia and surgery and the extremes of too high and too low pressure potentially have serious myocardial, cerebral and renal consequences. Although preoperative systolic blood pressure has been found to be a significant predictor of postoperative morbidity in numerous studies, there is no incontrovertible data showing that preoperative treatment of hypertension reduces perioperative risk. The drugs used to control blood pressure are not benign. Angiotensin-converting enzyme (ACE) inhibitors may have detrimental effects on glomerular filtration rate, while β-blockers may mask bleeding.

In view of the lability of blood pressure if left untreated, most clinicians agree that all hypertensives should be well controlled before surgery and that antihypertensive medication should be continued into the postoperative period as soon as is feasible.

Pulmonary disease

Between a quarter and a half of patients with vascular disease have co-existing pulmonary disease, many being heavy smokers. The consequences of anaesthesia and surgery on pulmonary function are extensive. Since most vascular patients are over 60 years, just the act of lying supine increases intrapulmonary shunting due to the change in the relative size of the functional residual capacity and the closing volumes of the lung. Induction of anaesthesia and the head-down position accentuate these changes and this is why anaesthetists always give at least 30% oxygen as the basis of the anaesthetic.

Preoperative assessment should include a comprehensive history in patients who present an obvious risk. This should include details of:

- dyspnoea;
- cough and sputum production;
- recent infection and treatment;
- wheezing and bronchodilator usage;
- smoking history;
- exercise limits;
- previous postoperative chest complications.

Clinical examination should be aimed at a functional assessment while at rest.

- Observation of the manner and rate of breathing and the shape of the chest are good indicators of likely function. For example, resting respiratory rates above 20/min, a barrel chest and pursing of lips with accessory muscle activity are highly suggestive of significant emphysema/bronchitis. These patients may also have an audible wheeze.

- Obesity, i.e. weight 30% above ideal increases the incidence of respiratory complications.
- Auscultation may reveal further evidence of chest disease but its main usefulness is to assess whether there is chest infection as indicated by coarse râles, rhonchi and evidence of consolidation. Quiet breath sounds are characteristic of emphysema in the absence of infection.

Further studies should be used to evaluate functional reserve. Investigations such as simple *spirometry* (FEV_1/FVC) and *arterial gases* provide specific data regarding the type of lung damage, e.g. whether restrictive or obstructive disease. Blood gases on air indicate the oxygenation deficit and whether carbon dioxide retention is a problem.

The data from these simple tests indicate to the anaesthetist whether to opt for regional or general anaesthesia and, if the latter, whether it would be safe to allow spontaneous ventilation. A reduced FEV_1/FVC is closely related to developing severe hypercapnia under anaesthesia if the patient is allowed to breathe spontaneously. These patients may also have highly reactive airways with a tendency to cough and wheeze unless deeply anaesthetized. However, unduly deep anaesthesia can result in further hypoventilation and poor respiratory ciliary activity. Significant hypoventilation may result in a need for mechanical ventilatory support while poor ciliary activity potentially increases the tendency for sputum retention and atelectasis. Many anaesthetists, if not using a regional technique, will opt for a technique that attempts to have a patient awake promptly at the end of surgery so that coughing is initiated early.

Preoperative preparation for these patients includes:

- controlling chest infections with antibiotics;
- breathing exercises such as incentive spirometry;
- bronchodilators and steroids for wheeze;
- cessation of smoking preferably >2 months before elective surgery.

Diabetes

Diabetes is a risk factor for ischaemic heart disease, peripheral vascular disease and renal impairment. Coronary artery disease is the commonest cause of death in diabetics and the incidence of silent infarcts is high. Diabetics are at risk of developing acute renal failure, particularly if there are simultaneous insults such as perioperative hypotension, recent radio-contrast studies or non-steroidal anti-inflammatory agent administration.

Many diabetics have an autonomic neuropathy which has important implications for the anaesthetist. Patients who demonstrate postural hypotension and a resting tachycardia are at particular risk of silent myocardial ischaemia, intraoperative hypotension and sudden death in the early postoperative period.

Insulin-dependent diabetics

On the day of surgery, the normal insulin regimen is suspended and intravenous soluble insulin titrated according to a sliding scale based on intermittent blood sugar measurements. The blood sugar should be maintained between 6 and 11 mmol/l; the most serious complication to be avoided is hypoglycaemia. Glucose is given as 5% dextrose throughout the perioperative period.

Non-insulin dependent diabetics

Oral medication should not be given on the day of surgery and, if the patient is undergoing minor surgery, there is no need for insulin. However, those undergoing major surgery should be also put on a sliding scale of insulin on the morning of their operation with a background infusion of 5% dextrose.

Renal dysfunction

Up to 15% of patients who present for vascular surgery have evidence of renal dysfunction from associated disease such as hypertension, diabetes, or the concomitant ingestion of non-steroidal agents or ACE inhibitors. Also, radiographic dye studies may precipitate acute renal failure, particularly if there has been an enforced period of 'nil by mouth' and the procedure has necessitated a sedative agent which is hypotensive.

It is important to note that 50% of glomerular filtration rate can be lost with no change in serum creatinine. Therefore, patients with creatinine concentrations at the upper end of normal may be at severe risk from even minor insults. During surgery, failure by the anaesthetist to maintain a stable blood pressure commensurate with the patient's normal values is an insidious insult to the kidneys which is most likely to reveal itself in patients with renal impairment. Direct renal trauma or cross-clamping the aorta above the renal vessels are more obvious insults that may lead to renal failure.

Preoperative, peri-operative and postoperative optimization of these patients with regards to volume is fundamental to maintaining renal function.

Electrolyte abnormalities

Patients with vascular disease often develop electrolyte abnormalities as a result of diuretic therapy. Hypokalaemia is the commonest abnormality.

If the serum level of potassium is <3 mmol/l and chronic hypokalaemia is suspected, potassium should be replaced orally over 3–4 days. In an emergency, potassium can be replaced intravenously at a rate of no more than 20 mmol/h.

It is important to note that most situations that cause potassium loss also result in low plasma magnesium concentrations. Low potassium and low magnesium independently make the myocardium more irritable and liable to supraventricular tachyarrhythmias which may reduce cardiac output by up to 30%. It may be necessary to supplement magnesium simultaneously with potassium.

Anaesthetic management

Carotid artery surgery

Anaesthesia for carotid artery surgery can be undertaken with either a general or regional technique. In both a light premed with benzo-diazepines may be justified to ameliorate anxiety and consequent tachycardia and hypertension. Patients should be given all their usual antihypertensive agents on the day of surgery.

General anaesthesia

The principles of general anaesthesia are no different from those for any other surgery, except that special attention is paid to those factors that are known to control cerebral blood flow, including those that:

● control intracranial pressure such as venous drainage and arterial carbon dioxide tension;
● maintain arterial pressure.

Induction of anaesthesia aims to avoid wild fluctuations of blood pressure. Intubation is usually undertaken with a normal tracheal tube, although some anaesthetists prefer a reinforced tube. Pretreatment with lignocaine, opiates or an infusion of esmolol (a short-acting β-blocker) helps to prevent surges in blood pressure or intracranial pressure during intubation. Standard monitoring should always include an arterial line, continuous ECG, end-tidal carbon dioxide and oxygen saturation measurements. Central venous or pulmonary artery catheterization are un-necessary unless there is a particular indication such as a markedly reduced ejection fraction.

The patient is positioned with his head up and slightly to the side. The legs are preferably placed horizontal or are slightly elevated so as to mini-mize postural hypotension. This head-up position does predispose the patient to air access via accidentally opened veins in the neck. If the patient is repositioned head down during extubation or recovery, this air may gain entry to the heart and provoke sudden hypotension and collapse.

When anaesthesia is maintained by a volatile agent, studies have shown a significant difference in the critical regional cerebral blood flow, i.e. the flow below which EEG changes characteristic of ischaemia develop, with different agents. Isoflurane is 'safer' than halothane or enflurane. This evidence goes hand in hand with the observation that isoflurane is able to depress cerebral metabolic rate to a greater degree than other agents.

Further aims during surgery include maintenance of normocapnia, normotension or mild hypertension and avoidance of hypovolaemia. Ideally, there should be no systolic arterial pressure decrease >40 mmHg from normal and upward surges in blood pressure, typically in response to clamping of the carotid, can be controlled by esmolol, alfentanil or application of local anaesthetic to the carotid sinus.

At the end of surgery, a smooth but rapid awakening is the aim to allow evaluation of the neurological status.

Patients should be transferred to a high-dependency unit post-operatively where they can be monitored and where oxygen can be administered. Nursing staff should be alerted to observe closely for fluctuations in arterial pressure outside pre-set limits, neurological deterioration and the presence of a wound haematoma which may compromise the airway.

Regional anaesthesia

Regional anaesthesia for carotid endarterectomy is popular in many countries since neurological assessment is immediate and there is some evidence of earlier hospital discharge. Other advantages such as lowered cerebral and cardiac complications are less apparent. However, regional techniques do allow the surgeon to apply the clamp and immediately to evaluate the adequacy of contralateral flow. This means that there will be a number of patients in whom a shunt is not required and in whom shunt-associated complications can be avoided.

Adequate analgesia is usually provided by blocking the dermatomes from C2 to C4. This can be done by a fan-shaped subcutaneous injection placed in the posterior border of the sternomastoid above and below the point at which the external jugular vein crosses the muscle. Alternatives include an interscalene approach to the cervical plexus to block deep and superficial cervical nerves. These blocks are associated with the risks of intrathecal and epidural injections and puncture of the carotid and vertebral arteries.

Peripheral vascular surgery

Restoration of peripheral blood flow is most frequently required in the presence of atherosclerotic or embolic arterial obstruction. Surgical trauma is usually limited and blood loss minimal.

The problems of anaesthesia are as for any operation in patients with severe atherosclerotic disease but also include those of impaired circulation and consequent generation of a metabolic acidosis. The latter clearly depends on the suddenness of onset. An embolus may cause a rapid fall in pH, whereas the development of acidosis is less aggressive when a vessel with poor run-off is clamped.

A controversial issue in this group of patients is the choice of regional versus general anaesthesia. Recent randomized studies have found that epidural anaesthesia was associated with a lower incidence of graft failure and no elevation of plasminogen activator inhibitor levels seen with general anaesthesia. No difference between regional and general anaesthesia was seen with respect to cardiac morbidity, respiratory and renal failure or major infections. However, there is a feeling among anaesthetists that regional techniques are less of an insult to patients with poor chests.

Regional anaesthesia is most effectively provided by continuous epidural local anaesthetic infusion. In many patients, anticoagulant or thrombolytic therapy precludes the use of an epidural technique as there appears to be a low but real risk of epidural haematoma. Additional problems with epidural techniques include development of hypotension due to increased venous capacitance, both peroperatively and in recovery. This is easily remedied by 500–1000 ml aliquots of volume. All patients should have a urinary catheter in place until the epidural infusion is stopped as retention is a common problem.

Elective aortic surgery

As outlined above, patients are likely to be elderly with significant co-morbidity. Aortic surgery presents a number of major insults:

- a large abdominal incision;
- significant blood and fluid loss;
- heat loss;
- a temporary period of interrupted perfusion to the lower limbs followed by a reperfusion injury.

The combination of a patient with poor cardiorespiratory and renal reserve and this series of major insults makes aortic surgery high risk. Anaesthesia management attempts to minimize the effects of these insults to the extent that the details of drug choices for anaesthesia itself almost becomes secondary.

Preoperative preparation

Preparation for surgery includes:

- generous premedication;
- large-bore peripheral cannula for fluid infusion;

- direct arterial pressure monitoring;
- central venous access usually with a multilumen catheter for simultaneous drug infusions;
- central and peripheral temperature monitoring;
- urinary catheter.

A pulmonary artery catheter may be placed in patients with a history of poor myocardial function. However, unless cardiac output is measured it provides very little additional useful information, particularly in those patients with ejection fractions above 50%. The latter may be more conveniently provided by an oesophageal Doppler probe. In view of the abdominal incision and the usually poor respiratory function, many patients will also have an epidural placed for postoperative analgesia.

Patients should always be placed on a warming blanket and, if possible, have at least their upper torso covered by a disposable warm air blanket. All fast infusions should go through a blood warmer and modern warmers can infuse up to a litre of blood at 37°C in 1 min. Cold infusions promote poor clotting, worsen myocardial contractility and accelerate the development of metabolic acidosis.

Inhaled anaesthetics, intravenous drugs or a combination of both as well as continuous epidural anaesthesia have all been used successfully to maintain anaesthesia during abdominal aortic surgery. Studies have suggested that there is decreased postoperative morbidity when a combination of epidural and light general anaesthesia is followed by postoperative epidural analgesia.

Peri-operative management

Two specific times during surgery may destabilize the patient: Cross-clamping and unclamping the aorta.

Clamping the aorta

Clamping the aorta causes a sudden increase in peripheral vascular resistance or myocardial afterload which may result in a rise in left ventricular end-diastolic pressure. Infrarenal cross-clamping may increase afterload by 40%, leading to a significant fall in cardiac output of between 15% and 35%.

If the patient is known to have poor left ventricular function, then surgical application of the clamp should be done slowly and in deliberate steps. Destabilization can in part be prevented by continuous infusion of vasodilators such as glyceryl trinitrate prior to clamping. This provides dilatation of potential collaterals so minimizing the expected surge in blood pressure as well as preserving normal myocardial blood flow, and thus maintaining contractility and containing the rise in left ventricular end diastolic pressure. Healthy hearts tend to produce a rise in blood pressure with little evidence of ischaemia.

Between 5% and 10% of patients develop acute renal failure after elective aortic surgery and it is particularly prevalent among those with diabetes or evidence of pre-existing renal impairment. Many anaesthetists administer mannitol prior to cross-clamping to achieve a brisk diuresis or run a dopamine infusion. However, these techniques are likely to be more successful if fluid status throughout tends to be in excess rather than deficit and if systolic blood pressures are maintained close to preoperative values. Dopamine infusions can be replaced by low-dose frusemide infusions but care should be taken to avoid volume depletion. A good guide to the latter is the ability of the patient to maintain his central and peripheral temperature during anaesthesia.

Aortic clamp release

Release of the aortic clamp results in a sudden decrease in afterload and reperfusion of the lower part of the body. Acid metabolites from the previously unperfused limbs enter the circulation causing vasodilatation and metabolic acidosis. It is therefore preferable that the clamp is released slowly. Release of the clamp is usually followed by a fall in blood pressure which can be minimized by prior reduction of the vasodilator infusion and by rapidly increasing fluid administration.

Postoperative management

Postoperatively patients who are haemodynamically stable, given adequate analgesia and warm can be extubated immediately and taken to a recovery or high-dependency unit.

Cold patients by definition have become hypovolaemic and as they warm require fluids to maintain a blood pressure. Fluid requirements can be frighteningly high, particularly in the absence of inotropes, if the goal is to avoid hypotension and oliguria. Cold patients may also shiver and increase their oxygen requirements three-fold. Since many of these patients have poor respiratory reserve, the demands on their respiratory system during this period of warming cannot be safely met. It is, therefore, common practice for such patients to undergo a few hours of ventilation in an intensive care unit. As a rule, if fluid management is aggressive in theatre, the need for postoperative ventilation is reduced except for those patients with compromised ventilatory function through chronic pulmonary disease.

With the modern use of packed cells for blood replacement it is important to provide adequate clotting factors. A rule of thumb is to provide 1 unit of fresh frozen plasma for every 2 units of blood. Some vascular teams have access to autotransfusion systems which allow blood retrieved by suction to be washed, filtered and retransfused. This blood retains the advantages of being warm, at normal pH and potassium content and perfectly matched.

Surgery for ruptured abdominal aortic aneurysm

Patients with a ruptured aortic aneurysm are best taken *immediately* to the operating theatre rather than resuscitated in the accident and emergency department as mortality is proportional to the time taken to achieve proximal control of the aorta (see Chapter 11). It is therefore imperative that the anaesthetist does not unnecessarily delay the start of surgery with over-enthusiastic resuscitation. Patients may survive initial rupture due to tamponade of the bleeding site by retroperitoneal haematoma; vigorous resuscitation may overcome this tamponade and result in fatal bleeding.

On transfer to the operating theatre, the patient should be given 100% oxygen and two large-bore peripheral lines should be inserted. Ideally, induction is started once the abdomen is prepared and draped with the surgeon standing by. ECG and pulse oximetry should be monitored together with non-invasive blood pressure measurement. Some fluids can be given to achieve a systolic of around 100 mmHg.

Once induced and intubated, systemic arterial pressure can be expected to drop precipitously as muscle relaxation slackens the tamponade. Immediate laparotomy and aortic clamping should follow. Once the aorta is cross-clamped, further monitoring can be instituted and anaesthesia can then proceed in the manner used for the elective operation.

Prognosis is much worse for these patients as they may have undergone a period of hypotension with resultant cerebral, myocardial, splanchnic and renal hypoperfusion. They may require a massive transfusion and usually have more difficult surgery and consequently a more prolonged period under anaesthesia. Metabolic acidosis, hypothermia, consumption and dilutional coagulopathy and oliguria are common immediate complications.

Blood transfusion

Patients undergoing vascular surgery frequently require blood transfusion to replace losses during surgery. To avoid the hazards of exposure to allogeneic blood, a number of strategies are in routine practice.

Predonation

Preoperative autologous donation of blood reduces the need for allogeneic transfusion. Studies have demonstrated that in patients undergoing surgical procedures with an anticipated blood loss of >1 litre, predonation of 3 or more units increases their chance of avoiding allogeneic blood to 85%. Administration of recombinant human erythropoietin enhances the preoperative collection of blood and may prevent preoperative anaemia. Predonation involves a patient coming to the blood bank once a week for 2–3 weeks and donating a unit of blood per visit. Therefore, it is time consuming and expensive and its cost-effectiveness has been questioned when compared to other strategies. Also, there is no time for donation if patients are undergoing emergency surgery which is particularly relevant for vascular surgery.

Haemodilution

Acute normovolaemic haemodilution is more convenient, less expensive and preserves blood components better than predonation. It can be performed immediately before or during surgery and it involves venesection of blood which is stored with citrate phosphate dextrose at room temperature, therefore ensuring a supply of fresh whole blood. As long as normovolaemia is maintained by the infusion of colloid, cardiac output and hence oxygen delivery are preserved. It has been suggested that moderate haemodilution (haematocrit of 28%) is safe in those over 60 years; however, it should be used with caution in those with co-existing disease such as coronary artery disease.

Salvaged blood

The use of cell-salvaging devices during vascular surgery significantly reduces the need for banked blood. Current machinery for performing these techniques is completely automated and consists of a regional heparinized collection system for retransfusion of washed red blood cells with an haematocrit >50. This machinery is initially expensive to buy, but the financial break-even point is when >2 stored units of blood are used. Salvaged red blood cells have a normal survival time and their main advantage over banked blood is that they have higher levels of 2,3-diphosphoglycerate. It should, however, be remembered that a dilutional coagulopathy can still occur as the coagulation factors are discarded during the cell-washing process.

Platelets and clotting factors

During surgery when blood loss is great, transfusion of platelets and clotting factors is also required, even though few studies have been performed to determine whether perioperative administration improves outcome. If there is continued bleeding, platelets should be transfused if the count is $<100 \times 10^9/l$. In some circumstances, platelet dysfunction may be more important than platelet count in explaining continued haemorrhage; therefore, if there is suspicion of platelet dysfunction, platelets should be transfused even if the count is normal.

Replacement of the entire blood volume leaves the patient with approximately one-third of the original concentration of clotting factors. Coagulopathy from dilution does not usually occur until replacement exceeds 1 blood volume or when the prothrombin and partial thromboplastin times exceed 1.5–1.8 times the control values. Under these circumstances, fresh frozen plasma should be transfused. It should be given in doses calculated to achieve 30% of plasma factor concentration (10–15 ml/kg). Cryoprecipitate should be given to massively transfused patients with fibrinogen concentrations <80–100 mg/dl.

Recovery following major vascular surgery

The majority of vascular patients require high-dependency care where they can be monitored adequately. Some vascular surgery patients, in particular those undergoing emergency repairs of abdominal aortic aneurysms or routine and emergency thoracic aortic repairs, require intensive care.

Patients undergoing major aortic surgery may require time for stabilization postoperatively and during this period they require ventilatory support. Adequate stabilization is characterized by a warm well-perfused periphery in a relatively pain-free patient, passing good volumes of urine and adequately oxygenated on <40% oxygen. The period to warmth and good perfusion can be accelerated by the use of external warmers and infusion of warm fluid or blood products. Alternatively, particularly if there is concern regarding myocardial function, a low-dose infusion of glyceryl trinitrate (2 mg/h) can be continued from theatre while warm blood products are given. The rationale for glyceryl trinitrate is to reduce venous tone and allow optimal volume administration without misleading surges in central venous pressures while the patient is patently hypovolaemic and reflexly oliguric.

Patients should not be extubated until they are awake, comfortable and stabilized as described above. *Failure to oxygenate adequately* may be due to basal collapse which can be treated by application of positive end expiratory pressure (PEEP). To qualify for extubation, patients should be able to achieve a tidal volume of 5 ml/kg.

Failure to pass adequate urine may be due to relatively low blood pressure, which ideally should be at its premorbid level. It may be low due to excessive sedation, the effects of the epidural or inadequate volume. Once these are corrected, it is usually unnecessary to give an inotrope to restore blood pressure. If hypotension is a problem, attention should be directed either to a myocardial problem or, particularly in emergency cases, to the presence of a pre-existing infection, usually involving the chest. If necessary, noradrenaline is titrated to achieve the desired blood pressure. If despite normovolaemia and normotension urine output remains inadequate, frusemide is administered as a 10 mg bolus and continued as an infusion (1–4 mg/h). The rationale for frusemide is to reduce oxygen consumption in the renal medulla. An alternative approach would be to infuse dopamine once volume and blood pressure are normal.

Postoperative pain control

Although conventional opiate analgesia will suffice for many of these patients, it is not as effective as an epidural with either local anaesthetics alone or supplemented with epidural opiates. Usually, patients who have received continuous epidural anaesthesia can be extubated earlier than patients who have received general anaesthesia alone. The benefits of epidural analgesia over intravenous infusions of opiates are:

- decreased sedation;
- better tolerance of physiotherapy;
- increased lung volumes;
- improved oxygenation;
- faster restoration of normal gut motility.

Summary

- Preoperative evaluation and optimization of the patient's chronic medical condition is vital prior to surgery in this high-risk group of patients.
- Carotid artery and aortic artery surgery have specific peroperative problems which have to be anticipated if serious cardiac, cerebral or renal sequelae are to be avoided.
- Close attention to the details of postoperative management is required to maintain adequate circulating volume, oxygenation and renal function in order to achieve early extubation and discharge to the ward.
- Good pain relief plays an integral role in facilitating effective physiotherapy and early ambulation.

Areas of controversy

- Regional versus general anaesthesia?
- Should regional anaesthesia be used in the anticoagulated patient?
- Method of preoperative optimization of oxygen transport in high-risk surgical patients?
- Bank blood versus predonation versus haemodilution?

Further reading

- Clark NJ, Stanley TH. Anesthesia for vascular surgery. In: Miller RD (ed) *Anesthesia.* New York: Churchill Livingstone 1990, pp 1851–1895.
- Garrioch MA, Fitch W. Anaesthesia for carotid artery surgery. *British Journal of Anaesthesia* 1993;**71**:569–579.
- Cordingley J, Palazzo M. Renal rescue: management of impending renal failure. In: Vincent JL (ed) *Yearbook of Intensive Care and Emergency Medicine.* Berlin: Springer-Verlag, 1996, pp 675–689.
- D'Ambra MN, Kaplan DK. Alternatives to allogeneic blood use in surgery: Acute normovolemic hemodilution and preoperative autologous donation. *American Journal of Surgery* 1995;**170**:49S–52S.
- American Society of Anesthesiologists Task Force on Blood Component Therapy. Practice guidelines for blood component therapy. *Anesthesiology* 1996;**84**:732–747.

8
Outcome Measures in Vascular Surgery

S Byford, AM Garratt, DJ Torgerson and AH Davies

Introduction

Outcome measures following the treatment of patients with vascular disease are wide ranging from patient survival following repair of a ruptured abdominal aneurysm to the cosmetic benefits of multiple avulsions under local anaesthetic for the treatment of varicose veins. To determine the benefit of any vascular treatment or intervention it is necessary to show improvement following treatment. This improvement needs to be sufficient to overcome the potential risks of the intervention. One further consideration is the cost benefit to the community as well as the individual from performing an intervention.

Standard clinical outcome measures

Mortality

Patient mortality following a procedure is a definite endpoint and can be looked at from two viewpoints: whether the intervention prevents mortality or is the cause of mortality. It must be acknowledged that the majority of patients on whom vascular surgery is performed are elderly and have atherosclerotic disease, factors which are associated with a significant mortality. The majority of papers published with respect to outcome measures and mortality use the Kaplan-Meier statistical calculation, which allows patients to be recruited and not all followed up to the final end point. The important feature of this calculation is the calculation of the number of patients at risk.

Improvement of symptoms

One of the main purposes of elective surgery is the improvement of symptoms and this is also the most objective outcome measure. However, in the majority of cases, there is no strict stratification of symptomatology prior to surgery and it is therefore difficult to record an accurate measure of improvement. For example:

- *Measurement of claudication distance.* Following an angioplasty, a patient may initially notice an improvement in his walking distance but is unlikely to be able to quantify this improvement.
- In patients who have significant symptoms prior to *varicose vein surgery*, it can be difficult to elicit an accurate measure of improvement.

Morbidity

There may be associated morbidity following any treatment intervention. This may range from pain or wound infection following a surgical procedure, to blockage of a femorodistal graft resulting in amputation, to death. It is probably important to look at morbidity in two ways.

- *Generalized morbidity* relates to any form of operative intervention and may be regarded more as a complication of anaesthesia.
- *Specific complications*, e.g. stroke from or during carotid endarterectomy or nerve damage at the time of varicose vein stripping.

Patency

A major outcome measure in vascular surgery is the patency of a blood vessel, i.e. that it is open. In large studies patency *is often calculated over the years* using lifetable analysis. Three terms that are often used with respect to patency are:

- *Primary patency* is patency without any intervention to keep the vessel open.
- *Primary-assisted patency* is patency achieved without any intervention and through some form of intervention based on intervening on a patent graft, i.e. the angioplasty of stenosis would still be regarded as a graft that is patent.
- *Secondary patency* includes any graft that is open even if it has had an angioplasty for stenosis or has been unblocked, i.e. by definition, secondary patency should be the higher result.

While there is a statistical difference between primary and secondary patency (Fig. 8.1), it must be accepted that there must be a certain degree of bias in this calculation by the simple definition. For example, if 30% of vein grafts are known to develop a stenosis and if these criteria for intervention are adopted, a 20/30% difference can be predicted in the primary and secondary patency rates.

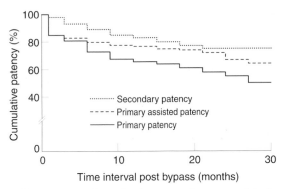

Fig. 8.1. **Life-table presentation of primary, primary-assisted and secondary patencies in a cohort of patients who have undergone femorodistal bypass.**

Follow-up

The aims of following up vascular patients are manifold and it has clinical and research implications. Obviously, the latter are dependent on the trial and the indication for follow-up.

The aims of clinical follow-up must be patient reassurance and to ensure by internal audit that interventions are giving satisfactory results. In the case of a vein graft there may be benefits in offering specific follow-up investigations such as duplex imaging. Similarly, patients who have small asymptomatic abdominal aortic aneurysms need to be followed up with ultrasound to determine if their condition is deteriorating and surgery is indicated. The benefit to the patient of follow-up in terms of reassurance has probably been underestimated; however, even in those units that do not follow-up the majority of their patients, it is accepted that patients should have easy/direct access to the clinicians who were involved in their care.

Audit

It is imperative for practitioners to audit their results with respect to outcome in order to ensure good clinical practice at all levels. If a problem is identified during the audit cycle, e.g. a high rate of wound infection or poor outcome from surgical intervention, it is beholden on clinicians to see if their clinical practice can be altered to improve outcome. Implementation of any revised procedure similarly needs to be audited.

Trials

The randomized controlled trial (RCT) is the 'gold standard' of research methods. However, relative to pharmaceutical interventions, there is a paucity of trials of surgical interventions. Furthermore, in both medical and surgical trials, few contemporaneous economic evaluations have been undertaken. This failing is an important omission because, as with estimates of effectiveness, the best evidence for cost-effectiveness will be usually gathered from a randomized trial.

A number of important design issues need to be considered when planning a trial which has a significant economic component.

Trial design

For a trial to produce optimum data for an economic analysis, a pragmatic approach is generally preferred to an explanatory one. In brief, an *explanatory trial* seeks to produce information on the underlying efficacy of a therapeutic intervention by testing theoretical hypotheses, whereas a *pragmatic trial* aims to choose between alternative treatments in clinical practice. Pragmatic trials provide information to enable health policy makers to identify those treatments which are most likely to be beneficial and cost-effective in routine clinical practice. These different philosophies often require different trial designs.

Blinding

One of the most important differences in trial design between pragmatic and explanatory studies is that patients and clinicians are blind to treatment allocation in the former. In drug trials this often means the use of placebos (although in comparisons of different drugs, efforts are made to make all the drugs look and taste the same). In surgical trials the patient can be blinded to the type of surgical intervention he receives, but this can be difficult.

There are three reasons for blinding:

- Any psychological effects of trial participation are the same in all arms of the trial, thereby allowing an unbiased comparison.
- The attitudes and perceptions of the clinicians involved in the trial are the same towards all treatment arms, such that a group receiving an active compound does not receive better or worse treatment than the control group.
- It allows the unbiased estimate of patient outcome by trial researchers.

Although these are powerful reasons for the use of placebos, strong counter-arguments exist. For the economic evaluation of a new treatment to be accurate, an unbiased estimate of outcome is required. This does not, however, have to be achieved by blinding patients and clinicians. Instead, independent assessors can be employed who are blind to the group allocation of the patient. With respect to patient and clinician attitudes across treatment groups, blinding may not lead to pragmatic estimates of effectiveness and this could lead to the most cost-effective therapy being rejected.

Sample size estimation

One of the first requirements of a trial design is to estimate the sample size necessary to show a difference in outcome which is either clinically or economically relevant or is important to the patient. From the economic perspective, there may be changes in clinical outcome which could lead to cost saving.

Economic evaluation techniques

There are three main methods of economic evaluation:

- cost–benefit analysis (CBA);
- cost–effectiveness analysis (CEA);
- cost–utility analysis (CUA).

All three involve the identification, measurement and comparison of relevant costs and benefits and all measure costs in monetary terms. The major differentiating feature is the method employed to measure the benefits, or outcomes, of health care.

Cost–benefit analysis

A CBA attempts to convert all the benefits of health-care interventions into monetary values; thus, costs and benefits are measured in the same units. This feature, peculiar to CBA, means that a single intervention can be evaluated in isolation; all other methods of economic evaluation require a comparator. If an intervention yields benefits whose sum is greater than the costs, it should be adopted, and vice versa. However, converting the myriad of important health-related benefits, such as life years gained or complications avoided, into monetary terms is a challenge which has never been fully met.

Cost-effectiveness analysis

For this reason, CEA is more commonly employed in the health-care sector. CEA avoids the thorny issue of converting health effects into monetary values by measuring benefits in terms of clinically relevant scales such as life years gained, or cancer avoided. The benefits of two or more interventions are combined with their respective costs, providing a measure of cost per unit of health improvement. Priority should be given to those interventions with the lowest cost per unit of health gained. CEA is not problem free; where the outcome measure employed is disease specific, comparisons between health-care programmes which generate very different forms of health benefit would be impossible. For example, how can you compare an intervention which values outcomes in terms of strokes averted with one in which outcomes are measured in terms of blood pressure level? Even when the results are expressed in terms of more general measures of effectiveness, such as cost per life gained, there is no generally accepted value beyond which a cost per life gained is deemed acceptable.

Cost-utility analysis

CUA, a variant of CEA, measures the health effects of all interventions in units of utility (well-being, satisfaction, etc.), and hence avoids the limitations of disease-specific scales. The most commonly employed method of CUA is the *quality adjusted life year (QALY)*. A QALY incorporates the effects of a treatment on both the quantity and quality of life by combining data on expected life years gained with the utility value of the resulting health state. For example, if an intervention realizes 10 life years per person but these years are lived in only 50% of full health, the outcome is a gain of 5 QALYs. Resources should be directed towards those interventions which involve the lowest cost per QALY gained. Criticisms regarding the quality of data and the methodology employed in the calculation of QALYs abound, but the importance of CUA is increasing as research in this area continues to improve.

Health outcome assessment

Two broad approaches to measuring patient perceptions of the outcomes of health care have been proposed:

- *specific instruments* that focus on a particular disease or client group;
- *generic instruments* that provide a summary of health-related quality of life (HRQL) (Table 8.1).

Both approaches have their strengths and weaknesses and there are potential advantages to using the two in conjunction.

Generic instruments

As generic instruments can take account of multiple conditions, they can measure wide effects such as the influence of co-morbidity on health. Their general nature makes them suitable for comparisons between different groups of patients and the general or disease-free populations.

Table 8.1. Taxonomy of measures of health outcome.

	Advantages	Disadvantages	Examples
Generic instruments			
Health profiles	Single instrument May detect different effects on different aspects of HRQL Enable comparisons across conditions/programmes Can be used in cost-effectiveness analysis	May not focus adequately on area of primary interest May not be responsive Do not take account of values attached to levels of HRQL	Short-Form 36-Item Health Survey
Utility measures	Single index representing HRQL Can be used in cost-utility analysis	Attribution problems of single index May not be responsive	Euroqol
Specific instruments			
Condition specific Disease specific Function specific Population specific Problem specific	Focus on primary area of interest Relevance to clinicians and clinical attribution May be more responsive	Not comprehensive and may miss side-effects Cannot compare across conditions/programmes	Aberdeen Varicose Veins Questionnaire Sabbatsberg Sexual Rating Scale Functional Status (II)-R Measure The Pain Perception Profile

The restricted nature of specific instruments can limit their ability to capture the side-effects of an intervention which may be detected by a responsive generic instrument. This makes the latter potentially useful for assessing the impact of new health-care technologies for which the range of effects is uncertain.

There are two major classes of generic instrument:

- health profiles;
- utility measures.

Health profiles measure HRQL across a number of distinct dimensions. Items within health profiles are summed and scored to reflect these individual dimensions. The short-form 36-item (SF-36) health survey is an example of a health profile that uses 36 items to measure HRQL across eight dimensions: physical functioning, social functioning, role limitations due to physical problems, role limitations due to emotional problems, mental health, vitality, pain and general health perception. Responses to individual items are summed to produce eight scale scores from 0 to 100, where 0 is the worst possible HRQL and 100 the best. Health profiles do not usually take account of values or preferences attached to HRQL states which limits their application in economic evaluation. These values are calculated for individual HRQL states derived from *utility measures* such as the Euroqol, which makes it suitable for use in a CUA. In the Euroqol, subjects are asked to complete five items covering mobility, self-care, main activity, pain/discomfort and anxiety/depression. Combinations of possible responses, or HRQL states, have been valued by the general public and on the basis of its responses to the five items, patients are classified into a number of categories each of which has a value associated with it.

Specific instruments

In theory, the narrow focus of specific instruments makes them more responsive or sensitive to clinically important changes in health resulting from health care. Specific instruments can be selected that reflect the areas of greatest importance and make them more suitable for the purpose of clinical attribution. Instruments can be specific to a particular condition, disease, function, population or problem. The Aberdeen Varicose Veins Questionnaire is a clinically-derived condition-specific measure of varicose vein severity. The aspects of varicose veins covered by the 13 items include pain and dysfunction, cosmetic appearance and complications.

To be of practical value a measure of outcome must satisfy the criteria of validity, reliability, responsiveness and acceptability. *Reliability* refers to an instrument's ability to measure a parameter in a consistent manner and can be assessed through internal consistency, i.e. the level of agreement between questions that measure related aspects of health, and test–retest, i.e. the stability of an instrument over repeated administrations. For instruments designed to measure outcome, it has been argued that test–retest is the most appropriate method of assessing reliability.

Validity refers to an instrument's ability to measure what is intended. In the absence of a 'gold-standard' measure of HRQL, validity is usually assessed through construct validity or how an instrument should behave in relation to some theory or construct.

Responsiveness refers to an instrument's ability to detect important changes in HRQL. A common approach to assessing responsiveness is to compare the change scores of instruments following the introduction of some intervention of known efficacy.

Finally, instruments must be *acceptable*, i.e. they should be easy to administer and simple for patients to complete. Acceptability depends on the application of the instrument, i.e. those intended for research purposes have to satisfy less stringent acceptability criteria than those that are to be used routinely.

The absence of suitable measures of patient outcome has been a major impediment to assessing the cost-effectiveness of surgical and other techniques in the management of varicose veins. The application of valid, reliable and responsive measures of outcome, and their use as end points in clinical trials, can provide clinicians with important information on the effectiveness of these procedures in terms of HRQL gains for patients presenting with varicose veins. Generic instruments, such as the SF-36, which can be administered across different patient groups, are useful for assessing the impact of interventions on overall HRQL and have greater potential to capture unforeseen side-effects associated with interventions. Generic instruments that incorporate explicit valuations, such as the Euroqol, are useful for purposes of economic evaluation, including the comparison of HRQL outcomes for different groups of patients, e.g. varicose vein surgery versus cholecystectomy. Specific instruments, such as the Aberdeen Varicose Veins Questionnaire, have greater potential to be more responsive to clinically important changes in HRQL and their narrow focus can make them useful for clinical attribution.

Summary

- Outcome measures and their assessment are important.
- A randomized controlled trial is the ideal method of evaluation of surgical procedures and should include a contemporaneous economic evaluation and appropriate measures of health outcome.
- Audit and alteration of practice is important.

Areas of controversy

- Is a randomized clinical trial needed if observational studies suggest markedly better results from a specific technique?
- What is the ideal timing of a randomized controlled trial with regard to a new interventional technique?

Further reading

- Pocock SJ. *Clinical Trials: A Practical Approach.* Chichester: John Wiley & Sons, 1983.
- Beattie DK, Golledge J, Greenhalgh RM, Davies AH. Quality of life assessment in vascular disease: Towards a consensus. *European Journal of Vascular and Endovascular Surgery* 1997;**13**:9–13.
- Russell IT. Evaluating new surgical procedures. *British Medical Journal* 1995;**311**: 1243–1244.
- Garratt AM, Ruta DA, Abdalla MI, Buckingham JK, Russell IT. The SF-36 health survey questionnaire: an outcome measure suitable for routine use within the NHS. *British Medical Journal* 1993;**306**:1440–1444.
- Torgerson DJ, Campbell MK. Economic Note – Cost effectiveness calculations to aid sample size estimation. *British Medical Journal* 1999 (in press).
- Torgerson DJ, Ryan M, Ratcliffe J. Economics in sample size determination for clinical trials. *Quarterly Journal of Medicine* 1995;**88**:517–521.
- Altman DG. *Practical Statistics for Medical Research.* London: Chapman & Hall, 1996.

9
Extracranial Carotid Disease

A Ross Naylor

Introduction

The extracranial carotid arteries are vulnerable to a number of atheromatous and non-atheromatous disorders. Stroke is the third commonest cause of death and permanent neurological disability with an annual UK incidence of 2 per 1000 population. Each year in the UK about 120 000 patients suffer their first stroke. Recent evidence suggests that overall stroke mortality has started to decline, a feature which is ascribed to improved acute care and patient survival rather than a fall in the overall incidence. However, because the proportion of elderly patients in the population is increasing, the overall incidence of stroke could increase quite significantly over the next two decades.

This chapter deals predominantly with atheromatous disease and stroke prevention in particular. It also summarizes practical and clinical aspects of fibromuscular dysplasia, aneurysm and carotid body tumour.

Aetiology

Atheromatous carotid disease

Stroke is defined as an acute loss of focal or occasionally global cerebral function with symptoms exceeding 24 h or leading to death which after due investigation has a vascular cause. A transient ischaemic attack (TIA) has the same definition except that the symptoms resolve within 24 h.

Recent epidemiological studies suggest that approximately 80% of all strokes are ischaemic while 20% are haemorrhagic. Three-quarters of all ischaemic strokes present with carotid territory features, 15% with vertebrobasilar features, while in 10% it is not possible to discriminate between the two on clinical grounds alone. The most important risk factors for stroke are:

- hypertension (60%);
- ischaemic heart disease (38%);

- a cardioembolic source (20%);
- a preceding TIA (15%);
- increasing age;
- diabetes (10%).

For every 100 patients who present with a carotid territory, ischaemic infarction, 50% is due to thromboembolism of either the internal carotid artery (ICA) or the middle cerebral artery (MCA) (Fig. 9.1), and 25% is secondary to small vessel disease affecting the lenticulostriate arteries (Fig. 9.2). An embolism from the heart is the underlying cause in 15% of patients, while a predisposing haematological disorder or non-atheromatous condition (fibromuscular dysplasia, arteritis, etc.) accounts for an acute stroke in 5–10% of patients. Thus, overall, the majority of stokes are *ischaemic*, the majority of ischaemic strokes affect the carotid territory and the largest single cause of carotid territory ischaemic stroke is thromboembolism of the ICA or MCA.

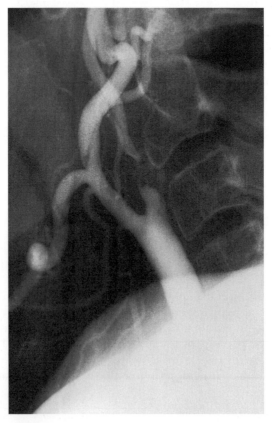

Fig. 9.1 Severe stenosis at the origin of the internal carotid artery.

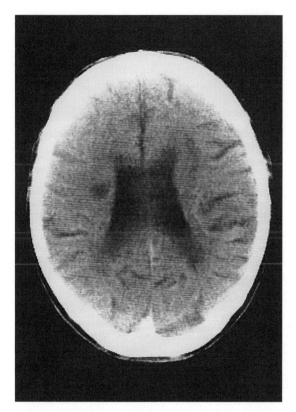

Fig. 9.2 Small lacunar infarction due to occlusion of a perforating end artery in a patient with diabetes and hypertension.

Non-atheromatous disorders

Fibromuscular dysplasia (FMD) is a rare condition affecting the renal (90%) and carotid (10%) arteries in young women. One-third of patients with carotid artery FMD have co-existing renal involvement, the majority have bilateral carotid involvement and co-existent intracranial aneurysms are not unusual. Pathologically, the condition is typified by fibrotic webs in association with dilatations due to focal mural degradation.

Aneurysms affecting the extracranial circulation are unusual and comprise <5% of all peripheral aneurysms. The commonest underlying aetiology is atherosclerosis. However, aneurysm formation in the younger patient should raise the possibility of unusual aetiologies such as FMD, post trauma, dissection and, rarely, mycotic causes.

A number of arteritic processes affect the extracranial carotid circulation and its principal branches, notably Takayasu's disease and giant-cell arteritis. *Takayasu's disease* is a rare condition where all the layers of the arterial wall are involved in the inflammatory process which is of a granulomatous nature and ultimately progresses to vascular occlusion. While Takayasu's disease tends to affect the younger female, *giant-cell arteritis* predominantly affects the older female patient. The latter is a systemic condition of unknown aetiology with the potential to involve any large artery, although the carotid artery and its branches are the commonest sites of involvement.

The carotid body (3 mm diameter) is located within the adventia of the posterior aspect of the carotid bifurcation and its physiological role is the maintenance of homeostasis with regard to blood gases and pH. Embryologically, it consists of cells derived from the neural crest ectoderm and is closely related to similar tissues found along the course of the vagus nerve, jugular vein, adrenal medulla, aortic arch and components of the autonomic nervous system. When a carotid body tumour (paraganglioma) develops, the bifurcation splays apart as the clumps of neoplastic epithelioid chief cells proliferate. There is preliminary evidence that a proportion of carotid body tumours may have an autosomal dominant inheritance.

Clinical features

Atheromatous disease

Extracranial occlusive carotid artery disease can present in two ways:

- symptomatic;
- asymptomatic.

Symptomatic carotid disease

Symptoms which are typically suggestive of a *carotid territory event* are:

- focal hemisensory/hemimotor deficits;
- amaurosis fugax (monocular visual loss likened to a shutter or curtain over the vision);
- evidence of higher cortical dysfunction (e.g. expressive dysphasia or visuospatial neglect).

Homonymous hemianopia is only seen in large carotid territory infarcts and only then in association with severe paralysis and higher cortical dysfunction.

Typical *vertebrobasilar symptoms* include:

- bilateral motor/sensory impairment;
- bilateral visual loss;
- dysarthria;

- nystagmus; problems with gait, stance and dizziness
- homonymous hemianopia.

Up to 10% of vertebrobasilar strokes, however, present with hemi-sensory/hemimotor signs, thereby making clinical differentiation from a carotid territory stroke more difficult. Isolated dizziness and vertigo are not due to carotid disease and should only be considered to be a vertebrobasilar symptom if accompanied by other more definite vertebro-basilar symptoms.

It is unwise to base clinical decision making or referral practice on the presence or absence of a *carotid bruit.* For example, up to two-thirds of patients with a 90–99% stenosis do not have a carotid bruit, while up to one-third of patients with a carotid occlusion still have an audible bruit. There are, however, two important high-risk subgroups to identify:

- crescendo TIA;
- stroke in evolution.

Crescendo TIAs involve repeated TIAs within a relatively short period of time. On each occasion, the neurological deficit will have fully recovered before the onset of the next event, and these may occur on a daily basis. In '*stroke in evolution*', the initial neurological deficit starts to improve but becomes acutely worse again and as that deficit begins to improve a further neurological deterioration ensues. Both of these phenomena should be considered medical emergencies and the patient admitted directly to hospital. It is generally considered that the underlying aetio-logy is an acutely unstable plaque with overlying thrombus and the patient is at high risk of stroke.

Asymptomatic carotid disease

About 10% of the population aged over 70 years has an asymptomatic internal carotid stenosis >50%, and this figure increases to 25% in patients with co-existent hypertension. Asymptomatic carotid stenoses present as an incidental finding during auscultation of the neck, follow-ing carotid ultrasound scanning of the contralateral symptomatic artery and occasionally as a work-up towards other surgical procedures. There is relatively little information available as to why the asymptomatic plaque can remain stable for many years before causing problems but it is assumed that an acute event precipitates a change within the structure of the plaque, causing overlying fissuring, rupture or thrombosis and there-after, clustering of symptoms.

Non-atheromatous disease

Fibromuscular dysplasia, the arterites, carotid aneurysm and carotid body tumours can present with symptoms or as an incidental finding. Because many of these conditions involve varying degrees of vascular occlusion and dilatation, symptoms can arise as a result of:

- thromboembolism (e.g. TIA or a stroke);
- rupture of an aneurysm;
- distal dissection;
- presence of a pulsatile mass or compressive symptoms such as hoarseness;
- neurogenic swallowing difficulties;
- Horner's syndrome.

The neurological symptoms in *Takayasu's disease* can develop as a result of occlusion of the carotid arteries alone or via renovascular hypertension.

Temporal arteritis is an important condition to diagnose early because of the potential for blindness. It tends to be preceded by general malaise, headache and muscle pains with tenderness over the superficial temporal artery.

Carotid body tumours usually present with a non-tender palpable mass which never regresses and is usually non-functional. However, if the tumour envelopes the bifurcation and extends towards adjacent structures, local compression can cause cranial nerve palsies, swallowing problems and/or Horner's syndrome. Overall, 5% of all carotid body tumours are bilateral and as a general rule 5% are locally invasive and 5% systemically malignant.

See Chapter 13 for further details on carotid artery aneurysms.

Diagnosis

Atheromatous disease

One of the major ultrasound developments of the last two decades has been the advent of colour Doppler. This gives clinicians a non-invasive means of evaluating the carotid artery without the risk of stroke associated with angiography. Duplex combines real-time (B-mode) imaging with Doppler waveform analysis. In addition, colour flow imaging has dramatically improved the accuracy and sensitivity of the investigation to 90% or more (Plate 4). Duplex is, however, very operator dependent and technical experience must be taken into account when interpreting duplex findings.

In Leicester, we have abandoned routine preoperative carotid angiography and perform a carotid endarterectomy based on colour Doppler assessment alone in 92% of patients using a combination of B-mode imaging and a peak systolic velocity >200 cm/s and an end diastolic velocity >120 cm/s to diagnose an internal carotid artery stenosis of >70%. Our main indications for performing selective carotid angiography include:

- inability to obtain satisfactory images of the bifurcation;
- inability to visualize the distal internal carotid artery;
- abnormal common carotid waveform suggestive of proximal disease;
- high resistance signal in the distal ICA suggestive of a syphon stenosis.

Carotid angiography is still, however, performed in about 50% of vascular centres prior to carotid endarterectomy. The rationale is that it is still the 'gold standard' and only angiography can allow accurate grading of a stenosis, delineation of upper and lower plaque end points and an image of the proximal common carotid artery origin, carotid siphon and intracranial circulation. However, there is no conclusive evidence that recognition of carotid siphon disease actually alters stroke risk during carotid endarterectomy and the overall incidence of intracranial occlusive disease and intracranial aneurysms found on routine angiography is <1%.

The fundamental problem with regard to carotid angiography is the risk of stroke, which overall, following any carotid angiogram, is 0.5%. In symptomatic patients with a stenosis >50% on duplex, angiography is associated with a 2% stroke rate. However, this risk can be minimized by non-selective arch arteriography. Selective carotid catheterization is rarely required with good quality digital subtraction equipment (Fig. 9.3).

Magnetic resonance angiography (MRA) has also been developed in the last 10 years and a number of centres use it in combination with duplex. Although there is considerable potential for the future, MRA still has problems with regard to interpretation of a severe stenosis because turbulence and vortex formation can reduce the signal which leads to overestimation of the degree of stenosis. In future, it may become the investigation of choice, although, as with angiography, an accurate and accepted method of determining degree of stenosis is still required.

The role of CT imaging in patients with extracranial carotid artery disease remains controversial. In Leicester we do not perform CT scans routinely as an internal audit of our previous experience showed that it rarely changed our clinical practice and led to unacceptable delays in getting patients to theatre. We would, however, advocate preoperative CT scanning and referral to a neurologist in any patient with atypical or non-hemispheric symptoms. Patients with persistent symptoms but no significant carotid disease should undergo cardiac investigation (24-h ECG and echocardiography).

Non-atheromatous disease

Fibromuscular dysplasia should be suspected in younger females with carotid territory symptoms, and if a bizarre beaded appearance is

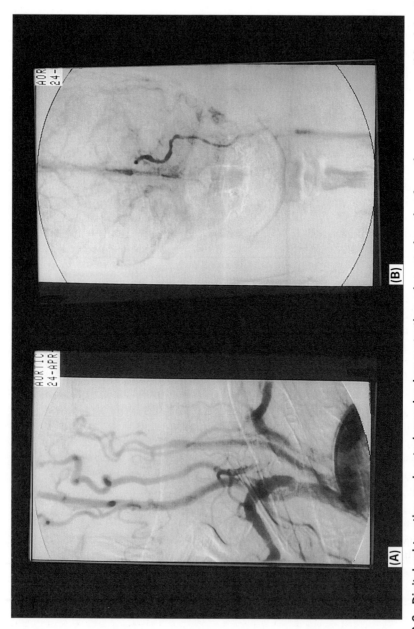

Fig. 9.3. Digital subtraction arch arteriography demonstrating adequate imaging from the common carotid origins to the circle of Willis. Note severe stenosis of (A) left ICA origin plus (B) disease of carotid siphon.

suspected on duplex, an angiogram should be performed which should include the intracranial circulation to exclude aneurysm.

Similarly, angiography is the investigation of choice in patients with *Takayasu's disease* because of the potential for involving the aortic arch and its branches and the abdominal aorta and its branches.

Giant-cell arteritis is primarily a diagnosis of suspicion with corroboration by elevated plasma viscosity, raised erythrocyte sedimentation rate and, most importantly, temporal artery biopsy.

Extracranial carotid aneurysms can be diagnosed using duplex ultrasound and if there is no evidence of extension above or below the limits of duplex, then it should be possible to treat these surgically without the need for angiography. If, however, there is any question of upper access problems, angiography should be performed.

Carotid body tumours can also be diagnosed using colour Doppler but it is still important to perform angiography in these patients in order to evaluate vascular anatomy and co-existent atherosclerotic disease, and to exclude bilateral tumours and other primary and secondary paraganglionomas. There is no consensus view on the role of CT/MRI scanning or radionuclide imaging but if there is any evidence of extension towards the base of the brain then some form of tomographic imaging is essential.

Management

Atheromatous disease

Symptomatic carotid artery disease

There is clear evidence from European and American randomized trials that in patients presenting with a severe (>70%) stenosis and appropriate ipsilateral carotid territory symptoms, carotid endarterectomy plus best medical therapy confers a 6–10-fold reduction in the long-term risk of stroke as compared with best medical therapy alone. Optimal medical care includes control of blood pressure, hyperlipidaemia, ischaemic heart disease and diabetes, cessation of smoking and commencing aspirin. For patients with a mild-to-moderate stenosis (<70%), carotid surgery has no definite role to play. However, patients with moderate stenoses (50–70%) and recurrent carotid territory symptoms despite best medical therapy should be considered for carotid endarterectomy provided optimal medical care has been implemented (Fig. 9.4). In the latter situation it is always useful to seek the additional input of a neurologist.

Patients with crescendo TIAs should have a CT scan to exclude haemorrhage and then go on to a heparin infusion prior to urgent endarterectomy. Patients with stroke in evolution but no significant residual deficit should also be considered for emergency carotid

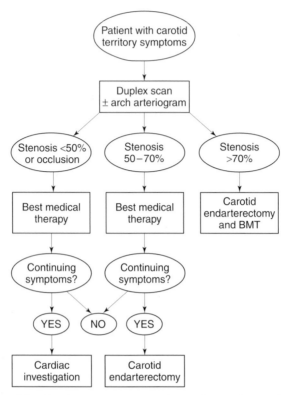

Fig. 9.4. Algorithm for the management of a patient with carotid territory symptoms. BMT = best medical treatment.

endarterectomy. There is no evidence of a role for emergency carotid surgery in the presence of an established severe acute stroke.

Asymptomatic disease

A number of trials, predominantly based in the USA, have evaluated the role of carotid surgery in asymptomatic carotid artery disease. The majority were either poorly designed or stopped prematurely. However, the Asymptomatic Carotid Artery Atherosclerosis Study now suggests that patients with an asymptomatic stenosis >60% have a projected 5-year stroke risk of about 12%, which can be reduced to about 6% with prophylactic endarterectomy. This equates to an actual risk reduction of about 6% and a relative risk reduction of about 50%. This trial has a number of important clinical implications, not least being the fact that 1% of the general population has a stenosis >60% and therefore prophylactic endarterectomy in all such patients would be impractical. Clearly, therefore, an element of case selection is required and our policy is to offer prophylactic endarterectomy to the dominant carotid artery in patients with severe (>70%) bilateral asymptomatic carotid stenoses and in those with one carotid artery occluded and the other stenosed >70%.

A further area of controversy is the role of synchronous carotid endarterectomy and coronary artery bypass surgery. Perioperative stroke complicates coronary surgery in about 2% of patients but certain risk factors predispose to an increase in the overall risk of operative stroke. For example, patients aged over 60 years who have a carotid stenosis >75% have a stroke risk of about 15% as compared with <1% in the remainder. As a consequence, our current policy is to undertake synchronous coronary and carotid reconstruction in patients with carotid stenoses >70%, with the endarterectomy performed immediately prior to the patient undergoing bypass.

Non-atheromatous disease

The management of fibromuscular dysplasia, arteritis, carotid aneurysm and carotid body tumours depends on presentation. In principle, up to the level of the styloid process, symptomatic stenoses associated with fibromuscular dysplasia can be treated by percutaneous angioplasty but for extensive dysplasia, including dilatation and/or aneurysm formation, resection and interposition bypass is recommended. Asymptomatic disease should be left alone.

Giant-cell arteritis is treated with steroid therapy following biopsy diagnosis.

Takayasu's disease is not amenable to endarterectomy or angioplasty and if symptoms are of sufficient severity, then bypass reconstruction is required. Because Takayasu's disease of the extracranial carotid arteries has the potential to involve the aortic arch, the collaborative input of a cardiac surgical team is usually necessary.

Carotid aneurysms preferably require excision and interposition vein bypass or resection and end-to-end anastomosis. Rarely, the most distal aspect of the ICA may be inaccessible and ligation may have to be considered.

Carotid body tumours are treated by excision with dissection usually being performed in the subadventitial plane. These tumours are very vascular and care must be taken when dissecting the tumour off the posterior aspect of the bifurcation where the arterial wall may be very thin. Bleeding may be reduced by preoperative embolization but there is no consensus on the role of this adjuvant technique. It is certainly not an alternative to surgery. In one-quarter of patients, the tumour entirely encircles the bifurcation, making preservation of the bifurcation impossible; these patients inevitably require resection plus interposition vein graft bypass.

Carotid endarterectomy

The carotid artery is exposed via an anterior sternomastoid incision dividing platysma and retracting sternomastoid laterally. An important landmark for finding the carotid bifurcation is the common facial vein which is divided and retracted laterally. The carotid bifurcation is then exposed, identifying and preserving the vagus and hypoglossal nerves.

The endarterectomy is performed under systemic heparinization and a longitudinal arteriotomy made across the bifurcation into the internal carotid artery above the upper limit of the disease. Cerebral perfusion can be maintained by insertion of a temporary indwelling shunt and the plaque is removed with an endarterectomy plane between the plaque and the media. It is important to remove all intimal fragments and achieve a smooth feathered or tapered distal intimal step. Alternatively, the distal intimal step can be tacked down for safety using interrupted prolene sutures. The arteriotomy is either closed primarily or as a patch angioplasty using long saphenous vein from the groin or a prosthetic material such as polytetrafluoroethylene (PTFE) or Dacron (Fig. 9.5). Flow is normally restored first up the external carotid artery and then up the internal carotid artery.

Although relatively straightforward in principle, carotid endarterectomy must be performed with meticulous attention to technical detail as any operation-related stroke is not readily amenable to correction. Accordingly a number of controversial issues relating to the practice of carotid endarterectomy have developed over the four decades of its practice. In many there is no consensus viewpoint and individual surgeons have evolved a personal practice with which they feel most comfortable.

Monitoring

Perioperative monitoring with transcranial Doppler is employed in many UK centres, but is by no means universally accepted. During the operation, blood flow in the ipsilateral middle cerebral artery can be continuously monitored using a 2-MHz fixed-head probe ultrasound system which permits early identification, and therefore correction, of unpredictable events such as embolization, shunt kinking malfunction and platelet embolization while the neck is being closed.

Quality control

The principle of quality control assessment is to identify abnormalities prior to restoration of flow and correct them where possible. A number of methods are available for this, including completion angiography, B-mode ultrasound, colour Doppler ultrasound, angioscopy and continuous-wave Doppler. In Leicester our current practice is to use continuous transcranial Doppler monitoring supplemented by completion

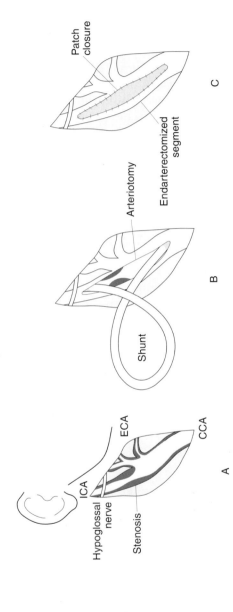

Fig. 9.5. **Basic technique of carotid endarterectomy using an indwelling shunt and patch closure. ICA = internal carotid artery; ECA = external carotid artery; CCA = common carotid artery.**

angioscopic assessment immediately prior to restoration of flow; this has resulted in a sustained reduction in risk of intraoperative stroke from 4% to 0.5%.

Shunting and patching

The question as to whether patients should be shunted or patched remains controversial. Preliminary evidence from overviews of available randomized trials suggests that routine patching may be associated with a significant reduction in the risk of perioperative stroke, carotid thrombosis and late restenosis as compared with primary closure.

Surgeons either routinely shunt, never shunt or selectively shunt. The latter is based on a direct or indirect assessment of the adequacy of cerebral perfusion during carotid clamping using either stump pressure, transcranial Doppler ultrasound, near infrared spectroscopy, EEG, evoked potentials or a subjective assessment of carotid backflow. There is, however, no universally accepted threshold upon which one can safely plan for selective carotid shunting because no 2 patients present with the same susceptibility and there are few randomized trials.

Carotid angioplasty

A new alternative to carotid endarterectomy is carotid angioplasty (Fig. 9.6). The potential advantages of this less invasive approach include lower cost, shorter hospital stay, avoidance of general anaesthetic and no risk of cranial nerve injury. The main risk remains thromboembolic stroke and the place of angioplasty in the management of symptomatic patients is the subject of ongoing randomized trials.

Outcome

Atheromatous disease

International trials have demonstrated that the 30-day mortality following carotid endarterectomy is between 0.6% and 1%. The risk of death and/or disabling stroke (defined as a Rankin score of 3 or more) is 3.5–5% and the risk of any stroke is 5–7.5%. Research suggests that two-thirds of perioperative strokes occur intraoperatively (i.e. the patient recovers from the anaesthetic with a new neurological deficit) while one-third occur postoperatively (i.e. the patient recovers normally from anaesthesia, but then develops a new neurological deficit).

The majority of intraoperative strokes tend to follow inadvertent technical error, the most important being residual luminal thrombus which embolizes following restoration of flow.

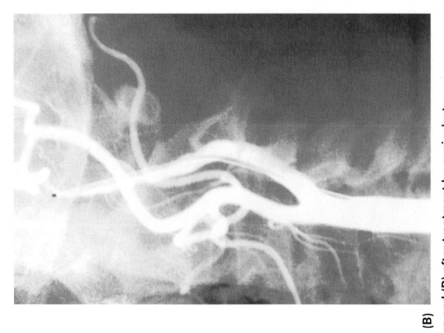

(B)

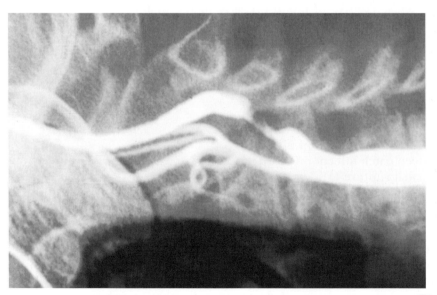

(A)

Fig. 9.6. **Severe carotid stenosis (A) before and (B) after treatment by angioplasty.**

Postoperative strokes are usually due either to postoperative carotid thrombosis (two-thirds) or intracranial haemorrhage (one-third). Carotid thrombosis may follow technical errors such as corrugation or kinking of the carotid artery or a residual intimal flap, but may also be due to an aggressive tendency for platelets to form within the endarterectomy zone. As a consequence, we now routinely monitor endarterectomy patients with transcranial Doppler for 3–6 h following restoration of flow. Any patient with sustained embolization is treated with intravenous Dextran-40 and, to date, this has abolished postoperative carotid thrombosis in the last 500 patients.

Reperfusion injury

Intracranial haemorrhage complicates about 1% of carotid endarterectomies and tends to be more prevalent in patients with severe bilateral carotid artery disease, poor collateralization via the circle of Willis and impaired cerebrovascular reserve. These patients appear to have impaired cerebral autoregulation which does not return to normal until about 5 days after the procedure. During this time, the brain is susceptible to high blood flow (hyperperfusion syndrome) and the risk of haemorrhage is increased. Intracranial haemorrhage is very difficult to treat and has a high morbidity and mortality following endarterectomy. Accordingly, the only treatment is prevention which requires very close control of blood pressure in the first 72 h of postoperative care.

There are a number of other recognized complications following endarterectomy:

- hypertension (66%);
- false aneurysm formation (<1%);
- cranial nerve injury (5%);
- wound infection (5%);
- myocardial infarction (4%);
- deep patch infection (<1%);
- patch rupture (1%).

The most important of these is *patch rupture* which is most commonly associated with the use of vein patches. The incidence appears to be higher in patients where the vein is harvested from the saphenous vein at the ankle rather than the groin, and it tends to occur on the 5th postoperative day with a transverse rupture through the central portion of the patch in female patients with a past history of hypertension. Vein patch rupture can be avoided by using a prosthetic patch but this is then susceptible to a 1% risk of deep graft infection which is also a very difficult condition to treat.

Restenosis

Long-term, the risk of restenosis appears to be higher in patients closed primarily as compared with those closed with a patch. The cumulative annual risk of developing an occlusion and/or recurrent stenosis of >70% in the operated artery is of the order of 2–3% per annum. However, the risk of suffering any late cerebral ischaemic events in the territory of the operated carotid is 3–6% per annum. The cumulative risk of ipsilateral stroke is about 1.5% per annum while the cumulative risk of stroke in the contralateral (non-operated) hemisphere is 2% per annum. In general, recurrent stenoses developing within the first 2 years following endarterectomy are due to neointimal hyperplasia and intervention is only warranted in patients who become symptomatic. Serial surveillance is therefore not justified.

Non-atheromatous disease

Evidence suggests that intraluminal dilatation of the webs and stenoses in *fibromuscular dysplasia* confer long-term protection against late stroke, but occasionally these patients may suffer subarachnoid haemorrhage from an undiagnosed intracranial aneurysm. There is no conclusive evidence of the safety of long-term percutaneous angioplasty in fibromuscular disease.

Any vein bypass performed on the carotid vessels is susceptible to vein graft stenosis which probably occurs in up to one-third of patients. This can be treated by percutaneous balloon angioplasty and accordingly we now enter all our carotid bypass patients into a programme of surveillance.

It is possible to perform resection of a *carotid aneurysm* plus distal reconstruction in three-quarters of patients, although the higher the procedure, the higher is the risk of cranial nerve injury. Ligation of the carotid artery carries a significant risk of stroke and should only be performed as a last resort in patients where some method of monitoring (e.g. transcranial Doppler or awake testing) suggests it will be safe.

About 5% of *carotid body tumours* are locally malignant and about 5% systemically malignant. Any recurrent tumour tends to be slow growing and quite marked infiltration into the neck structures can be present by the time it becomes clinically apparent. In the majority, complete removal of the carotid body tumour results in cure and the overall risks of recurrence are very small. The risk of cranial nerve injury may be as high as 20%; the operative stroke rate is about 5%.

Summary

- The majority of strokes are ischaemic, involve the carotid territory and the largest single cause is thromboembolism of the internal carotid artery and/or middle cerebral artery.
- Carotid endarterectomy has an important role in the management of selected patients with symptomatic, severe carotid stenoses.
- Carotid endarterectomy confers a 45% reduction in the long-term risk of stroke but if the perioperative morbidity could be reduced to 0, the overall long-term risk reduction in stroke would increase to 75%.
- Optimal medical care is equally important in long-term stroke prevention.
- The number of strokes prevented by carotid endarterectomy is small in comparison to the overall problem of stroke in the UK.

Areas of controversy

- Is carotid endarterectomy a cost-effective means of stroke prevention for the population as a whole?
- What is the role of endarterectomy in patients with asymptomatic carotid artery disease?
- Should carotid endarterectomy only be performed by vascular surgeons with an adequate workload and audited results?
- What is the role of patch angioplasty and shunting in carotid endarterectomy?
- Does perioperative monitoring and quality control assessment improve clinical outcome?
- Is carotid angioplasty a safe and durable alternative to carotid endarterectomy in the prevention of stroke?

Further reading

- Moore WS (ed). *Surgery for Cerebral Vascular Disease*, 2nd edn. Philadelphia: WB Saunders, 1996.
- Naylor AR, Ruckley CV. Complications after carotid surgery. In: Campbell B (ed). *Operative Complications in Vascular Surgery; A Practical Approach to Management.* Oxford: Butterworth Heinemann, 1996, pp 73–88.
- Bamford J, Sandercock P, Dennis M, Burn J, Warlow CP. A prospective study of acute cerebrovascular disease in the community. The Oxfordshire Community Stroke Project 1981–1986 (No. 1) Methodology, demography and incidence cases of first ever stroke. *Journal of Neurology, Neurosurgery and Psychiatry* 1988;**51**:1373–1380.
- European Carotid Surgery Triallists Collaborative Group. MRC European Carotid Surgery Trial; Interim results for symptomatic patients with severe (70–99%) or with mild (0–29%) carotid stenosis. *Lancet* 1991;**337**:1235–1241.

- European Carotid Surgery Triallists Collaborative Group. MRC European Carotid Surgery Trial: Endarterectomy for moderate symptomatic carotid stenosis; Interim results. *Lancet* 1996;**347**:1591–1593.
- North American Symptomatic Carotid Endarterectomy Trial Collaborators. Beneficial effect of carotid endarterectomy in symptomatic patients with high grade stenosis. *New England Journal of Medicine* 1991;**325**:445–453.
- Executive Committee for the Asymptomatic Carotid Atherosclerosis Study. Endarterectomy for asymptomatic carotid artery stenosis. *JAMA* 1995;**273**:1421–1461.
- Council C, Salinas R, Warlow CP, Naylor AR. A comparison of different types of patch in carotid patch angioplasty; A systematic review of the randomised trials. In: Warlow CP, van Gijn J, Sandercock P (eds) *Stroke Module of the Cochrane Database of Systematic Reviews.* London: BMJ Publishing Group, 1996.
- Council C, Salinas R, Warlow CP, Naylor AR. The role of carotid artery shunting during carotid endarterectomy; A systematic review of the randomised trials of routine and selective shunting and the different methods of intraoperative monitoring. In: Warlow CP, van Gijn J, Sandercock P (eds) *Stroke Module of the Cochrane Database of Systematic Reviews.* London: BMJ Publishing Group, 1996.

10

Subclavian and Upper Limb Disorders

JF Thompson

Introduction

Occlusive or aneurysmal disorders affecting the subclavian artery and upper limb vessels present rare but demanding challenges to vascular specialists.

Acute upper limb ischaemia is a true emergency, as collateral vessels, due to chronic, progressive, obliterative disease are usually less well developed than in the lower limb. The resultant ischaemia is consequently more profound and revascularization must be achieved within 2–4 h before irreversible muscle necrosis takes place. As upper limb ischaemia represents only 5% of an average vascular surgeon's experience, and often presents out of normal working hours, surgeons in training see it less frequently and should take careful note of the lessons learnt, particularly in these days of shorter training programmes.

Acute upper limb ischaemia

Aetiology

The causes of upper limb ischaemia are best considered anatomically (Table 10.1).

Acute thrombosis *in situ* is a relatively rare cause of acute upper limb ischaemia but may affect the subclavian and axillary arteries in several special situations:

- In *acute aortic dissection* the patient is usually elderly and hypertensive. The dissection is usually felt as an excruciating, tearing, interscapular pain which can radiate along the axial branches of the aorta to the right arm, head, left arm, trunk and both legs. The left arm is more often affected than the right as the entry point of the dissection is usually within the arch of the aorta. A more proximal dissection, which

Table 10.1. **Causes of acute upper limb ischaemia.**

Heart and great vessels	Emboli from mural thrombosis, especially following myocardial infarction, cardiac arrhythmia, artrial myxoma, vegetations or atherosclerotic embolus from proximal plaque
Subclavian artery	Occlusive disease leading to chronic upper limb ischaemia or disordered cerebral circulation
Subclavian/axillary system	Compression syndromes such as thoracic outlet syndrome, poststenotic aneurysm formation, radiation endarteritis or trauma
Peripheral vessels	Fractures of the long bones causing direct intimal damage, transection or false aneurysm formation. More distally, the vessels of the hand may be affected by trauma, vibration, vasospasm or thermal injury

disrupts the coronary circulation and aortic valve along with the cerebral vessels, is often fatal.

● *Axillary artery thrombosis due to trauma* (either a fracture of the surgical neck of the humerus or pressure from a chair back or crutch are easily identified factors).

● *Acute deterioration in patients with chronic occlusion of the great vessels* in Takayasu's disease, giant cell arteritis and similar conditions (see Chapter 9).

● *Thrombosis of an axillo-subclavian artery aneurysm* due to poststenotic dilatation in thoracic outlet syndrome.

Clinical features

Occlusive disease leading to *in situ* thrombosis is rare in the upper limb; *emboli* are by far the commonest cause of acute upper limb ischaemia. The ischaemia leads rapidly to the classical clinical picture of severe pain, pallor, coldness with loss of pulses, function and sensation and is a true surgical emergency.

The origin of the embolus is usually cardiac, and as the population affected by juvenile rheumatic fever diminishes, the commonest cause is atrial fibrillation secondary to ischaemic heart disease or ventricular dyskinesia due to recent myocardial infarction. This is reflected by the operative mortality which, although high at 11%, is less than half that described in most lower limb series. This may reflect the widespread use of local rather than general anaesthesia during upper limb embolectomy. It also reflects the poor overall medical state of these elderly patients.

Athero-embolus may also arise from occlusive disease of the innominate, subclavian or axillary systems, or aneurysmal dilatation of these vessels. Several special circumstances may lead to acute upper limb ischaemia:

- accidental injection of drugs into the brachial artery causing acute vasospasm thrombosis or embolus (see below);
- ingestion of drugs causing vasospasm and trauma;
- Motorcycle injury often leads to severe traction at the root of the neck as the arm flails or the victim falls on the shoulder tip.

As in lower limb injuries, a careful multidisciplinary assessment is vital, for irretrievable damage to the brachial plexus may make a good functional outcome impossible, and in the presence of a contused brachial plexus, primary amputation should be considered. If, on the other hand, there is clean avulsion or severing of the nerve trunks, reconstruction should be followed by early microsurgical repair of the plexus.

Diagnosis

The history and examination usually yield a clear diagnosis in acute upper limb ischaemia, by revealing the medical predisposition and precise site of the ischaemic block. Ninety percent of cases will be due to emboli resulting in an occlusion at the upper axillary artery (where the circumflex humeral artery arises) or at the brachial artery trifurcation, with proximal clot propagating back to the distal brachial artery. There may be a history or ECG changes suggestive of acute myocardial infarction or arrhythmia.

As with lower limb ischaemia, the contralateral limb provides a good idea as to the condition of the affected limb's arteries before the embolus occurred; clear, palpable pulses are the norm in the upper limb and anything less should raise the suspicion of pre-existing, more generalized arterial disease.

Ischaemia affecting the digits is usually due to local trauma such as frostbite or severe vasospastic disease. It may be due to a large shower of small emboli, as in subacute bacterial endocarditis, drug injection or embolism from a subclavian aneurysm, and the treatment is usually supportive as the vessels involved are too small for surgical intervention.

Trauma is usually associated with obvious injury. Compression in thoracic outlet syndrome is considered below.

Very few investigations are required before treating most cases of brachial embolus. Full blood count, urea and electrolytes, ECG and urine for glucose are mandatory. Plain X-rays may reveal associated structural anomalies such as cervical rib or fracture.

Careful pulse palpation at the axillary, brachial and distal vessels and a comparison with the unaffected side may enable the position of the lesion to be determined with surprising accuracy. Hand-held continuous wave Doppler, using an 8-MHz probe, can map the level of the occlusion. A completely normal bi- or tri-phasic Doppler signal should be expected. Modern instruments are very sensitive and may pick up tiny collateral vessels or low rates of flow distal to subocclusive thrombus, so a high degree of suspicion is essential. Duplex scanning can give accurate images of the lesion, e.g. an intimal flap due to direct arterial trauma.

Angiography is rarely needed except in unusual cases, such as where thrombolysis is to be considered or in trauma where a bypass or other reconstruction may be required (see below).

Management

Brachial embolectomy is an important surgical 'set piece'. The collateral supply to the arm means that the limb remains viable but embolectomy may still be required to prevent subsequent claudication. Except in the case of aortic dissection or trauma, immediate heparinization with 5000 iu of unfractionated heparin is the norm. The patient should be taken to theatre without delay. An anaesthetist *must* be present throughout the procedure. Good quality intravenous access via the contralateral limb, ECG monitoring, pulse oximetry and supplemental oxygen are mandatory. Intravenous sedation is seldom required and must be given in small incremental doses as the patients are often frail. Analgesia in the form of fentanyl or diamorphine may be helpful and, if embolectomy is painful, 5–10 ml of 1% plain intra-arterial lignocaine can be instilled during the procedure to good effect.

The whole limb is prepared with undyed chlorhexidine solution and draped. The hand is placed in a transparent plastic 'bowel' bag and abducted to 90° on an arm board. The line of the proposed incision is infiltrated with 10 ml of plain 1% lignocaine solution and after sufficient time, the incision is made in a 'lazy S' configuration, starting at the posterior border of the biceps muscle, passing laterally across the skin crease of the antecubital fossa and extending distally. The distal brachial artery is exposed by dividing the flexor retinaculum and is crossed by the median nerve. Additional local anaesthetic is often required during the dissection and a degree of median nerve palsy is to be expected postoperatively. The radial and ulnar artery origins should be exposed and controlled with fine silastic slings.

The principles of balloon–catheter embolectomy are covered in Chapter 14, except that here a smaller 2 or 3F catheter is usually required.

Although the degree of ischaemia is often such that there appears to be time for low dose intra-arterial thrombolysis, local anaesthetic embolectomy is so safe, quick and effective, that it is probably not reasonable to expose the patient to the increased risk of stroke associated with thrombolytic therapy.

Following successful surgery, the patient is kept on an infusion of heparin, 1000 iu/h, and warfarin. Careful postoperative observations are instituted. 'Coronary care' may be appropriate.

Chronic upper limb ischaemia

The extensive proximal collateral circulation around the head, neck and shoulder can mask the progressive symptoms of arterial occlusive disease affecting the upper limb. Elderly patients tolerate surprisingly poor perfusion in the arm due to decreased metabolic demand and the smaller muscle bulk.

Aetiology

Chronic upper limb occlusive disease may be caused by:

● atherosclerotic occlusion;
● aneurysm with chronic athero-embolism;
● thoracic outlet syndrome;
● the arteritides;
● fibromuscular hyperplasia;
● scleroderma and related connective tissue disorders.

Clinical features

In contrast to the lower limb, twice as many patients affected by occlusive disease of the upper limb are female. Subclavian artery occlusion is more common on the left. As well as the expected symptoms of muscular fatigue (termed 'claudication', although patients do not of course walk on their hands), there may be disordered cerebral circulation or both. Proximal subclavian artery occlusion may result in the so-called *subclavian steal syndrome*, where blood reaches the affected arm via the ipsilateral carotid artery, the circle of Willis and by retrograde flow down the vertebral artery to the distal subclavian artery (Fig. 10.1). Vigorous use of the arm 'steals' blood from the posterior cerebral circulation causing dizziness, vertigo or even syncope, as well as claudication in the affected limb.

More central atheroma from stenoses or aneurysm may embolize and mimic microvascular vasospasm. *Unilateral Raynaud's phenomenon* points to a local rather than a systematic cause – usually a cervical rib. Chronic digital ischaemia is seen in severe (primary) Raynaud's disease, or Raynaud's phenomenon secondary to a long list of conditions, the commonest of which are the autoimmune syndromes such as CREST (calcinosis, Raynaud's phenomenon, oesophageal dysmotility, scleroderma and telangectasia) or local causes such as non-freezing cold injury or vibration white finger (see Chapter 22).

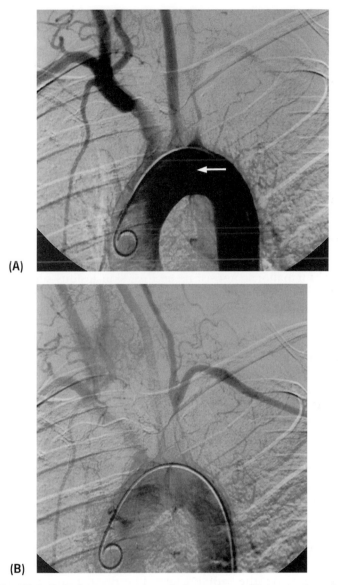

(A)

(B)

Fig. 10.1. (A) Subclavian artery stenosis (arrow) and (B) Later view showing contrast filling from vertebral to subclavian artery.

Diagnosis

A careful history often leads to a surprisingly accurate diagnosis. It is rare for the digital manifestations of severe vasospasm to be present without more obvious features of the systemic disease such as the telangectases of

CREST syndrome. The exception is Takayasu's disease where diffuse cerebral and upper limb involvement leads to presentation with progressive upper limb ischaemia (hence the older term 'pulseless disease'). Insidious, occult renal artery involvement may lead to hypertension; rarely, pulmonary and mesenteric artery stenoses lead to postprandial angina and pulmonary hypertension. The hypertensive disease often goes unrecognized due to the upper limb involvement and patients may present with secondary effects of hypertension such as headache, visual disturbance or even stroke.

In contrast, patients with atherosclerotic occlusive disease of the upper limb frequently have evidence of severe arterial disease at other sites, especially the lower limbs, coronary and extracranial carotid circulation. The common risk factors associated with atherosclerosis (a family history, cigarette smoking, hypertension, diabetes and hyperlipidaemia) are usually present.

Clinical examination should be directed towards:

- *Inspection* for pallor, cyanosis, tissue loss, skin lesions such as splinter haemorrhages or telangectases, arteriovenous malformations or the tapered digits of scleroderma. The subclavian artery often rides high in the supraclavicular fossa in thoracic outlet syndrome, due to upward displacement over a cervical rib. In all cases, a comparison with the contralateral limb is useful.

- *Palpation* for cervical rib or aneurysm in the supraclavicular fossa Tenderness over the brachial plexus with reproduction of symptoms may be found in patients with thoracic outlet syndrome. The ulnar nerve should be palpated above the medial epicondyle and the wrist examined for median nerve compression using Tinel's and Phalen's tests.

- *Pulses* should be checked at the axillary, brachial, radial and ulnar sites for presence, delay, or diminution and the Allen's test should be used to assess the palmar inflow. In this test, the patient's fist is clenched in a neutral position and the examiner's index and second fingers are used to occlude both radial and ulnar arteries. The fist is released and the palmar capillary bed inspected. Release of the ulnar artery compression results in normal, sluggish or absent filling. The process is then repeated for the radial artery. The distal radial artery can be damaged by previous arterial cannulation or as a result of trauma (including parasuicide). Pulse palpation is important for the diagnosis of thoracic outlet syndrome. The radial pulse is carefully palpated as the arm is elevated to 90° and then externally rotated into the 'surrender' position (Fig. 10.2). It is important not to exaggerate this position by protruding the head and neck as many normal individuals occlude their radial pulses during this manoeuvre. Auscultation in the deltopectoral triangle may reveal an infraclavicular bruit due to pro-

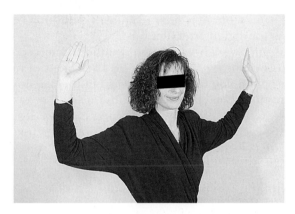

Fig. 10.2 'Surrender' or 90° AER (abduction external rotation) position. The Roos test involves *slow* repetitive finger clenching and, although a 3-min test is advocated, most patients reproduce their symptoms much sooner.

gressive compression of the subclavian artery in arterial thoracic outlet syndrome. Repeated slow finger flexion in this position over a period of several minutes will provoke the patient's primary symptoms in cases of thoracic outlet syndrome (Roos test).

- *Blood pressure* should be measured in both arms and if reduced, an 8-MHz Doppler probe used to determine the systolic arterial pressure at the wrist. *Subclavian steal syndrome* may be provoked by inflating a blood pressure cuff on the upper arm at a pressure just above systolic in order to provoke brachial ischaemia. The vertebral artery may be insonated over the transverse processes on the affected side. After 3–4 min the cuff is rapidly deflated leading to reactive hyperaemic flow in the limb and the patient may complain of giddiness or light headedness. In some cases, bidirectional Doppler may reveal reversal of flow during the hyperaemic flow.
- *Continuous wave Doppler* can be used to map the digital artery flow and to localize occlusion or stenoses.
- *Duplex ultrasound* is helpful in localizing stenoses or aneurysms in the larger, more proximal vessels and can replace angiography in the diagnosis of thoracic outlet syndrome. The subclavian artery is scanned in the neutral position via the supraclavicular window and the arm is elevated to the 90° abduction/external rotation position. This is a dynamic investigation and the arm can be scanned in positions corresponding to the patient's symptoms, such as driving or reading a newspaper.
- *Angiography* is usually required to demonstrate proximal occlusion, segmental blocks or distal vessel disease. Biplanar digital subtraction angiographic views are required to demonstrate the origins of the

supra-aortic trunks, but non-subtracted high definition films are useful when looking for digital artery lesions.

- *Special investigations* such as capillary nailfold microscopy, cold and vibratory provocation are helpful in the assessment of vasospastic disorders. Neurophysiological testing may aid in the diagnosis of thoracic outlet syndrome, where neurological and arterial symptoms co-exist and help to exclude other entrapments, e.g. cervical spondylosis and carpal tunnel syndrome. Specific blood tests for the systemic vasculitides are considered in Chapter 22.

Management

The primary aim in treatment of chronic arm ischaemia is to relieve the patient's symptoms, so oral analgesia is given. Low-dose aspirin (75 mg) should be started immediately. The correction of risk factors is important, especially stopping smoking, dealing with hypertension and hypercholesterolaemia. Many surgeons are reluctant to proceed with invasive investigations until patients have stopped smoking for a period of approximately 3 months so as to allow the hypercoagulable state associated with cigarette smoking to settle, unless tissue loss is a danger.

In any event, patients should not undergo angiography with a view to intervention unless their symptoms are severe enough to warrant it; this is especially true of the elderly, who may only require reassurance, and those with subclavian steal syndrome, which is often mild, or an incidental finding at angiography.

It is vital that the patient should be informed as to the importance of stopping smoking as well as the details, strengths, weaknesses and possible complications of any intervention. This should be documented in the notes (often in the form of a letter to the general practitioner). Stroke and major amputation are devastating complications and patients and their families should understand the risks involved.

Angioplasty

In cases of *proximal arterial stenosis or occlusion*, such as subclavian steal syndrome, percutaneous transluminal angioplasty (PTA) is often successful (Fig. 10.3); stenting is not normally required unless the lesion recurs. If access for PTA is difficult, a retrograde approach via the brachial artery may be helpful.

Surgery

If PTA fails or is thought to be too hazardous, reconstruction can usually be achieved without opening the chest. Carotid/subclavian bypass using saphenous vein or polytetrafluoroethylene (PTFE) or (in the author's view preferable) transposition of the subclavian artery origin to the

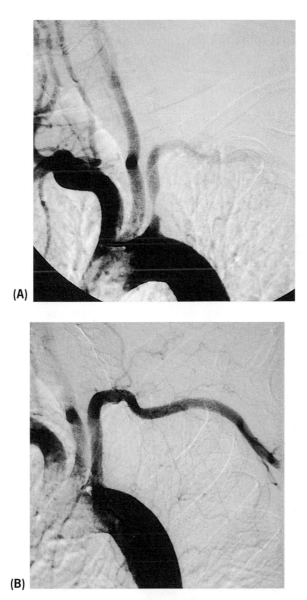

(A)

(B)

Fig. 10.3. Proximal subclavian artery occlusion (A) before and (B) after treatment by transluminal balloon angioplasty.

common carotid, are durable operations with patency rates of up to 100% at 5 years. Subclavian–subclavian bypass is used less frequently, but axillary cross-over grafting or femoroaxillary bypass are useful alternatives.

If cross-over grafting is not feasible, the aortic arch can be exposed through a median sternotomy in suitable patients and an inverted Dacron bifurcation graft used to restore brachial or cephalic perfusion.

Axillary or subclavian arterial occlusion can be bypassed using reversed saphenous vein grafting from the common carotid to the brachial artery. To avoid precipitating steal syndromes or stroke, both carotid arteries should be duplex scanned – carotid endarterectomy may be required either synchronously or as a staged procedure.

In cases of *radiation arteritis*, careful assessment may be required as radiation osteonecrosis of the humerus and contractures around the capsule of the shoulder joint are common. Percutaneous treatment of these lesions avoids operating in a hostile field (Fig. 10.4). Surgical reconstruction of the subclavian arteries in cases of giant cell arteritis or Takayasu's disease should be deferred until the disease is inactive or under control with steroids.

In cases of *distal brachial ischaemia*, the cephalic vein can be used as an *in situ* bypass as its anatomical course closely follows the arterial tree. A small jump graft of vein (either from the arm or the long saphenous vein) is required to bridge the gap between the subclavian or carotid inflow site and the cephalic vein origin at the deltopectoral triangle.

As long as the Allen's test has been carried out (see above) and the continuity of at least one distal artery has been confirmed, it is accept-

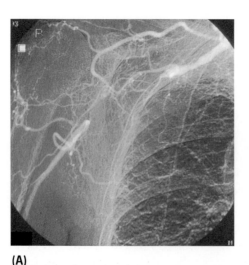 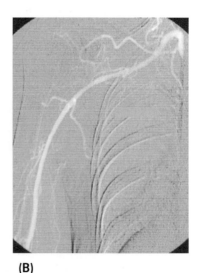

(A)   **(B)**

Fig. 10.4. **Axillary artery occlusion following (A) radiotherapy and (B) treatment with a Wallstent.** (Reproduced from Beard JD, Gaines PA (eds). *Vascular and Endovascular Surgery.* London: WB Saunders, 1998, with permission.)

able to leave isolated lesions of the radial or ulnar arteries alone, except in young symptomatic individuals such as musicians or sportsmen.

Intra-arterial injections

Inadvertent arterial injection of drugs results in widespread intravascular thrombosis and can be limb threatening. This condition is best treated by systemic heparinization along with oral aspirin, placement of an epidural catheter for continuous brachial plexus blockade and iloprost infusion. Thoracoscopic sympathectomy seems a sensible option but is as yet unproven.

Outcome

Because of the good collateral supply, even conservative treatment of chronic arterial occlusion in the upper limb, with heparinization, gives reasonable results with a good return of perfusion within 24–48 h. Optimal outcomes are obtained by careful reassessment and reconstruction of suitable patients using the techniques described above.

Upper limb embolectomy is a very satisfying operation with results that are technically satisfactory in the majority of cases – primarily because the embolectomy catheter can be steered with ease into the distal run-off vessels. Most clinical disappointments are associated with co-morbidity, such as coincident myocardial infarction.

Thoracic outlet syndrome

Compression of the constituent structures of the neurovascular bundle at the root of the neck (Fig. 10.5) by a cervical rib or fibrous band, normal clavicle, first rib, or a wide variety of anatomical anomalies of the scalenus anterior and related muscles, gives rise to thoracic outlet syndrome. Patients may have venous, arterial or neurological symptoms, or any combination of these. Symptoms are characteristically related to posture and are provoked by activities involving the elevated limb.

Venous thoracic outlet syndrome

In venous thoracic outlet syndrome the subclavian vein is usually compressed by the normal clavicle or an hypertrophied subclavius muscle. Patients often give a history of body building or repetitive upper limb activity at work. Venographic studies may demonstrate intrinsic venous abnormalities but it is probably necessary to have both extrinsic and intrinsic compression before severe problems arise. Initially, patients complain of congestion, swelling and cyanosis but eventually thrombosis

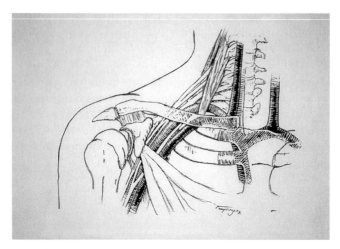

Fig. 10.5. Thoracic outlet. The components of the neurovascular bundle pass through a narrow space bordered by the scalene muscles, clavicle and upper border of the first rib.

of the axillosubclavian system (Paget Schroetter syndrome) may supervene.

Arterial thoracic outlet syndrome

Arterial thoracic outlet syndrome is usually associated with a bony anomaly such as a cervical rib, or costoclavicular compression between the lower border of the clavicle and the upper border of the first rib. The patient complains of symptoms of ischaemia, aching and early fatigue, especially on working with the arm elevated. The female : male ratio is approximately 3:1 and the median onset is at 36 years. Patients may also describe episodic unilateral vasospasm not provoked by cold or other stimuli. Poststenotic aneurysm formation may occur and thrombosis of such an aneurysm may threaten the limb. Asymptomatic cervical ribs are best left alone but the patient should be made aware of the diagnosis.

Neurological thoracic outlet syndrome

Neurological thoracic outlet syndrome affects either the lower (C8/T1) or upper (C5/6) trunks of the brachial plexus. Because the lowest trunk of the plexus lies close to the subclavian artery, brachial ischaemia often accompanies symptoms of paraesthesia in the ulnar nerve distribution, along with occasional vasospasm. For this reason, North American surgeons emphasize the neurological features of the symptoms whereas European specialists concentrate on the vascular compression. In advanced cases, there may be dramatic muscle wasting involving the intrinsic musculature of the affected limb. Upper plexus thoracic outlet syndrome leads to symptoms of aching and paraesthesia in the median and sometimes radial nerve distribution. The pain often affects the area over the trapezius muscle with the side of the face and head. As well as a cervical rib, this variant of thoracic outlet syndrome may be caused by anomalies of the scalene muscle group, fibrous bands or trauma due to stretching following severe hyperextension injuries of the cervical spine.

Patients often complain of a characteristic headache which is unilateral and occurs in an occipitofrontal distribution, settling behind the eyes. This is due to spasm in the rectus capitus muscles which in part inserts directly into the dura.

Neurological thoracic outlet syndrome often co-exists with a more distal nerve entrapment syndrome such as carpal tunnel compression. This 'double crush' syndrome occurs where one disorder sensitizes the nerve and gives rise to symptoms due to the other. Peripheral neuropathy, as seen in diabetes, may also sensitize the peripheral nerves.

Management

Treatment depends on the variant (venous, arterial or neurological), severity of the symptoms and response to conservative management.

Venous variant

Venous engorgement may respond to a decrease in repetitive upper limb exercises with postural advice, but if subclavian thrombosis supervenes

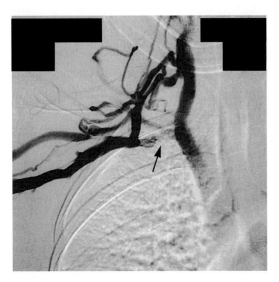

Fig. 10.6. Axillosubclavian vein thrombosis in Paget Schroetter syndrome. Successful lysis has demonstrated the focal lesion just medial to the first rib (arrow). The extensive venous collaterals are also shown.

(Fig. 10.6), good results can be obtained by early catheter-directed low-dose intravenous thrombolysis. This should be done via the brachial vein as the cephalic system may bypass the primary thrombosis. After the vein has been opened by lysis, the patient may be given warfarin for 2–3 months; however, rethrombosis may recur.

We recommend immediate duplex scanning to confirm the diagnosis by demonstrating ipsilateral subclavian arterial compression (the vein *must* therefore be compressed as well) or direct venous compression with variation of the normal venous flow in response to ventilation. The asymptomatic side is often affected. The patient is heparinized and placed on the next elective operating list for transaxillary first-rib resection. As the upper border of the first rib is the fulcrum about which costo-clavicular compression takes place, this operation effectively removes the venous compression. Often a thick rind is found round the vein due to chronic compression. This is carefully removed.

If the vein is palpably damaged the options are to leave it alone, so that collaterals may develop; to perform patch venoplasty or bypass; or to complete the operation and go on to employ postoperative balloon veno-plasty. This often reveals a tight web which does not 'pop' open like an atherosclerotic plaque and may represent a valve or embryonal anomaly of venous fusion. Stenting of this lesion is universally unsuccessful if the rib has not been previously removed as the stent is fractured by the per-sisting costoclavicular scissors mechanism.

In patients with chronic venous hypertension due to subclavian venous thrombosis secondary to thoracic outlet syndrome or central line throm-bosis, bypass, by means of a jugular vein swingdown operation or superficial femoral venous graft, has been advocated. The results of these operations are variable and we would advocate the creation of a brachial artery to cephalic vein fistula to increase collateral circulation. The fistula is disconnected 6-months later.

Arterial variant

Patient with arterial compression respond well to decompression. If the subclavian artery is damaged as a result of aneurysm formation or intimal trauma leading to distal embolus from thoracic outlet compression, first rib resection is mandatory. Although some surgeons perform a transaxil-lary first-rib resection and then reconstruct the artery via a separate supra-clavicular incision, a combined supra/infraclavicular approach is also useful and avoids the need to reposition the patient. Vein grafting may be used but externally reinforced PTFE with end-to-end anastomosis is a resilient procedure.

In patients with mild or moderate ischaemia due to arterial thoracic outlet syndrome, a referral should be made to a physiotherapist or osteopath who understands the condition. A programme of increased aerobic fitness, attention to posture, sleeping position and an analysis of the ergonomics of working, driving and other daily activities is affective in 60% of cases in our experience.

If surgery is undertaken, a combination of a good clinical history and examination, positive duplex scan and an absence of secondary diagnoses, such as cervical spine osteoarthritis, are rewarded by cure in up to 90% of cases. Transaxillary first-rib resection should be employed for primary arterial and lower trunk neurological thoracic outlet syndrome. If a cervical rib is present, it can be resected from below and as long as the first rib and any associated fibrous band is removed, cure is assured.

Neurological variant

Neurological thoracic outlet syndrome is approached in the same way except that upper plexus thoracic outlet syndrome is better treated by supraclavicular exploration. In this way subtle anatomical anomalies can be demonstrated and dealt with. Results of a thorough supraclavicular scalenectomy are equivalent to first-rib resection over the long term – an adequate operation is more important than the route employed.

Outcome

Following successful thoracic outlet decompression surgery, there is a 5% incidence of recurrent symptoms, usually of the neurological type. This is due to a failure to make the correct diagnosis in the first place (where symptoms are persistent rather than truly recurrent) or technical failure during the operation (usually because of an inadequate clearance of the posterior stump of the first rib). True postoperative scarring with reattachment to the brachial plexus is less common. The operation is difficult but usually successful if performed by an expert.

Summary

- Acute upper limb ischaemia (usually due to embolic disease) is rarer than lower limb ischaemia and is a surgical emergency. Treatment is by emergency local anaesthetic thromboembolectomy and anticoagulation, or low-dose intra-arterial thrombolysis.
- Chronic upper limb ischaemia is a relatively benign condition. Selected cases will benefit from proximal angioplasty. Vein grafting is technically demanding but usually successful.
- Unilateral vasospastic symptoms usually have a local cause.
- Carefully selected patients with thoracic outlet syndrome can respond well to surgical decompression.

Areas of controversy

- Role of primary intra-arterial thrombolysis versus embolectomy for the treatment of upper limb emboli.
- Role of surgery for thoracic outlet syndrome if there are no objective symptoms or signs.
- Management of the asymptomatic cervical rib.
- Role of thrombolysis and first-rib excision for axillary vein thrombosis.

Further reading

- Bell PRF, Jamieson CW, Ruckley CE (eds). *Surgical Management of Vascular Disease.* London: WB Saunders, 1992.
- Earnshaw JJ (ed). *Practical Peripheral Arterial Thrombolysis.* Oxford: Butterworth Heinemann, 1994.
- Darke SG, Chant ADB, Barros D'Sa AAB. Acute deep venous thrombosis of the upper extremity. In: *Emergency Vascular Practice.* London: Edward Arnold 1987, pp 150–160.
- Mackinnan SE (ed). Thoracic outlet syndrome. *Seminars in Thoracic and Cardiovascular Surgery* 1996;**8**:175–228.

11
Abdominal Aortic Aneurysms

Michael G Wyatt

Introduction

Aneurysms of the abdominal aorta usually arise below the renal arteries. They have been recognized for thousands of years and are potentially lethal if allowed to rupture. Modern management concentrates on their detection and repair prior to rupture in an attempt to improve patient survival.

Aortic aneurysms have been implicated as the thirteenth commonest cause of death in the UK. They account for approximately 1.2% of male and 0.6% of female deaths. In a population aged over 60 years, about 5% will have abdominal aortic aneurysms.

The incidence of death due to aortic aneurysm has steadily increased over the last 30 years. This might be due in part to a progressive increase in the number of elderly in the population, but age-specific death rates have also increased. Much of this apparent change may be due to increased awareness of the disease, improved diagnosis and altered referral patterns.

Aortic aneurysms are almost exclusively confined to the elderly population. Few patients die from rupture prior to the age of 60, and the disease becomes more common with advancing years. Men are more commonly affected than women. At the age of 67, a man is 10 times more likely to die from a ruptured aortic aneurysm than a woman.

Aetiology

The aetiology of most aneurysms is difficult to define and is usually multifactorial. Nevertheless, several distinct types of aneurysmal disease can be recognized, each with a clearly distinct aetiology. These include:

- atherosclerotic (see Chapter 1);
- inflammatory;
- infective; ⎫ (see Chapter 13)
- traumatic. ⎭

Although most aortic aneurysms are thought to occur as a direct consequence of atherosclerosis, the molecular biology is complex. An alternative theory is that aneurysms form as a distinct disease process, with atherosclerosis being a secondary phenomenon due to abnormal flow patterns within the aneurysmal sac.

In addition, aortic aneurysms can be associated with connective tissue diseases such as Marfan's syndrome and Ehlers-Danlos type IV. This association suggests that genetic factors may predispose to aneurysmal disease.

Inflammatory aortic aneurysms are an uncommon variant of atherosclerotic aneurysms and account for between 5% and 10% of all aortic aneurysms and occur primarily in male patients (Fig. 11.1). Their true aetiology is unknown.

Clinical features

Most abdominal aortic aneurysms are asymptomatic and are discovered incidentally during abdominal examination or by ultrasonography. Many patients present with a pulsatile abdominal mass and the true extent of the aneurysm is often not appreciated prior to investigation.

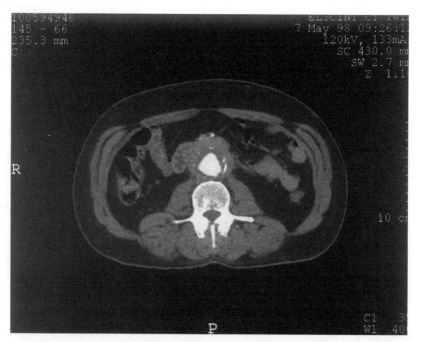

Fig. 11.1. CT scan showing an inflammatory abdominal aortic aneurysm. Note the dense mass of inflammatory tissue surrounding the aorta.

When symptoms arise, they are usually related to:

- posterior erosion into the vertebral bodies;
- distal embolization;
- thrombosis;
- rupture.

Posterior erosion presents with back pain, whereas thrombus embolizing from the aneurysm sac presents with acute ischaemia of one or both legs. Similar symptoms arise if an aneurysm thromboses.

If a patient presents with sudden-onset abdominal and back pain associated with pallor, hypotension, tachycardia and hypovolaemic shock, a rupture must be suspected. If this occurs, the results of emergency operative intervention are poor. Occasionally, a rupture may be contained locally within the retroperitoneal structures, which may allow adequate time to stabilize the patient prior to urgent repair. These patients with contained ruptures have a better outlook.

Rarer presentations of abdominal aortic aneurysms include fistulation into the duodenum or inferior vena cava. An aortoduodenal fistula presents with sudden-onset upper gastrointestinal bleeding, which is usually episodic over a number of days. The diagnosis can be made on endoscopy. An aortocaval fistula is usually associated with retroperitoneal rupture. At laparotomy the surgeon is faced with massive venous bleeding on opening the aorta. If the diagnosis is not made, the patient will rapidly exsanguinate and die. Very rarely, an aortocaval fistula will develop in isolation. These patients present with high output cardiac failure.

Diagnosis

Clinical

Most aortic aneurysms (90%) can be diagnosed clinically by manual examination of the abdomen. The exceptions include small aneurysms in obese patients when specific imaging is often required. The differential diagnosis of a pulsatile abdominal mass includes pancreatic and gastric neoplasm, but in these conditions the pulsation is transmitted and not pulsatile. Normal aortas may be palpated in thin individuals and tortuous or ectatic aortas can be made more prominent by lumbar lordosis. By pressing the fingers of both hands down on either side of the aorta, some idea of aortic size can be obtained; this should not exceed 3 cm.

The upper extent of most aortic aneurysms can be assessed by placing a hand between the pulsatile mass and the costal margin. If this is possible, the aneurysm is usually infrarenal. Occasionally this is not possible, and these aneurysms can still be infrarenal but must be suspected to arise above the renal arteries.

Plain-film radiography

Plain-film radiography is widely available, but rarely helpful in the diagnosis of an abdominal aortic aneurysm. The radiographic signs of arterial aneurysms involve either calcification of the wall of the artery (Fig. 11.2) or displacement of adjacent structures by the aneurysm. Often, the main value of a plain film is to demonstrate an alternative diagnosis.

Intravenous pyelography (IVP) can be used to demonstrate the relationship of the ureters to the abdominal aortic aneurysm but must only be used in a stable situation.

Ultrasound

If an aortic aneurysm is suspected on clinical examination, a simple ultrasound examination will often confirm or refute the diagnosis. Ultrasound

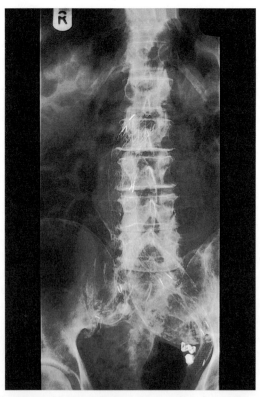

Fig. 11.2. Plain abdominal film showing a large calcified aortoiliac aneurysm, which has been repaired using an intra-luminal aortic stent graft.

is widely available and usually requires no patient preparation. It is safe, non-invasive and in suitable patients provides good definition of the upper abdomen, allowing accurate diagnosis of the presence of an abdominal aortic aneurysm.

Ultrasound imaging usually provides good sectional images of the aneurysm and colour Doppler can distinguish low echogenicity thrombus from slowly flowing blood (see Chapter 4). Abdominal imaging is best achieved using low-frequency transducers (2.5–3.5 MHz.). These machines are mobile allowing their use with sick patients who cannot be moved.

Unfortunately, in some patients, images obtained from an ultrasound scanner are of poor quality due to poor acoustic windows. This is particularly true in the presence of excessive bowel gas or in obese or ventilated patients. In addition, ultrasound alone is often unable accurately to define the upper extent of such an aneurysm or predict visceral involvement.

Ultrasound can visualize the aorta in 97% of cases and has been proposed as a screening tool to identify patients with asymptomatic aortic aneurysms who might be at risk of rupture. Population screening programmes are running in several regions within the UK and initial findings suggest that they can reduce the incidence of rupture and death in the male population. However, a large multicentre trial is required to obtain sufficient numbers for statistical analysis with the power to demonstrate conclusively the cost-effectiveness or otherwise of screening for abdominal aortic aneurysm.

Computerized axial tomography

This is the investigation of choice for patients with non-ruptured aortic aneurysms (Fig. 11.3). It can accurately predict the size and the extent of the aneurysm and also to some degree the extent of visceral and renal artery involvement. In addition, conventional CT scanning can produce a series of parallel sections which can subsequently be reconstructed to help define complex anatomy.

To demonstrate aortic aneurysms satisfactorily, it is necessary to give relatively large volumes of iodinated contrast media (70–150 ml). This can be a problem in patients with hypertension, renal impairment or allergies to contrast media. Conventional CT scanners are only able to produce uniplaner transverse images and the precise upper limit of the aneurysm is often difficult to predict. This is especially true when the aneurysm is large and there is a degree of tortuosity and overlap just below the true neck. A further limitation to CT is its inability to detect visceral and renal artery origin stenosis and the presence of multiple renal arteries.

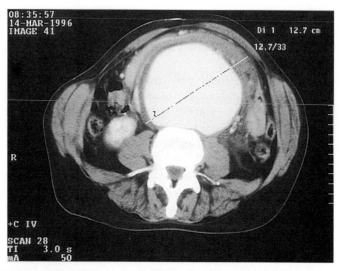

Fig. 11.3. CT scan showing a large aortic aneurysm with little contained thrombus. This aneurysm is at significant risk of rupture.

The new generation of fast (spiral CT, helical CT) or ultrafast (ultrafast CT, electron beam technology) scanners can overcome many of these problems. They can acquire 3D information with better spatial resolution during a single breath-hold. Three-dimensional image reconstruction is easier with these scanners and evaluation of the branch vessel anatomy is much clearer (see Chapter 5). New generation CT scanners are rapidly replacing conventional arteriography in the assessment of complex aneurysmal disease.

Magnetic resonance imaging

MRI can overcome many of the problems encountered with ultrasound or CT imaging (see Chapter 5). It is non-invasive and completely safe. It has an ability to image in multiple planes and can precisely map anatomical structures. This allows for accurate 3D reconstruction and accurate preoperative assessment of not only the upper limit of the aneurysm, but also its shape and possible aetiology (i.e. inflammatory) (Fig. 11.4).

Arteriography

Arteriography is invasive and carries potential renal and embolic complications when used for the assessment of patients with aortic aneurysmal disease. It is not performed routinely for infrarenal aneurysms, but is

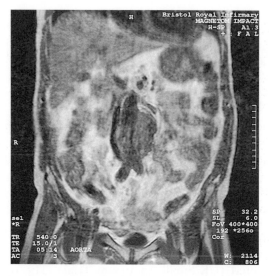

Fig. 11.4. MRI showing an abdominal aortic aneurysm. Note the presence of a good length of normal aorta (aortic neck) between the renal arteries and the aortic sac.

essential when an aneurysm extends towards the renal arteries. Until recently, it was the only investigation able accurately to detail visceral artery occlusive or stenotic disease. It can also give an accurate representation of the exact relationship between renal and mesenteric vessels and the aneurysm. In addition, it can visualize anatomic variation, including the presence of multiple renal arteries. An arteriogram can be used to interpret CT results and define renal artery involvement in patients with tortuous aortas. A lateral view is often helpful to appreciate the full extent of aortic tortuosity and to visualize superior mesenteric and coeliac origins.

Arteriography is essential when there is associated lower limb occlusive disease or popliteal aneurysms (see Chapter 5).

Initial management

Asymptomatic aortic aneurysms

In a non-ruptured abdominal aortic aneurysm, the decision whether to recommend elective surgical repair must always be taken advisedly. The surgeon must balance the operative risk of morbidity and mortality against the risk of rupture and premature death associated with conservative treatment. Factors to consider when making this decision include:

- size of the aneurysm;
- proximal extent of the aneurysm;
- general health of the patient;
- individual surgeon's audited results.

Aneurysm size

The most important factor determining rupture of an abdominal aortic aneurysm is its size. Aneurysms grow at a rate of approximately 4.5 mm a year and, in general, as their size increases, so does their chance of rupture. The 5-year risk of rupture of a small aneurysm (<4 cm) is less than 15%, at 7.0 cm, this risk rises to 95%.

Some small aneurysms can also rupture, particularly in patients with hypertension and chronic obstructive pulmonary disease.

A multicentre randomized controlled trial comparing surgical repair with regular ultrasound surveillance of small aortic aneurysms has recently completed (UK Small Aneurysm Trial). The results were published in the *Lancet* in November 1998. They suggest no survival benefit for early surgical repair of asymptomatic infrarenal abdominal aortic aneurysms between 4.0 cm and 5.5 cm when compared to a programme of regular ultrasound surveillance with surgery performed:

- when the aneurysm size reaches 5.5 cm
- if the expansion rate is >1 cm per year
- or if the aneurysm becomes symptomatic or tender.

The annual rupture rate for patients included in this study was 1%.

In a modern surgical centre, the overall mortality for elective aneurysm repair should be around 5%. However, with the advent of new technologies such as aortic stenting (see later), many centres are now treating sicker patients. This has resulted in a rise in mortality to around 8–9%. If high risk cases are excluded, the mortality rate for uncomplicated abdominal aortic aneurysm repair approaches 2%.

A suggested management regime is given in Table 11.1.

Table 11.1. **Management of abdominal aortic aneurysms according to size.**

Size	Management
Less than 4 cm	No treatment/yearly ultrasound scans
4–5.4 cm	No treatment/6 monthly ultrasound scans
5.5 cm or greater *or* rapid expansion *or* symptomatic	Open surgical/endovascular repair

Proximal extent of aneurysms

Occasionally, the upper extent of the aneurysmal sac will either involve or extend above the renal arteries. Juxtarenal aneurysms are defined as aneurysms that originate immediately below the renal arteries, allowing no space for infrarenal aortic clamping and suture placement. These are sometimes called pararenal aneurysms. Suprarenal aneurysms are aneurysms that originate above the renal arteries. These may also involve the superior mesenteric and coeliac trunks. Aneurysms which extend above the coeliac trunk are correctly classified as being thoracoabdominal (see Chapter 12).

General health of the patient

The repair of an asymptomatic abdominal aortic aneurysm is an elective procedure and should not put the patient at unnecessary additional risk to life or quality of life. It is essential that any co-existing medical problems are identified and if possible corrected prior to surgery. Patients with advanced malignancy or neurological degenerative diseases are clearly not candidates for aneurysmal repair. The main risk factors in these patients, however, will be cardiac and/or respiratory (see Chapter 7).

Audit of results

Early series reporting the results of elective aortic aneurysm repair quoted mortality rates as high as 15%. In major centres, this mortality rate has begun to fall with improvement in operative and anaesthetic technique, in addition to improvements in postoperative care. Increased specialization in vascular surgery is producing continued reduction in reported mortality rates for aortic surgery. In many specialist vascular units, the operative mortality is <5%. Unfortunately, in some district general hospitals where abdominal aortic aneurysm are repaired by general surgeons without specialist knowledge, mortality rates >10% are still reported. In is important that each surgeon offering elective abdominal aortic aneurysm repair is aware of his mortality rate prior to exposure of patients to this additional risk.

Symptomatic and ruptured aortic aneurysms

The preoperative assessment of a patient with a ruptured abdominal aortic aneurysm is different from that employed for elective repair. Patients presenting with a pulsatile mass, hypotension and abdominal, back or flank pain should be taken directly to the operating room for repair of a presumed abdominal rupture. The surgeon should only consider withholding surgery in the following circumstances:

- patient was refused elective surgery;
- history of widespread malignancy;
- history of a severe degenerative neurological disorder;
- known suprarenal or thoracoabdominal aneurysm;
- severe cardio/respiratory disease;
- prolonged hypotension and anuria;
- Unconscious patient with fixed, dilated pupils.

Once a decision to operate has been made, there should be no hesitation for diagnostic work-up. At the time of presentation, the initial rupture is frequently 'contained' by a combination of the patient's hypotensive state and the surrounding retroperitoneal tissues. Vigorous fluid resuscitation with elevation of blood pressure should be delayed until the patient is in the anaesthetic room and the aorta has been controlled above the rupture.

Mortality figures for ruptured abdominal aortic aneurysm are high (>80%). Direct arterial bleeding into the peritoneal cavity is usually fatal. These patients present with sudden collapse, hypotension and loss of consciousness. If a rupture is contained allowing controlled elective repair, the mortality may be as low as 20%.

Surgical management

Essential technical advances in the repair of abdominal aortic aneurysms include:

- specific cardiopulmonary preoperative work-up;
- specialist vascular anaesthetists;
- specifically designed retractors (i.e. Omnitract);
- minimal dissection techniques;
- no circumvention of vessels;
- simple front clamps;
- inlay grafting;
- tube grafting;
- coated knitted grafts.

Despite these evolutions, the surgery for abdominal aortic aneurysms remains a challenge and technical expertise is the factor which has the greatest influence on subsequent outcome.

Asymptomatic aortic aneurysms

In elective surgery for abdominal aortic aneurysm, the exposure must be adequate to obtain both proximal and distal control. If the iliac arteries are not involved, some surgeons prefer to use a transverse abdominal incision. For most abdominal aortic aneurysms, however, a full length midline incision will suffice. Occasionally, aortic aneurysms are repaired using a retroperitoneal approach, thus avoiding the need for a laparotomy. An operative technique combining both a transperitoneal and a retroperitoneal dissection has also been described.

Most aneurysms are repaired under general anaesthesia, often with the addition of an epidural catheter. This can lessen the amount of inhalation agents used and decrease the amount of systemic analgesia required in the postoperative period. Invasive cardiovascular monitoring with a radial artery catheter and in high-risk patients a pulmonary artery catheter is standard practice in most circumstances. The bladder is catheterized to allow the accurate measurement of urine output both in theatre and in the postoperative recovery phase. A nasogastric tube is used to decompress the stomach. Prior to surgery, all patients receive prophylactic antibiotics. Systemic heparin (5000 iu) is often administered just prior to aortic cross-clamping.

The peritoneum is incised in the midline and the aneurysm exposed. Both iliac arteries are exposed over their anterior surface and the proximal neck of the aneurysm is dissected free. Each vessel is clamped in turn and the sac incised longitudinally. Bleeding is often encountered from patent lumbar vessels and the inferior mesenteric artery. These are oversewn from within the sac. An inlay synthetic graft is sutured with 2/0 or 3/0 vascular sutures, taking deep bites. A straight or tube graft can be used for 60% of patients. If the iliac arteries are involved in the aneurysmal process, the distal vascular clamps can be placed on the external and internal iliac arteries. This allows for aneurysm repair using a bifurcated graft onto the common iliac arteries or below. It is desirable to preserve blood flow to at least one internal iliac artery, because in some patients this might be a critical part of the blood supply to the colon and cauda equina. Following successful haemostasis, the aneurysm sac is closed over the graft, the peritoneum repaired and the abdomen closed.

Postoperatively, the patient is managed on an intensive care unit or in a high-dependency unit depending on availability. Discharge is usually possible within 10 days to 2 weeks.

Inflammatory aneurysms

The principles of treatment for inflammatory aneurysms are identical to those for atherosclerotic aneurysms. However, dissection and clamping of the aortic neck of an inflammatory aneurysm may be more difficult.

Proximal aortic clamping is often hampered by the presence of retroperitoneal fibrosis. This results in plastering of the duodenum onto the aneurysmal surface and often the left renal vein and ureters become embedded within the inflammatory tissue. An attempt may be made to dissect these structures free but the incidence of damage is increased, as is the chance of opening the aneurysmal sac prior to adequate proximal control.

Various techniques have been described to lessen these risks:

- dissection of duodenum along with a layer of the aneurysmal sac ('onion-skinning' the aneurysm);
- temporary suprarenal or supracoeliac clamping;
- retroperitoneal/extraperitoneal dissection;
- ureteric stenting.

Despite these operative 'tricks', the mortality (3–19%) and morbidity (7–15%) rates for inflammatory aneurysm repair are greater than those for the repair of the more commonly encountered atherosclerotic aneurysm.

Ruptured aortic aneurysms

When an aortic aneurysm ruptures, surgery should be performed without delay. It is important not to 'crash clamp' the aorta. The haematoma around the neck should be carefully dissected and the clamp carefully placed below the renal arteries, taking considerable care to avoid damage to the left renal vein. If free bleeding is encountered or if a contained leak ruptures, the aorta can be compressed manually to obtain initial control. A temporary supracoeliac clamp can often allow incision of the sac and more precise infrarenal clamp placement prior to repair. In a desperate situation, the surgeon's fingers or an intraluminal balloon can be used to obtain control. Following successful aortic and iliac control, an inlay graft is used as for the elective situation.

Heparin is not usually given to these patients. Adequate administration of blood, fresh frozen plasma and platelets will improve patient survival (see Chapter 7).

Complications

The complications associated with aortic surgery can be divided into three groups (Table 11.2).

Technical and operative

Both arterial and venous *bleeding* can cause serious problems during aneurysm surgery. Following control of the aorta and iliac arteries, arterial bleeding usually arises from patent lumbar arteries or the inferior mesenteric artery. Small arteries at the edge of the aneurysm sac can also bleed and should be sealed with diathermy or oversewing. Following completion of the graft it is important to confirm haemostasis prior to

Table 11.2. **Complications following abdominal aortic aneurysm repair.**

Technical and operative	Bleeding
	Embolism
	Thrombosis
	Technical errors
Early postoperative	Cardiac
	Respiratory
	Renal
	Stroke
	Gastrointestinal
	Deep venous thrombosis
	Pulmonary embolus
	Spinal cord ischaemia
	Wound (infection/dehiscence)
Late postoperative	Graft infection
	Anastomotic aneurysms
	Sexual dysfunction

abdominal closure. Arteries that were dry with the aorta clamped may start to bleed when flow is restored due to re-establishment of arterial flow. Venous bleeding during aneurysm repair is often much more difficult to control than arterial and can be catastrophic. Great care must be taken to avoid damage to the iliac veins, inferior vena cava and left renal vein. If any of these structures are damaged, repair must be immediate and effective. Other sources of venous bleeding during aneurysm repair include lumbar veins, retroaortic left renal vein and aortocaval fistulas. Re-bleeding in the early postoperative phase is the commonest reason for re-laparotomy following aortic surgery. These explorations are associated with increased mortality.

Limb ischaemia as a complication of aortic surgery is usually due to distal *embolus*. This usually involves laminated thrombus from the inside of the aneurysm sac and can result in a condition called 'trash foot'. This occurs when the debris enters the small vessels of the foot from where it can not be recovered.

A rarer cause of leg ischaemia is *arterial thrombosis*. This usually follows prolonged aortic clamping in the absence of heparin. Occasionally, the patient will be found to have a hypercoagulable state, the commonest being thrombocythaemia.

Technical errors include intimal flaps, twisting or compression of bifurcated graft limbs, and clamp damage to native arteries.

Early postoperative

Cardiac complications account for the majority of deaths following aortic aneurysm repair. These include arrhythmias, congestive cardiac failure and myocardial infarct.

Minor *chest problems* are also common and a proportion of patients will develop pneumonia.

Although acute renal failure is uncommon following infrarenal aneurysm repair, many patients show minor impairment to their *renal function*. This may well be a function of pre-existing renovascular disease. Prolonged periods of hypotension during surgery also exacerbate renal dysfunction and may precipitate overt renal failure. Other causes of renal failure following aortic surgery include:

- renal artery occlusion;
- renal vein ligation;
- ureteric injury;
- nephrotoxic agents;
- transfusion reactions;
- products of muscle necrosis.

Occasionally a patient may suffer a *stroke* following aneurysm surgery. The results of this can be devastating and often no cause can be found.

The most serious *gastrointestinal complication* following aortic surgery is bowel infarction. If not recognized early, the patient will die. Other complications include:

- acute peptic ulcer bleed/perforation;
- acute gastric dilatation;
- duodenal damage/aortoenteric fistula;
- prolonged paralytic ileus;
- mechanical obstruction;
- pancreatitis;
- cholecystitis.

Deep venous thrombosis and *pulmonary embolus* can occur after any abdominal procedure, but prolonged aortic clamping may increase their incidence. If heparin is used, this increase is probably not apparent. Rarely, a patient will develop *spinal cord ischaemia*, due to interference with the cord blood supply. This is more frequent the higher the aorta is clamped, but can occur with infrarenal clamping.

Late postoperative

Graft infection is the most devastating complication to occur in the late postoperative period. It is thankfully rare, occurring in 1–2% of patients, but the results can be fatal. When diagnosed, treatment is directed towards removal of the infected aortic graft and replacement with an extra-anatomic graft. More recently, antibiotic-soaked grafts have been used '*in situ*' with good result.

Anastomotic aneurysms are most commonly found in the groins following aortobifemoral grafting. Most can be treated surgically with minimal additional risk.

Sexual dysfunction can occur due to disruption of the preaortic autonomic plexuses. Manifestations include failure to ejaculate, impotence and inability to sustain an erection.

Endoluminal repair

One of the most exciting areas of development in the treatment of abdominal aortic aneurysms involves the deployment of aortic stent–graft combinations within the aneurysm sac in an attempt to exclude the sac from the systemic circulation (Fig. 11.5). These stent–graft combinations are continually being updated and although endovascular aortic aneurysm repair appears feasible, the long-term results are awaited before this becomes the preferred method of treatment for abdominal aortic aneurysms.

There are three types of endograft available for aortic aneurysm repair. These are straight, bifurcated and aorto-uni-iliac grafts (Fig. 11.6). The last of these requires a surgical cross-over procedure following either radiological or surgical ablation of one common iliac artery.

The indications for endovascular treatment are not yet agreed, but available data suggest that endovascular repair of abdominal aortic aneurysms results in morbidity and mortality figures similar to those of open repair.

Complications include:

- development of endoleaks (immediate, early, late);
- continued aneurysm expansion;
- stent–graft migration, dislocation and displacement.

The *advantages* include:

- minimal patient discomfort;
- less reliance on intensive care, high-dependency facilities;
- a shorter hospital stay.

The major *disadvantage* is the expense of both the stent–graft combinations and the additional radiological facilities required within the operating theatre to facilitate their insertion.

Aortic stents are suitable for the treatment of approximately 5% (straight), 30% (bifurcated) and 70% (uni-iliac) of infrarenal aortic aneurysms. The long-term results are awaited and a UK multicentre randomized trial of stent–graft repair versus open repair (EVAR trial) is to commence in 1999.

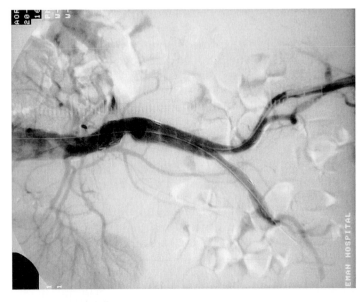

(A)

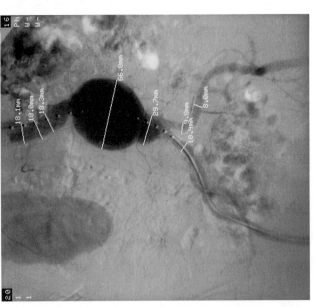

(B)

Fig. 11.5. (A) Arteriogram showing an abdominal aortic aneurysm. Note the measurements taken to allow for accurate stent–graft sizing. (B) Operative arteriogram taken after succesful bifurcate stent–graft placement. This shows complete exclusion of the aneurysmal sac from the arterial circulation (the right femoral artery remains clamped).

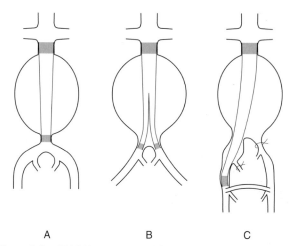

Fig. 11.6. (A) straight, (B) bifurcate and (C) aorto-uni-iliac stent–graft systems. Note for the aorto-uni-iliac graft, one common iliac artery must be occluded and an extra-anatomical bypass is required.

Summary

- Most abdominal aortic aneurysms arise secondary to atherosclerosis.
- The incidence of abdominal aortic aneurysm is increasing.
- The incidence of rupture increases as the size of the aneurysm increases.
- Modern management concentrates on detection and repair prior to rupture.
- Mortality for elective repair must not exceed that of conservative treatment.
- The major risk factors for aneurysm repair are cardiac, respiratory and renal.
- Symptomatic aneurysms should be repaired urgently in suitable patients.

Areas of controversy

- Should elective aortic aneurysm surgery be performed outside of specialist vascular centres?
- Should general surgeons be repairing ruptured aortic aneurysms?
- Should all patients with a ruptured aneurysm be offered surgery?
- Should aortic aneurysm stenting procedures be performed?

Further reading

● Collin J. Aneurysms. In: Galland RB, Clyne CAC (eds). *Clinical Problems in Vascular Surgery*. London: Edward Arnold, 1994, pp 89–96.

- Horrocks M (ed). *Arterial Aneurysms. Diagnosis and Management.* Oxford: Butterworth Heinemann, 1995.
- Greenhalgh RM, Mannick JA (eds). *The Cause and Management of Aneurysms.* London: WB Saunders, 1990.
- Silva MB, Hobson RW. Infrarenal aortic aneurysms. In: Ouriel K (ed). *Lower Extremity Vascular Disease.* Philadelphia: WB Saunders, 1995.
- The UK Small Aneurysm Trial Participants. Mortality results for randomized controlled trial of early elective surgery or ultrasonographic surveillance for small abdominal aneurysms. *Lancet.* 1998;352:1649–1655.

12

Descending Thoracic and Thoracoabdominal Aneurysms

Hans O Myhre, Jan Lundbom and Petter Aadahl

Introduction

Aneurysms of the descending thoracic and the thoracoabdominal aorta account for about 10% of all aortic aneurysms. Modern management has improved the outcome following surgical treatment, and early detection is important to allow treatment of these conditions before rupture occurs. Even ruptured aneurysms can be treated successfully, but at a significantly higher mortality rate. Recently, endovascular surgery has been introduced, offering new possibilities for treating aneurysms of the descending thoracic aorta.

Aetiology

Most descending thoracic and thoracoabdominal aneurysms are so-called atherosclerotic aneurysms. They usually occur in patients over the age of 50 and men are more frequently affected than women. Most patients have concomitant atherosclerotic arterial disease including coronary artery disease. Aneurysms are often multiple and it is not uncommon for patients who have been operated on for an infrarenal aortic aneurysm to later develop an aneurysm with more proximal location (Fig. 12.1). Rarer causes are:

- dissection (secondary aneurysm);
- trauma (false aneurysm);
- bacteraemia (mycotic aneurysm);
- collagen disorders, e.g. Marfan's syndrome;
- syphilitic aortitis;
- Takayasu's disease.

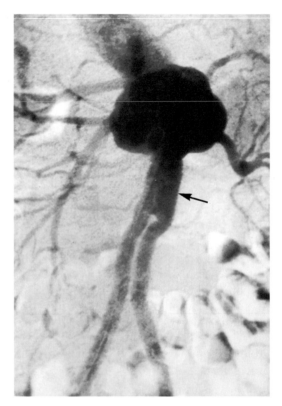

Fig. 12.1. **Arteriogram showing a suprarenal aneurysm in a patient previously operated on for infrarenal abdominal aortic aneurysm using a bifurcated Dacron graft (arrow). In this case, the proximal suture line was intact.**

Clinical features

As for infrarenal abdominal aortic aneurysms, it seems practical to divide the aneurysms into the following categories:

- asymptomatic aneurysms;
- aneurysms giving rise to pain, but without blood outside the aneurysm wall;
- ruptured aneurysms where blood is present outside the aneurysmal wall.

Most descending thoracic aneurysms are asymptomatic and detected on chest X-rays ordered for other conditions.

Chest pain, often radiating to the upper part of the back, is probably the commonest symptom, followed by symptoms related to compression of intrathoracic structures, such as the recurrent laryngeal nerve or the bronchial tree, causing hoarseness, dysphonia or stridor. Expansion of the aneurysm may also cause pain, probably from stretching the surrounding tissue.

Rupture into the tracheobronchial tree can cause haemoptysis and rupture into the oesophagus can lead to gastrointestinal bleeding. Following rupture into the pleura or retropleural space, the patient will often become haemodynamically unstable. Rupture will lead to death if left untreated, but in some cases the rupture is temporarily sealed, giving time for hospitalization and surgery.

In patients with descending thoracic aneurysms, the physical examination is usually negative. However, they should be investigated for associated cardiovascular diseases. Blood pressure should be measured at both upper extremities and the possibility of aneurysms in other arterial segments should be investigated. The differential diagnosis of aortic dissection should be kept in mind. Transoesophageal echocardiography is an excellent method of differentiation between the two conditions.

Some thoracoabdominal aneurysms can be detected during palpation of the abdomen if the abdominal part of the aneurysm is significant. When the size of an aneurysm does not decrease at the level of the costal margin, one may suspect that it is extending above the renal arteries.

Diagnosis

A standard chest X-ray will usually show expansion on the left side of the chest due to a descending thoracic aneurysm (Fig. 12.2). Calcification of

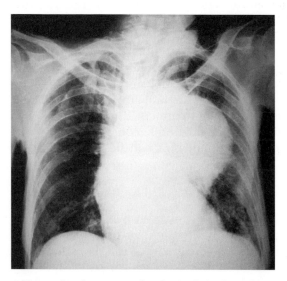

Fig. 12.2. Chest X-ray showing expansion in the left pleural space from an aneurysm of the descending thoracic aorta.

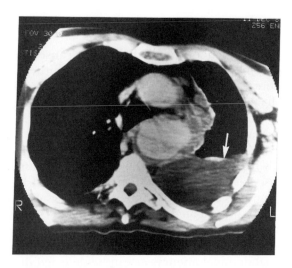

Fig. 12.3. CT scan of a patient with a ruptured aneurysm of the descending thoracic aorta. Blood is present in the left pleural space (arrow).

the aorta may be observed in about one-third of patients. There is a widening of the mediastinum and the aortic contour may be less pronounced than normal.

In haemodynamically stable patients, a CT scan is usually indicated and will give a good impression of the aneurysm's diameter and extension (Fig. 12.3). An important question is the relationship between the aneurysm and the subclavian artery as well as the anatomy of the aorta above the orifice of the visceral arteries. With modern spiral CT, the vascular anatomy can usually be described in sufficient detail.

We perform arteriography to obtain further information about the extent of the aneurysm, its relationship to major branches arising from the aorta and to exclude any visceral artery stenoses. These investigations are important for planning treatment, and can be supplemented by MRI in case more detailed information becomes necessary.

Thoracoabdominal aneurysms can be divided into four categories (Fig. 12.4).

- Type I includes the descending thoracic aorta to the visceral arteries;
- Type II includes most of the aorta from the subclavian artery to the bifurcation;
- Type III leaves the proximal part of the thoracic aorta relatively unaffected;
- Type IV is limited to the abdominal aorta, but includes the renal arteries, the coeliac and the superior mesenteric arteries.

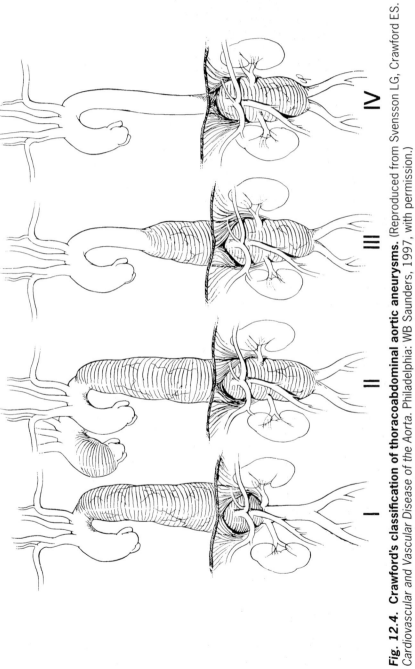

Fig. 12.4. Crawford's classification of thoracoabdominal aortic aneurysms. (Reproduced from Svensson LG, Crawford ES. *Cardiovascular and Vascular Disease of the Aorta.* Philadelphia: WB Saunders, 1997, with permission.)

Management

It has been reported that only 15–20% of patients with thoracoabdominal aneurysms were alive following 5 years of observation. The size of the aneurysms is important, since the tendency to rupture is significantly higher in aneurysms with a diameter of >6 cm compared to those <6 cm. However, it should be noted that even small saccular atherosclerotic aneurysms may rupture.

Associated cardiovascular disease increases the mortality. Patients with hypertension have a more serious prognosis than those without, and asymptomatic patients do better than symptomatic ones. About 50% of deaths are due to rupture, whereas the other half are caused by cardio-vascular disease.

Indications for surgery

In patients with pain caused by aneurysmal expansion or rupture, the indication for operation is usually straightforward since the outcome is fatal without surgery. However, old age, debility or diseases indicating a decreased life-expectancy as well as serious concomitant cardiovascular diseases may contraindicate surgery.

In patients with asymptomatic aneurysms, the operative morbidity and mortality must be weighed against the risk of rupture associated with non-operative treatment. In general, we advise surgery if the maximum diameter of the aneurysm is ≥6 cm or less for saccular aneurysm.

Preoperative preparation and monitoring

Prior to elective surgery, the patient should undergo a thorough cardio-logical investigation with stress ECG or stress echocardiography. If these investigations are positive, coronary angiography is indicated to identify coronary artery obstructions amenable to balloon angioplasty or surgery prior to elective aneurysm repair. Aortic valvular insufficiency is a relative contraindication to direct aortic cross-clamping.

Lung function tests, including FEV, should be carried out. FEV_1 should preferably be >1.0 L/s and increased pCO_2 is also a relative contraindication to surgery.

Decreased renal function is a major risk factor.

Operative technique

Descending thoracic aneurysm

For repair of descending thoracic aneurysms the operation is carried out through a left thoracotomy in the 4th interspace using a double-lumen endotracheal tube. Control of the descending thoracic aorta is usually achieved by cross-clamping below the left subclavian artery.

The operation can be performed using direct aortic cross-clamping, circulatory assist using atriofemoral bypass with a centrifugal pump or femorofemoral bypass using a heart–lung machine. If direct cross-clamping is applied, heparin is usually unnecessary. The use of shunting or bypass is controversial, but should probably be used if the aorta is expected to be cross-clamped for longer than 30 min.

Expedient surgery is of major importance in these procedures. A woven low porosity graft or a coated graft is usually used to reduce blood loss. Most intercostal arteries are oversewn with the exception of major arteries usually located at the T10–T12 level, which should be anastomosed to the graft, thus retaining the arterial blood supply to the spinal cord. An inlay technique is used and the graft covered with the aneurysmal sack.

Endovascular repair

Stent–grafts have been designed to treat descending thoracic aneurysms. Z-stents covered with uncrimped polyester seem to be advantageous and have been used by our group (Fig. 12.5). The introducer system has a

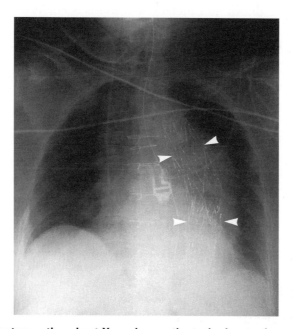

Fig. 12.5. **Postoperative chest X-ray in a patient who has undergone endovascular repair for an aneurysm of the descending thoracic aorta. The Z-stents of the graft are visualized (arrowheads).**

24 F diameter and can be inserted via the femoral artery, iliac artery or a side arm of the graft if an abdominal aneurysm is repaired simultaneously. An aneurysmal neck at least 2–3 cm from the subclavian artery is preferred. The graft can be placed across the subclavian artery which must then be reconstructed, either by reimplantation into the left common carotid artery or by a carotid–subclavian artery bypass.

The operative trauma is significantly lower than in open surgery, but long-term results are required.

Thoracoabdominal aneurysm repair

For thoracoabdominal aneurysm repair a thoraco-laparotomy is used. In Types I and II aneurysms (see above), we prefer extracorporal circulation using either atriofemoral or femorofemoral bypass, allowing perfusion of the distal part of the body while sequential clamping and the upper anastomosis are performed. Prior to aortic cross-clamping, 25–30 g of mannitol is given for renal protection. Cross-clamping of the aorta without shunting or bypass increases afterload. Immediately before clamping, vascular resistance is reduced either by inhalation of anaesthetics or vasodilators like nitroglycerine or sodium nitroprusside (SNP). During cross-clamping we prefer to maintain the systolic blood pressure in the range of 120–140 mmHg using SNP and nitroglycerine. Repeated blood gas samples are drawn and metabolic acidosis is corrected with sodium bicarbonate.

Most surgeons prefer to reimplant major intercostal arteries in the T10–L2 region. During repair of descending thoracic and thoraco-abdominal aneurysms, several adjuncts have been used in an attempt to decrease the risk of paraplegia or paraparesis. Expedient surgery and reimplantation of major intercostal arteries is probably of major importance.

Spinal fluid drainage has been applied by several centres to decrease the spinal fluid pressure which will usually increase during cross-clamping of the aorta. We prefer to perfuse the kidneys with Ringer's solution at 4°C containing 1000 iu of heparin/L whilst the proximal anastomosis is performed. The orifices of the visceral arteries are then anastomosed to one or more side holes in the main graft (Fig. 12.6). If the distance between the renal arteries is considerable, a separate graft to the left artery is preferred. The perfusion catheters are left until the anastomosis is almost completed. The catheters are then removed, the anastomosis completed and the blood flow to the visceral organs is re-established as soon as possible via the main graft. The bowel and liver should have first priority regarding revascularization.

Declamping of the aorta has to be done carefully in order to avoid a deleterious drop in blood pressure. Inotropic agents like dopamine are often necessary during this stage of the procedure. Although there is no

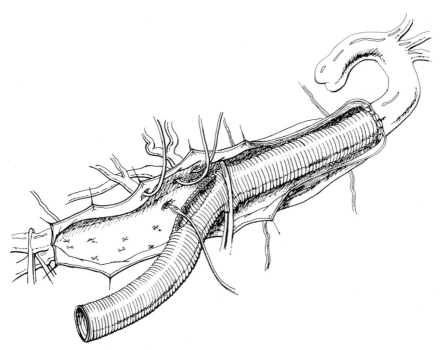

Fig. 12.6. Schematic illustration of Crawford's technique for replacement of thoracoabdominal aortic aneurysms. Catheters are placed into the orifices of the visceral arteries. The orifices are anastomosed to an opening in the main graft.

clinical evidence for the prophylactic use of dopamine to avoid renal failure, we routinely use a small dose (2–5 μg/kg/min). Finally, the distal anastomosis at the aortic bifurcation or the iliac arteries is made.

Maintaining body temperature will aid haemostasis but plasma and platelets are often required. Usually, the patient requires ventilatory support until the next morning. Pulmonary, hepatic and renal function is usually affected for 2–3 days and is then normalized.

Complications

Respiratory problems may occur after 2–3 days. They are especially seen in patients where the ischaemia time to the bowel has exceeded 45 min–1 h. Dialysis may become necessary in about 10% of patients, especially in those who had preoperative renal insufficiency.

The risk of complications including paraplegia and paraparesis should be discussed with the patients. There is a higher risk of paraplegia or paraparesis following operations for Types I and II aneurysms (15–25%) compared to Types III and IV (4–7%). One-third of the cases of paraplegia or paraparesis occur in the postoperative period, usually following an episode of hypotension. Therefore, monitoring of blood pressure is important.

Outcome

Significant variation in reported mortality rates may be due to patient selection, and if a series includes a high proportion of symptomatic patients or ruptures, one can expect the complication and mortality rates to be relatively high.

Following elective replacement of Types III and IV aneurysms, the mortality is usually in the order of 5–8% and >10% for Types I or II aneurysms. The mortality following operation for ruptured aneurysms is significantly higher; at between 40% and 60%. After surgery the prognosis is usually excellent and a 5-year survival of about 60% is usually obtained.

Summary

- Aneurysms of the descending thoracic and thoracoabdominal aorta comprise about 10% of all aortic aneurysms.
- The risk of rupture is significantly higher in patients with hypertension, larger aneurysms and in those who are symptomatic.
- Surgery should be offered to suitable patients with an aneurysm >6 cm.
- Major complications include haemorrhage, cardiac insufficiency, respiratory failure, paraplegia or paraparesis and renal failure.
- Patients with rupture or impending rupture should undergo emergency repair unless they have significant co-morbidity.

Areas of controversy

- Use of extracorporeal circulation and heparin for thoracic and thoraco-abdominal aneurysm repair.
- Use of shunting of visceral arteries.
- Intraoperative protection of the kidneys by irrigation with cold fluid.
- Monitoring of spinal cord function and spinal fluid drainage.
- Indications for surgery in patients with ruptured thoracoabdominal aneurysms.
- Role of stent grafting for descending thoracic aortic aneurysms.

Further reading

- Svensson LG, Crawford ES. *Cardiovascular and Vascular Disease of the Aorta.* Philadelphia: WB Saunders, 1997.
- Greenhalgh RM, Mannick JA. *The Cause and Management of Aneurysms.* Philadelphia: WB Saunders, 1990.
- Weimann WI (ed). *Thoracic and Thoracoabdominal Aortic Aneurysms.* Bologna: Monduzzi Editore, 1994.
- Hopkinson B, Yusuf W, Whitaker S, Veith F. *Endovascular Surgery for Aortic Aneurysms.* Philadelphia: WB Saunders, 1997.

13
Peripheral and Splanchnic Artery Aneurysms

Shane TR MacSweeney

Introduction

The majority of arterial aneurysms involve the abdominal aorta, but less often the aneurysmal process can affect:

- peripheral arteries;
- arteries arising from the aortic arch;
- splanchnic arteries (visceral/renal).

Their presentation is often unusual.

Peripheral arterial aneurysm

Popliteal aneurysm

The popliteal artery is the commonest site of a peripheral arterial aneurysm. Elderly men are most frequently affected. Popliteal aneurysm is normally associated with atherosclerosis but rare causes which should be considered, particularly when a popliteal aneurysm presents in younger patients, include popliteal artery entrapment syndrome, trauma and mycotic aneurysms. The aneurysms are fusiform or saccular in shape and larger aneurysms typically are lined with concentric layers of thrombus. Approximately 50% are bilateral and an aortic aneurysm is present in 25%.

Clinical features

Popliteal aneurysms may be detected while asymptomatic as an incidental finding or may present with symptoms of ischaemia, local pressure or rupture.

Ischaemia

This is the commonest clinical presentation. It can occur due to distal embolization of clot from within the aneurysm and/or thrombosis of the aneurysm sac itself. Symptoms may be acute or chronic depending on the rate of onset and adequacy of the collateral circulation. The propensity of popliteal aneurysms to present acutely with thrombosis in combination with an obliterated distal circulation due to recurrent embolization has led to their reputation as 'a sinister harbinger of sudden catastrophe'. This situation is difficult to salvage by conventional surgical methods and historically has been associated with an amputation rate of 28–69%.

Pressure on surrounding structures

Large aneurysms may present as a pulsatile mass or with symptoms due to compression of surrounding structures in the popliteal fossa. Compression of the popliteal vein may cause obstruction to venous return and limb swelling, although venous thrombosis is unusual. Compression of adjacent nerves may cause local or referred pain.

Rupture

Unlike aortic aneurysms, a popliteal aneurysm rarely presents with rupture. However, when it does occur, rupture is associated with a high probability of limb loss.

Management

Acute ischaemia

Intra-arterial thrombolysis has been an important advance in the management of acute ischaemia complicating a popliteal aneurysm. It has the potential to clear the distal circulation, converting an emergency operation with poor run-off into an urgent elective operation with good run-off. It is preferable to restrict lysis to the circulation distal to the aneurysm sac to reduce the risk of distal embolization due to lysis of the large volume of clot within the aneurysm itself (Fig. 13.1). Once the distal circulation is cleared, whether by lysis or surgical embolectomy, the aneurysm should be excluded by conventional surgical methods (see below).

Although thrombolysis is a useful technique it does have significant limitations in some patient groups: patients may present with advanced ischaemia and require primary amputation. Others with neurosensory deficit may be unable to tolerate the delay imposed by conventional infusion techniques; pulse spray or on-table lysis may be useful in this group. Thrombolysis may only be partially successful or fail completely. In a recent prospective study, 16/23 (70%) patients treated with thrombolysis alone or in combination with surgery had a successful outcome; the remainder (30%) required an amputation. Even in those in whom the limb is successfully salvaged, morbidity is high.

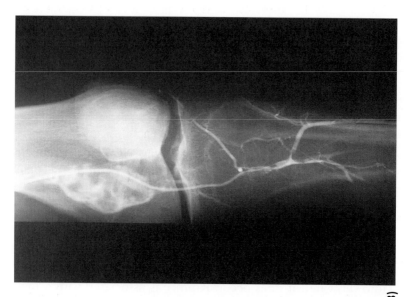

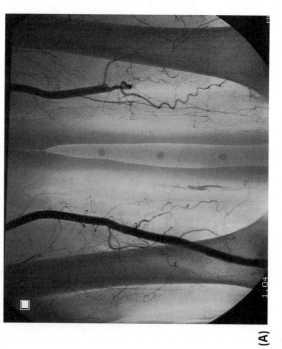

(A)

(B)

Fig. 13.1. (A) Initial angiogram of a patient who presented with an acutely ischaemic leg due to thrombosed popliteal aneurysm, showing an occluded distal superficial femoral artery. (B) Follow-up angiogram showing a thrombolysis catheter distal to the large volume of clot within the aneurysm with early clearance of the run-off vessels.

Chronic ischaemia

Chronic ischaemia may be associated either with a thrombosed aneurysm or a patent aneurysm with distal embolization. If the aneurysm is thrombosed, then further deterioration is unlikely as there is no flowing blood to carry emboli into the distal circulation. The aneurysm can be managed conservatively or surgically according to the severity of symptoms. If blood continues to flow through the aneurysm, then impairment of the circulation has already occurred and is likely to progress unless the aneurysm is excluded. Unless the patient is unfit for surgery, intervention should be carried out promptly.

Asymptomatic aneurysm

The management of asymptomatic popliteal aneurysms continues to generate controversy. Decisions are based on assessment of the balance of risks and benefits of a conservative versus an operative approach, i.e. the nature of the aneurysm and the condition of the patient. Traditionally, popliteal aneurysms have been treated aggressively on the basis of high morbidity rates in reported series. These retrospective reports of cases collected over many years probably overestimate the dangers of popliteal aneurysm. Conversely, recent anecdotal reports of successful treatment of acute ischaemia resulting from popliteal aneurysm by thrombolysis underestimate the dangers (see above). No randomized studies are available.

Aneurysmal factors associated with the development of symptoms in an asymptomatic aneurysm are:

- increasing diameter (symptoms increasingly common >3 cm);
- intraluminal thrombus (embolus source);
- loss of foot pulses (silent embolus);
- aneurysmal distortion.

Patients with a popliteal aneurysm have a decreased life expectancy due to associated cardiac and cerebrovascular disease. The 'high-risk' group is probably best managed conservatively as these patients are more likely to die from intercurrent disease before developing complications from their aneurysm, and they tolerate surgery poorly.

Surgical management

The principle of the procedure is to exclude the aneurysm from the circulation and to maintain the arterial supply to the lower limb. This may be done via a medial approach by ligating the aneurysm above and below and bypassing it, or by using a posterior approach, opening the aneurysm and inserting an inlay graft, similar to the repair of an aortic aneurysm (see Chapter 11). The saphenous vein is the conduit of choice. Excellent patency rates can be achieved by either technique, particularly if the run-off vessels are patent. Recently, endovascular techniques have been used but concerns over the long-term effect of repeated flexion of the prosthesis as it crosses the knee joint are a limitation.

Femoral aneurysm

Femoral aneurysms can be classified as either true or false. The femoral artery is a very common site for false aneurysm, usually secondary to a medical intervention such as cardiac catheterization. This discussion is restricted to true aneurysm.

The femoral aneurysm is the second commonest peripheral aneurysm after popliteal aneurysm and affects mainly elderly men. They are found in approximately 2–3% of patients with aortic aneurysm and are classified as:

- *Type 1.* Aneurysm restricted to the common femoral artery and not involving the common femoral bifurcation.
- *Type 2.* Involving the bifurcation of the common femoral artery and the origins of the profunda femoris and superficial femoral artery.

True femoral aneurysms are often bilateral and can be associated with aortoiliac and popliteal aneurysms, systemic hypertension and coronary artery disease. Isolated superficial femoral or profunda aneurysms have been reported but are very rare.

Their aetiology includes:

- atherosclerosis;
- trauma (blunt, penetrating, iatrogenic);
- inflammatory (Takayasu's, polyarteritis nodosa, systemic lupus erythematosus, Behçet's);
- infection (mycotic, syphilitic);
- connective tissue disorders (Marfan's, Ehlers-Danlos).

Clinical features

Asymptomatic femoral aneurysms are usually an incidental finding on clinical examination but may present with symptoms due to a pulsatile mass causing local pain and rarely compression of the femoral vein. Embolization or thrombosis may cause acute ischaemia.

Management

The management of asymptomatic true femoral aneurysms remains controversial. There are no natural history studies on femoral aneurysms and the indications for operative repair are unknown. In general, aneurysms >4 cm and those found in association with an aortic aneurysm should probably be repaired. In addition, symptomatic femoral aneurysms should receive prompt attention.

Repair consists of the insertion of a Dacron/PTFE interposition graft with appropriate modification if the profunda femoris artery is involved. The long-term results are good.

Iliac aneurysms

Iliac aneurysms are rare and usually present in association with aortic aneurysms. Isolated iliac aneurysms account for only about 1% of all aortoiliac aneurysmal disease. They are usually large, measuring between 4 and 8 cm in diameter, but their natural history is relatively unknown. They expand at a similar rate to aortic aneurysms (4 mm per annum) but little information exists as to their rupture rate.

Most iliac aneurysm present in men over 70 years of age and are atherosclerotic in nature. Other aetiologies include:

- congenital;
- syphilitic;
- tuberculous;
- pelvic fracture;
- gynaecological trauma;
- osteomyelitis;
- Behçet's disease;
- cystic medial necrosis.

Clinical features

Their clinical presentation is often fairly benign due to the capacity of the human pelvis, which often hides even large iliac aneurysmal dilatation. Suspicion should be raised if a pulsatile mass is found on abdominal, rectal or vaginal examination especially with a history of trauma or major pelvic surgery.

Management

Common iliac aneurysms

These should be treated conservatively if small (<3 cm) or kept under 6-monthly review if medium sized (3–4 cm). Patients with common iliac aneurysms >4 cm should be offered intervention. This can either involve endoluminal graft repair or open surgery using interposition grafts or ligation with cross-over grafting (Fig. 13.2).

Internal iliac aneurysms

These may be unilateral or bilateral. Small *unilateral* internal iliac arteries can be successfully treated using coil embolization techniques. For larger aneurysms, surgery consists of ligation of the proximal neck, incision of the sac and oversewing of the distal vessel or vessels.

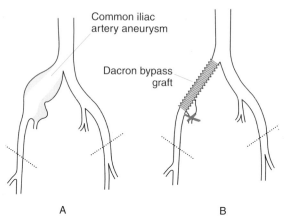

Fig. 13.2. **(A) Large right common iliac artery aneurysm with a small internal iliac aneurysm. (B) Operative treatment is with a straight Dacron iliac graft and tying off the internal iliac artery.**

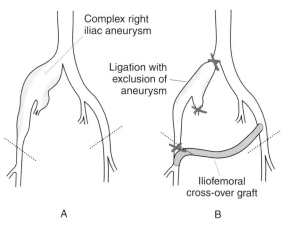

Fig. 13.3. **(A) A large right iliac aneurysm involving common, external and internal iliac vessels. (B) Operative treatment is ligation of the aneurysmal compex and an iliofemoral cross-over graft.**

Bilateral internal iliac aneurysms are more difficult to treat as bilateral ligation may result in vasculogenic impotence, buttock claudication or colonic ischaemia. For these patients it is important to attempt to maintain patency of at least one vessel and often a short Dacron graft is required.

Aneurysms involving the aortic arch arteries

Axillosubclavian aneurysms

These aneurysms are rare. True aneurysms of the proximal subclavian artery are usually associated with atherosclerosis; other occasional causes include cystic medial necrosis, syphilis and involvement by local inflammatory processes, such as tuberculous lymphadenopathy. By contrast, aneurysms of the distal subclavian/proximal axillary artery are almost always due to thoracic outlet syndrome, usually due to a cervical rib or band.

Aneurysms may be detected incidentally as pulsatile masses, although the commonest cause of an apparent aneurysm is a tortuous vessel of normal calibre. This can be determined rapidly by ultrasound. Symptoms may be due to local pressure causing pain, compression of the brachial plexus, hoarseness due to pressure on the right recurrent laryngeal nerve, and pressure on the trachea causing stridor. Vascular complications include embolization, usually into the hand and occasionally into the cerebral circulation. Rupture is rare but may be fatal.

Thoracic outlet syndrome

Aneurysm due to *thoracic outlet syndrome* is caused by post-stenotic dilatation. Presentation may be as a pulsatile mass or with recurrent episodes of microembolization which in the initial stages appear to resolve spontaneously. However, during this period, progressive cumulative damage to the run-off vessels occurs. Eventually severe ischaemia ensues, by which time the run-off vessels are often obliterated and there is a risk of limb loss.

If diagnosed prior to the development of ischaemic complications, resection of the cervical rib/band may be sufficient and regression of the dilatation may occur. If the artery is dilated to more than double its normal diameter or if ischaemic complications occur, then in addition the aneurysm should be resected and the artery anastomosed end-to-end, or more usually a Dacron/PTFE interposition graft inserted. Intimal damage is usually more extensive than is apparent on angiography or exterior inspection. Embolization may require embolectomy or on-table thrombolysis.

Extracranial carotid artery aneurysm

Aneurysms of the extracranial carotid artery are rare. Local sepsis may result in a mycotic aneurysm and trauma, whether accidental or following surgery, is a well recognized cause of false aneurysm. Carotid dissection may occur spontaneously or following trauma. True aneurysm typically involves the internal or common carotid artery (Fig. 13.4).

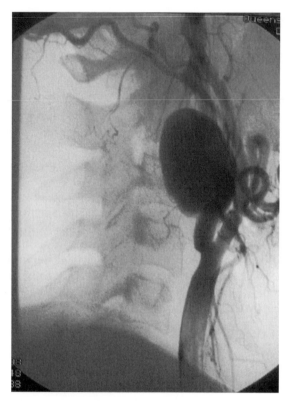

Fig. 13.4. Large dysplastic aneurysm of the internal carotid artery.

Data on the natural history of carotid aneurysm are scanty but there is a well recognized risk of stroke and transient ischaemic attack. Local pressure symptoms are common. Rupture is rare except in mycotic aneurysm when it may be fatal.

Treatment is by inlay grafting or ligation and bypass of the aneurysm. Ligation alone may be necessary when reconstruction is impossible. The use of covered stents is an alternative option which requires evaluation.

Splanchnic artery aneurysm

Aneurysmal dilatation of the splanchnic arteries is rare. However, with the increased use of computerized tomography, ultrasound and selective visceral arteriography, they are being discovered more frequently, although the majority are 'incidental findings' and of little consequence. Although their true incidence is unknown, their relative incidence is shown in Table 13.1.

Table 13.1. **Relative incidence of visceral artery aneurysms.**

Visceral artery	%
Splenic	60
Hepatic	10–20
Renal	22
Superior mesenteric	5–11
Pancreaticoduodenal	2
Gastroepiploic	4
Jejunal/ileal/coeliac	4–7
Gastroduodenal	1.5
Inferior mesenteric	Rare

Splenic artery aneurysm

Splenic artery aneurysms are the commonest visceral artery aneurysm and the commonest intra-abdominal aneurysm after aortic aneurysm. It affects women 4-fold more commonly than men.

Fragmentation of elastin fibres and smooth muscle disruption are associated with:

- medial fibrodysplasia;
- portal hypertension with splenomegaly;
- pregnancy.

Clinical findings

Most splenic artery aneurysms are asymptomatic and pass undetected. Non-specific epigastric and left flank pain may occur and rarely a mass is palpable. The most serious complication is rupture and is particularly prone to occur in the third trimester of pregnancy. Fetal death is usual (75–95%) and maternal death is common (50–75%).

Management

All symptomatic aneurysms warrant prompt intervention, particularly if discovered during pregnancy. Asymptomatic aneurysms in women of child-bearing age should probably be treated and this is essential in pregnancy or if further pregnancies are planned.

Most splenic artery aneurysms are detected in older patients as incidental findings, often due to the presence of calcification within the aneurysm sac (Fig. 13.5). Most are small (<2 cm diameter) and rupture rates are low (2%). Most asymptomatic splenic artery aneurysms can be managed conservatively. Intervention should be considered for large asymptomatic aneurysms >2 cm diameter and simple ligation without reconstruction is sufficient. Transcatheter embolization is an alternative to open surgery.

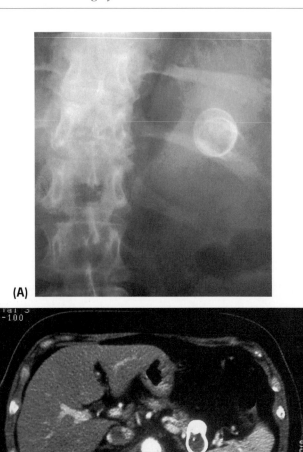

(A)

(B)

Fig. 13.5. (A) Plain abdominal radiograph showing calcification in an asymptomatic splenic artery aneurysm. (B) CT scan of the same patient showing the aneurysm with calcification clearly visible in the wall. The patient was successfully treated by transcatheter embolization.

Hepatic aneurysms

Hepatic artery aneurysms occur over a wide age range and are twice as common in men as women. Causes include:

- medial degeneration;
- trauma;
- inflammatory arteriopathies.

Atherosclerosis is common but may be a secondary phenomenon. Mycotic aneurysms now account for 10% of cases and are commoner in IV drug abusers and the immunosuppressed. The extrahepatic arteries are involved in 75% and the aneurysm is usually solitary.

Clinical findings

Most hepatic aneurysms are asymptomatic and physical examination is usually normal. Symptoms include vague upper abdominal and right upper quadrant pain which may occasionally be severe. Rupture is the presenting feature in 20%. This occurs with equal frequency into the abdominal cavity producing abdominal pain and shock, or into the biliary tree. Diagnosis may be difficult: ultrasound, CT and MRI are helpful and coeliac axis angiography is definitive.

Management

The mortality of rupture is 35%. Aggressive surgical treatment is recommended in otherwise fit patients. Aneurysms proximal to the gastroduodenal artery can usually be excised and ligated; aneurysms distal to the gastroduodenal artery should be excised and an interposition vein graft used to restore continuity. Good results have been reported for transcatheter embolization of intrahepatic aneurysms.

Other visceral aneurysms

Aneurysms of the superior mesenteric artery and its branches are often mycotic and present with non-specific abdominal pain and fever. Non-mycotic aneurysms may present with mesenteric angina or rupture into the peritoneal cavity.

Coeliac, gastroduodenal and pancreaticoduodenal aneurysm is very uncommon. Patients often present with vague upper gastrointestinal symptoms including:

- dyspepsia;
- nausea;
- anorexia;
- weight loss.

They can rupture into the stomach, duodenum or pancreatic duct and can present with pancreatitis, haematemesis or malaena.

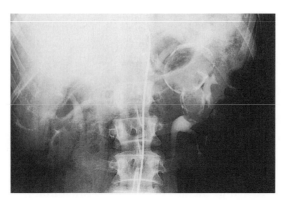

Fig. 13.6. X-Ray showing two calcified left renal artery aneurysms.

Renal artery aneurysm

These occur in 0.015% of autopsy series and in 0.3% of a large angiographic series (Fig. 13.6). They are almost always incidental findings. Most (85%) are saccular aneurysms which occur in the 'crotch' of arterial bifurcations and are associated with a deficient internal elastic lamina. Fusiform aneurysms occur in association with proximal stenoses. Fibromuscular disease may produce multiple small aneurysms giving a 'string of beads' appearance (see Chapter 24).

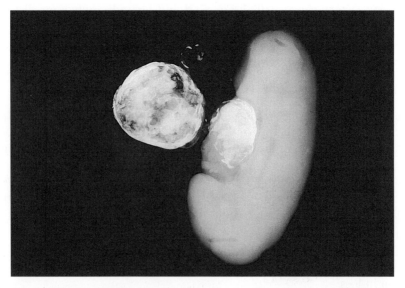

Fig. 13.7. X-Ray of nephrectomy specimen showing the two calcified aneurysms from Fig. 13.6.

Aneurysms may be associated with hypertension but are not necessarily causal. Careful evaluation is required before considering intervention as a treatment for renovascular hypertension.

The prognosis for saccular aneurysms is usually benign. Rupture appears to be very unusual except in pregnancy when it is associated with high fetal and maternal mortality.

Controversy exists as to whether asymptomatic aneurysms 2–4 cm should be repaired. It is recommended that aneurysms of >4 cm should be repaired. Aneurysms should be treated aggressively in pregnancy and probably in women of child-bearing age. Surgical treatment consists of excision of the aneurysm with reconstruction and carries a 5% risk of nephrectomy (Fig. 13.7).

Summary

- Any aneurysm may cause local pressure symptoms, ischaemic complications or rupture.
- The commonest site for a peripheral aneurysm is the popliteal artery.
- The incidence of false and infective peripheral artery aneurysms is increasing due to cardiological complications and drug abuse.

Areas of controversy

- Surgical treatment of asymptomatic aneurysms.
- Role of thrombolysis for acute ischaemia due to a popliteal aneurysm.
- Use of catheter-directed embolization or stenting for aneurysm exclusion.

Further reading

- MacSweeney STR. Thrombus as a prognostic indicator in popliteal aneurysms. In: Greenhalgh RM, Powell JT (eds) *Inflammatory and Thrombotic Problems in Vascular Surgery*. London: WB Saunders, 1997 pp 147–157.
- Horrocks M (ed) *Arterial Aneurysms: Diagnosis and Management*. Oxford: Butterworth-Heinemann, 1995.
- Stanley JC, Zelenock GB. Splanchnic artery aneurysms. In: Rutherford RB (ed) *Vascular Surgery*, 4th edn. Philadelphia: WB Saunders, 1995, pp 1124–1138.
- Milazzo VJ, Hobson RW. Axillo-subclavian artery aneurysms. In: Yao JST, Pearce WH (eds) *Aneurysms, New Findings and Treatment*. Boston: Appleton and Lange, 1994, pp 451–458.
- Van Way III CH. Renal artery aneurysms and arteriovenous fistulae. In: Rutherford RB (ed) *Vascular Surgery*, 4th edn. Philadelphia: WB Saunders, 1995, pp 1438–1443.
- Mansfield AO, Gilling Smith GL. Unusual presentations of aneurysms. In: Greenhalgh RM, Mannick JA (eds) *The Cause and Management of Aneurysms*. London: WB Saunders, 1990, pp 105–116.

14

Acute Leg Ischaemia

Jonathan D Beard and Peter A Gaines

Introduction

Acute ischaemia of the leg is an uncommon problem, the average District General Hospital serving a population of 250 000 seeing about 20 cases each year. However, the incidence in the elderly appears to be increasing and if treatment is delayed or unsatisfactory, many will lose a leg if not their life. There is good evidence that morbidity and mortality are reduced when patients are managed by a vascular service that provides 24-hour cover.

Aetiology

In the UK, the commonest causes of acute leg ischaemia are emboli of cardiac origin and thrombosis of atherosclerotic arteries (Table 14.1).

Embolism

Rheumatic heart disease used to be the cause of most peripheral emboli but now ischaemic heart disease is the main culprit and the majority of patients (80%) are in atrial fibrillation. Emboli tend to lodge at the bifurcation of a vessel, the commonest site being the bifurcation of the common femoral artery (50%). This is a very unusual site for thrombosis to occur and helps in the radiological differentiation of the two conditions (Fig. 14.1). With the passing of rheumatic heart disease, few emboli are now large enough to produce the classic saddle embolus of the aortic bifurcation.

Thrombosis

Due to the increasing age of the population, thrombosis of an atherosclerotic stenosis, typically of the superficial femoral and popliteal artery (50%), is now the commonest cause of acute leg ischaemia (Fig. 14.2). This may be compounded by other factors that further reduce flow (e.g. cardiac failure or immobility) or increase the viscosity of the blood (e.g. dehydration or polycythaemia).

Table 14.1. **Causes of acute leg ischaemia.**

Embolism	Cardiac arrhythmia
	Mural thrombus
	Valvular vegetations
	Atrial myxoma
	Aortic aneurysm
	Atherosclerotic plaque
Thrombosis	Atheromatous stenosis
	Popliteal aneurysm
	Graft stenosis
	Cardiac failure
	Thrombotic states
Other	Aortic dissection
	Arterial trauma
	External compression
	Compartment syndrome
	Popliteal entrapment
	Cystic adventitial disease

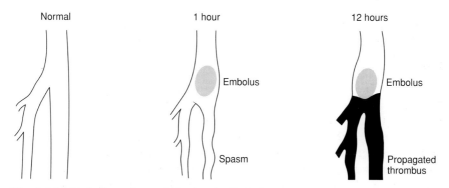

Fig. 14.1. Embolism. An embolus typically lodges at the bifurcation of an artery. The distal arteries go into spasm and if flow is not restored, thrombosis occurs.

Graft occlusion

Thrombosis of prosthetic bypass grafts is usually due to intimal hyperplasia at the anastomoses, or later, by progression of distal atherosclerosis. Vein graft occlusion may also be caused by the development of stenoses within the graft itself.

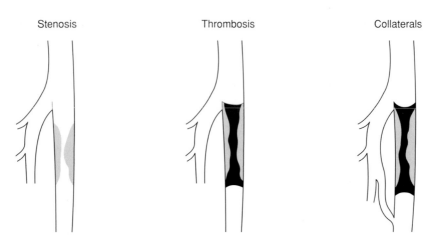

Stenosis   Thrombosis   Collaterals

Fig. 14.2. Thrombosis of an atherosclerotic artery occurs at a critical stenosis. Existing collaterals may be sufficient to maintain distal perfusion.

Popliteal aneurysms

The mechanism by which popliteal aneurysms cause leg ischaemia deserves special mention. Thrombus lining the sac may embolize to the tibial arteries and the resultant decrease in flow, especially in the aneurysm itself, results in extensive thrombosis of the aneurysm and the distal vessels.

Clinical features

Severe acute ischaemia

Severe acute ischaemia, as may occur with embolism of the common femoral artery or thrombosis of a popliteal aneurysm, results in the classic symptoms and signs of:

- pain;
- paralysis;
- paraesthesia;
- pallor;
- pulseless;
- perishing cold.

The pain is often severe and is due to vascular spasm. The paralysis and paraesthesia are due to ischaemia of the nerves and muscles. Initially the leg is marble white and the veins are empty and guttered. After 6–12 h vasodilatation occurs and the capillaries fill with stagnant deoxygenated blood, resulting in a mottled appearance with blanching on digital pressure. If flow is not rapidly restored, the arteries distal to the occlusion fill with propagated thrombus and capillary rupture occurs, resulting in fixed blue staining of the skin. Another sign of irreversible ischaemia is a tense calf with fixed plantar flexion of the foot and a bulging anterior compartment indicating muscle necrosis.

Moderate ischaemia

More often the ischaemia is less severe, e.g. when an embolus does not cause complete occlusion or when a thrombosis occurs. The gradual, more gentle onset of symptoms, sometimes over several days, is due to the prior development of collaterals around the offending stenosis. The foot is usually dusky with slow capillary return, and there may be patches of fixed skin staining or early gangrene affecting the toes and heel.

Diagnosis

A previous history of claudication and the absence of contralateral foot pulses both make the diagnosis of atherosclerotic thrombosis more likely (Table 14.2). Palpation of the contralateral popliteal pulse is vital as this may be the only clue to the presence of a thrombosed popliteal aneurysm.

Differentiation between thrombosis and embolism has been stressed in the past because of the poor results obtained for thrombosis treated by embolectomy. However, the clinical and radiological picture is often unclear and management should be dictated more by the severity of

Table 14.2. **Differences between embolism and thrombosis.**

	Embolism	Thrombosis
Incidence	Decreasing	Increasing
History	Arrhythmia, myocardial infarct	Claudication
Examination	White leg	Dusky foot
	Sensorimotor loss	Absent contralateral pulses
Arteriography	Occlusion of femoral bifurcation	Occlusion of iliac or superior femoral artery
	Multiple emboli	Collateral formation
	Normal arteries	Diseased arteries

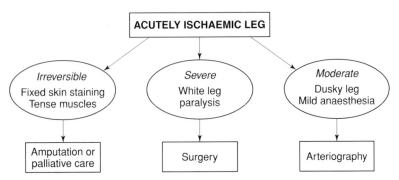

Fig. 14.3. Initial management of the acutely ischaemic leg.

ischaemia (Fig. 14.3). Doppler examination is of little help in assessment as often no signal is detectable. Arteriography is not always required (see below).

Management

Initial management

General measures

Pain should be treated with adequate amounts of morphine, an intravenous infusion of 5% dextrose begun, 5000 units of heparin given intravenously to reduce propagated thrombus and mask oxygen commenced. Blood should be taken for a full blood count, urea, electrolytes and glucose plus a chest X-ray and ECG. Appropriate treatment should be started for associated illness, e.g. digoxin for rapid atrial fibrillation and frusemide for cardiac failure.

Irreversible ischaemia

A minority of patients will be moribund at presentation, refuse intervention or have an irreversibly ischaemic leg. Whether or not to perform a primary amputation in the latter group will depend on the patient's general condition and likely quality of life. Amputation should be delayed to permit demarcation, if possible, but performed before systemic toxicity occurs. Attempted revascularization of a dead leg may result in a dead patient due to reperfusion injury.

Severe ischaemia

The severely ischaemic leg with sensorimotor loss requires emergency surgery. Thrombolysis may not act quickly enough and embolectomy is likely to be successful as the cause is often embolic, especially if there is no history of claudication and atrial fibrillation is present. Arteriography in this situation may waste time but should be performed if there is no femoral pulse as the problem might be an iliac thrombosis. An urgent duplex ultrasound scan is the best way to confirm a thrombosed popliteal aneurysm.

Moderate ischaemia

If there is no paralysis and only mild sensory loss, then arteriography with a view to thrombolysis should be performed as the cause is more likely to be a thrombosis. More time is available and if an arteriogram cannot be obtained immediately, it may be better to wait until a vascular radiologist is available, or transfer the patient, rather than risk inappropriate surgery.

Radiological management

Arteriography should be performed via the contralateral femoral artery and the volume of contrast kept to a minimum to avoid exacerbating cardiac or renal failure. If an embolus is demonstrated, then it may be possible for the radiologist to aspirate it through a large 9F catheter. If not, then embolectomy is usually required.

Percutaneous thrombolysis

Percutaneous thrombolysis should be considered for all patients with thrombotic occlusion and it is vital that this decision is made before the catheter is withdrawn (Fig. 14.4). The method depends on embedding

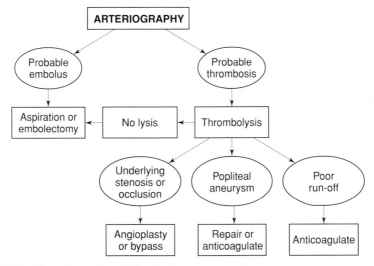

Fig. 14.4. Flow chart of radiological management.

the tip of the catheter in the thrombus which results in high local concentrations of lytic agent whilst minimizing any systemic effect.

For iliac and femoral occlusions the same contralateral puncture used for the diagnostic arteriogram can be employed. For popliteal and tibial occlusions, another ipsilateral, antegrade, femoral puncture is performed because catheter manipulation is easier and the risk of pericatheter thrombosis is reduced. Occluded grafts may require direct puncture.

The usual dose of streptokinase is 5000 unit/h which can be administered via a volumetric pump by dissolving a 100 000 unit vial in 1000 ml normal saline and setting an infusion rate of 50 ml/h. A syringe pump can be used but the smaller infusion volume risks unreliable drug delivery and increased pericatheter thrombosis. Adjuvant heparin 500 unit/h can reduce this latter problem but may increase the risk of bleeding.

Once in position the catheter should be securely fastened to the skin with a clear adhesive film dressing and the infusion commenced before the patient leaves the X-ray department. The patient should be nursed on a high-dependency or intensive care unit, according to a written protocol, and kept nil-by-mouth with adequate intravenous fluids and analgesia.

Repeat arteriograms are performed every 6–12 h to assess the degree of lysis and it is vital that the infusion is not stopped during transfer. As lysis occurs, the catheter is either advanced or withdrawn into the remaining thrombus, depending on the technique used (Fig. 14.5).

Thrombolysis should be complete within 24–36 h. Longer times are associated with an increased risk of serious bleeding and so treatment should be discontinued if there is little progress after 12 h. Lysis is successful in about two-thirds of cases, including grafts, and a similar proportion require either angioplasty or surgery to treat the underlying stenosis or occlusion.

When a popliteal aneurysm is revealed, surgical repair is usually required and there is little point in attempting to clear all the thrombus at the expense of delaying surgery.

If the arteries are diffusely ectatic, the best treatment is probably anticoagulation with heparin, followed by long-term warfarin. Anticoagulation is also employed after successful graft lysis, especially if the distal run-off is poor.

Complications

Haemorrhage may occur in up to half of patients during treatment but usually consists of local bleeding at the puncture site and requires only local compression. Direct graft punctures often require suture. Major bleeding, including gastrointestinal and cerebral haemorrhage, occurs in 5% of cases and patients with a recent history of bleeding disorders

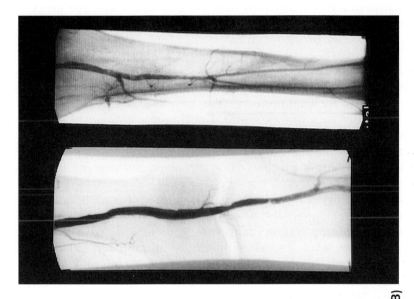

(A)

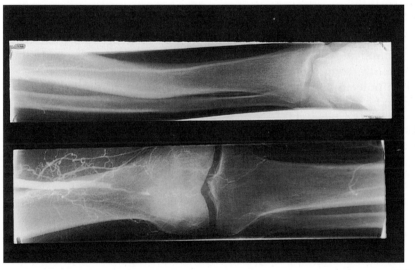

(B)

Fig. 14.5. Arteriogram showing (A) occlusion of the popliteal artery and (B) the diffuse ectasia revealed after percutaneous thrombolysis. The patient was susequently treated with warfarin.

should not be treated. Monitoring coagulation indices does not help predict haemorrhagic complications but it is worth checking the activated partial thromboplastin time (APPT) and fibrinogen every 6 h, especially if adjuvant heparin is used.

Advances

In an attempt to improve lysis rates and/or reduce complications, other agents and administration techniques have been introduced.

Streptokinase is cheap but may cause anaphylaxis or be inactivated by antibodies after previous exposure. Urokinase is a direct plasminogen activator but is very expensive. Tissue plasminogen activator (tPA) is a product of recombinant DNA technology and although it is more expensive, it is neither pyrogenic nor allergenic and may result in faster lysis.

Intermittent high-dose bolus injections, e.g. three 5 mg boluses of tPA injected at 10-min intervals, accelerate the rate of lysis but the risk of haemorrhagic complications may also be increased. With the pulsed spray technique, small, high-dose pulses are injected as a high pressure spray throughout the thrombus via a special catheter which has multiple side holes. The catheters and pumps are expensive, but the rapid lysis times mean that more severely ischaemic legs can be treated by thrombolysis.

Surgical management

With the increasing age of the population, underlying atherosclerosis often complicates ischaemia even if the cause is primarily embolic. Consequently, complex secondary procedures may well be necessary if initial embolectomy fails (Fig. 14.6). It is therefore advisable that this operation be performed by a vascular surgeon.

Anaesthesia

Local anaesthesia may be preferred in a slim patient with a clear-cut embolus and high cardiac risk. However, an anaesthetist should always be present to monitor the ECG and oxygen saturation, administer sedation or analgesia and convert to general anaesthesia if required. Obesity, confusion and the likelihood of additional procedures are good reasons for general anaesthesia.

Balloon catheter embolectomy

Both groins and the entire leg should be prepared to permit surgical access and arteriography. The foot is placed in a sterile transparent bag for ease of inspection. The common femoral artery bifurcation is exposed and controlled with silastic slings via a vertical groin incision.

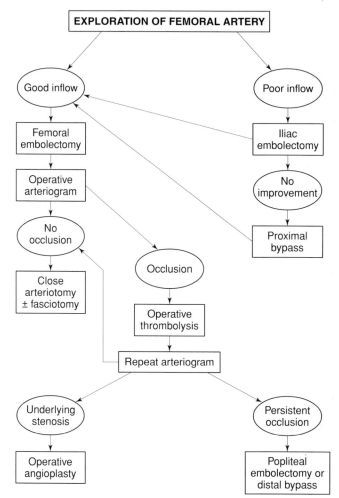

Fig. 14.6. Flow chart of surgical management.

Clamps should be avoided, if possible, because they can fragment a thrombus that may otherwise be removed intact.

An arteriotomy is made in the common femoral artery, avoiding any obvious plaque (Fig. 14.7). A transverse arteriotomy is easier to close without narrowing and can be converted to a diamond if a bypass is required. Any thrombus at the bifurcation can be removed by gentle suction or forceps and by momentarily releasing the sling.

If good pulsatile inflow is not present, then a 4 or 5F balloon catheter should be passed proximally up into the aorta, inflated and withdrawn. Pressure should be applied to the contralateral femoral artery during this procedure to prevent embolization. If good inflow cannot be achieved,

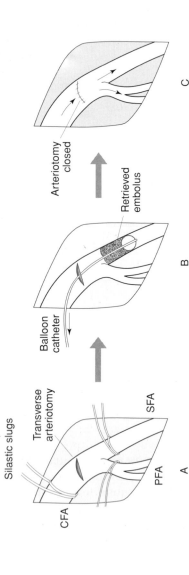

Fig. 14.7. Femoral embolectomy. (A) The femoral bifurcation is exposed and controlled with silastic slings. A transverse arteriotomy is made in the common femoral artery (CFA) and a 3 or 4F balloon catheter is passed down the superior femoral artery (SFA) and profunda femoral artery (PFA). (B) The balloon is gently inflated as the catheter is withdrawn to extract the clot. (C) After completion angiography the arteriotomy is closed.

then a femorofemoral or axillofemoral bypass is required. A saddle embolus can usually be retrieved by bilateral femoral embolectomy. A 3 or 4F balloon catheter should then be passed as far distally as possible down both the deep and superficial femoral arteries. Force should not be used if resistance is met as dissection or perforation may result. The balloon should be inflated only as the catheter is withdrawn and the amount of inflation adjusted to avoid excessive intimal friction. The procedure is repeated until no more thromboembolic material can be retrieved. Conventional embolectomy is performed blind and the surgeon has no control over the direction of the catheter past the popliteal trifurcation. End-hole balloon catheters permit selective catheterization of the tibial arteries, over a guidewire, under fluoroscopic control (Fig. 14.8).

Completion arteriography

A completion arteriogram should always be performed because persistent thrombus may be present even if the catheter passes to the foot and backbleeding is of no prognostic value. A film cassette, wrapped in a sterile towel is placed under the leg, 20 ml contrast medium infused down the superior femoral artery via a Tibbs cannula or an umbilical catheter and the film exposed. An image intensifier is better as real-time images are obtained and catheter manipulation can be controlled (Fig. 14.8C). The distal arteries should then be irrigated with 100 ml heparin saline and if no thrombus is present on the arteriogram, the arteriotomy can be closed with 5/0 prolene. On removing the clamps, the foot should become pink with palpable pulses.

Failed embolectomy

If the arteriogram shows persistent occlusion, then 100 000 units of streptokinase or 10 mg tPA in 100 ml heparin saline should be infused via the umbilical catheter over 30 min and the arteriogram repeated (Fig. 14.9). This often results in complete lysis of residual thrombus and reduces the need for popliteal exploration. The technique may also be used to lyse residual thrombus in the tibial arteries during repair of a popliteal aneurysm. If an underlying stenosis of the superior femoral artery is revealed, then on-table transluminal angioplasty may be attempted if the surgeon has experience of this technique. Persistent distal occlusion will require exploration of the below-knee popliteal artery and either popliteal embolectomy or femorodistal bypass.

Further management

Revascularization of the ischaemic leg results in a venous efflux of low pH and high potassium. The anaesthetist must be prepared to correct

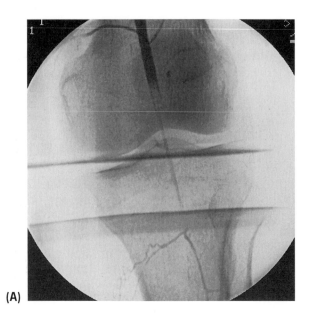

(A)

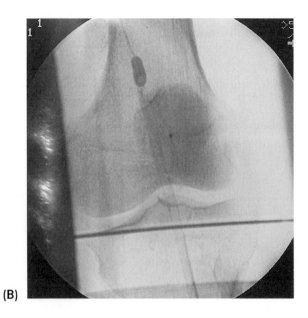

(B)

Fig. 14.8. (A) Operative arteriogram showing embolic occlusion of the popliteal artery. (B) A balloon catheter was passed under image intensifier control and the embolus retrieved.

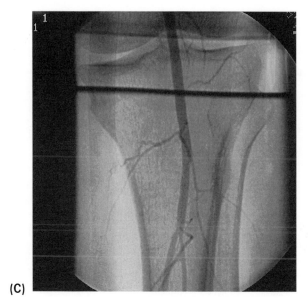

(C)

Fig. 14.8 (contd.). (C) The completion picture confirms patent vessels.

these as hypotension and arrhythmias may occur. Revascularization of ischaemic muscle may result in the release of free myoglobin. Myoglobinuria can cause acute renal failure which may be prevented by a good diuresis. Central venous pressure monitoring is important as many of these patients are easily tipped into heart failure and pulmonary oedema.

Compartment syndrome

Reperfusion may cause considerable muscle swelling within the fascial compartments of the lower leg. This compartment syndrome will lead to further muscle and nerve damage, resulting in foot drop or worse if not relieved. All muscle compartments should be decompressed by a fasciotomy if any muscle tenseness is present at the time of embolectomy or develops subsequently. Anterolateral and posteromedial incisions of skin and fascia from knee to ankle should be performed. A split-skin graft can be applied to the defects later.

Anticoagulation

Following embolectomy, anticoagulation with heparin and then warfarin is continued as this reduces the risk of recurrent embolism, especially if atrial fibrillation is present. If atrial fibrillation is not present, then other causes of embolism should be sought, including:

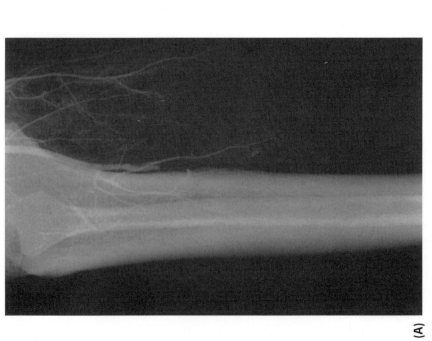

(A)

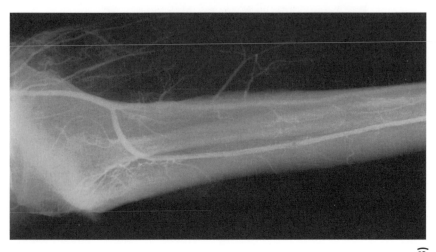

(B)

Fig. 14.9. Completion arteriogram showing persistent thrombus occluding the popliteal trifurcation despite passage of (A) an embolectomy catheter to the ankle and (B) complete lysis following intraoperative thrombolysis.

- serial cardiac enzymes to exclude myocardial infarction;
- echocardiography for valvular lesions;
- 24-h ECG monitoring for paroxysmal arrhythmias;
- ultrasound scan for abdominal aortic aneurysm;
- thrombotic screen for thrombophilia.

Outcome

Over the years, there has been little change in overall outcome because the improvements in radiological and surgical techniques have been balanced by increasing atherosclerotic arterial disease in ever older patients. Only 60–70% of patients admitted with an acutely ischaemic leg leave hospital with an intact limb. The 30-day mortality rate is 15–30% and 15% of survivors undergo an amputation. Patients with embolism have a high mortality due to their underlying cardiac disease. By contrast, those with thrombosis are at increased risk of amputation.

Patients with a high mortality are characterized by:

- cardiac failure;
- associated peripheral vascular disease;
- subsequent amputation.

Summary

- The management of the acutely ischaemic leg is often complex and prompt management by both vascular surgeons and radiologists is required if good results are to be obtained.
- The majority of patients can now be treated by percutaneous thrombolysis, aspiration and angioplasty.
- Surgery, including embolectomy, fasciotomy and bypass should be reserved for those with severe ischaemia or failed lysis.
- Completion arteriography is essential after embolectomy and intraoperative thrombolysis may reduce the need for more distal procedures.

Areas of controversy

- Should acute limb ischaemia ever be treated by general surgeons?
- Should preoperative arteriography always be performed?
- Is pulsed-spray thrombolysis, combined with clot aspiration, quick enough to treat all cases of acute leg ischaemia?
- Which thrombolytic regimen and agent is the safest and most cost-effective?

Further reading

- Bell PRF. The management of acute ischaemia of the limbs. In: Bell PRF, Jamieson CW, Ruckley CV (eds) *Surgical Management of Vascular Disease.* London: WB Saunders, 1992, pp 409–422.
- Section V: Lower extremity vascular emergencies. In: Greenhalgh RM, Hollier LH (eds) *Emergency Vascular Surgery.* London: WB Saunders, 1992, pp 411–424.
- Beard J. Embolectomy and operative thrombolysis for acute ischaemia of the lower limb. In: Strandness DE, Van Breda A (eds) *Vascular Diseases: Surgical and Interventional Therapy*, vol 1. New York: Churchill Livingstone, 1994, pp 303–420.
- Earnshaw JJ (ed). *Practical Peripheral Arterial Thrombolysis.* Oxford: Butterworth Heinemann, 1994.
- Chant ADB, Barros d'SA AB (eds). *Emergency Vascular Practice.* London: Edward Arnold, 1997.

15
Chronic Leg Ischaemia

Clifford P Shearman and Jonathan D Beard

Introduction

Peripheral vascular disease (PVD) commonly affects the abdominal aorta and lower limb arteries. Although PVD may produce embolization, or be associated with aneurysm formation, its main effect is restriction of limb blood flow. However, at rest the degree of luminal narrowing of a blood vessel has to be marked (80% area reduction) to produce a pressure fall and so many subjects with widespread atheroma will be completely asymptomatic.

Blood flow velocity through a stenosis is also a major determinant of the pressure gradient. During exercise the vascular bed of the lower limb muscles dilates, producing a fall in resistance accompanied by an increased blood flow velocity through the narrowed segment. A distal pressure fall may then occur which was not apparent at rest.

Pain on walking is most often the earliest clinical manifestation of PVD. If the perfusion of the lower limb continues to deteriorate, then the patient will suffer foot pain at rest followed by ulceration and gangrene which, if uncorrected, will result in limb loss. The Fontaine score is a useful clinical classification of the severity of ischaemia (Table 15.1).

Aetiology

The commonest cause of PVD is atherosclerosis (see Chapters 1 and 2).

Table 15.1. **Fontaine classification of chronic leg ischaemia.**

Stage I	Asymptomatic
Stage II	Intermittent claudication
Stage III	Ischaemic rest pain
Stage IV	Ulceration and/or gangrene

Intermittent claudication

Clinical features

A history of cramp-like pain on walking in the muscles of the leg, passing off within minutes on resting, and the absence of peripheral pulses is strongly supportive of the diagnosis

It is generally held that *calf claudication* is caused by disease of the superficial femoral artery and this will be associated with absent popliteal and foot pulses. The popliteal pulse can be difficult to palpate in muscular subjects: a bimanual examination helps. The position of the dorsalis pedis artery on the dorsum of the foot varies considerably and the posterior tibial artery can lie deep to the flexor tendons behind the medial malleolus. Many normal subjects possess only one palpable foot pulse.

Thigh and buttock claudication is associated with aortoiliac disease; the femoral pulse will be weak or absent and there may be a femoral bruit. This 'rule of thumb' may be a useful aid in the clinical diagnosis, but is not infallible; many patients with aortoiliac disease will present with calf claudication. The femoral artery is large and, if occluded by atheroma, should be palpable even if there is no pulse. If it cannot be felt then you are probably in the wrong place!

Best technique for palpation of peripheral arteries is described in Chapter 3.

Differential diagnosis

Pain due to *nerve root compression* and *arthropathy* is commonly mistaken for vascular claudication although this error can usually be avoided by a careful history. Whilst sciatic pain due to lumbosacral root compression is usually characteristic, cauda equina compression due to spinal stenosis can be difficult to differentiate especially in the presence of aortoiliac disease. The pain usually radiates down both legs and, although made worse by walking, may also be precipitated by prolonged standing and is not rapidly relieved by rest. The compartment syndrome or shin splints affect the anterior compartment of athletic individuals, usually after repetitive exercise such as road running.

A good history of claudication in a young patient should be taken seriously as some uncommon non-atherosclerotic conditions may progress to acute ischaemia if not diagnosed promptly. *Cystic adventitial disease* is due to a cystic abnormality, resembling a ganglion, in the adventitia of the popliteal artery. *Entrapment of the popliteal artery* occurs when the artery courses round the medial head of the gastrocnemius, rather than between the two heads. *Fibromuscular hyperplasia* usually affects the renal arteries but can affect the iliac artery, more often in women.

Investigation

Ankle brachial pressure indices

There are many causes for leg pain on walking in patients who happen also to have asymptomatic PVD. Conversely, the presence of pulses does not exclude claudication. Because of these problems it is best to submit all patients suspected of having intermittent claudication to simple non-invasive testing to assess the severity of disease.

The use of a hand-held Doppler ultrasound probe to measure the ankle brachial systolic pressure (ABPI) is simple, inexpensive and can be carried out in outpatients. A good history together with an ABPI of <0.9 confirms the diagnosis.

Exercise test

Exercise testing provides an objective measurement of walking distance and detects other exercise-limiting conditions such as breathlessness. However, exercise testing can be time consuming and many patients find it difficult or impossible to walk on a treadmill. In practice, exercise testing is only required for patients with a good history of claudication but normal resting ABPIs, or when another diagnosis, such as spinal stenosis, is suspected (Fig. 15.1).

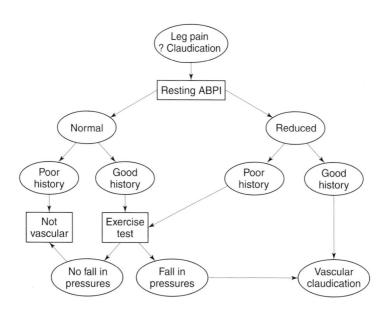

Fig. 15.1. Algorithm for the investigation of pain on walking. ABPI = ankle brachial systolic pressure index.

Further investigations

Colour Doppler ultrasound has become the first-line method of delineating the anatomical site of disease in the lower limb and, in particular, the suitability for intervention. This approach reduces the number of diagnostic angiograms undertaken in patients who are subsequently found unsuitable for intervention.

Diagnostic intra-arterial digital subtraction angiography (IADSA), is still widely used instead of duplex ultrasound or when the results are equivocal.

Invasive and/or expensive investigations should not be performed unless a decision has been made to proceed with interventional treatment.

Management

Claudication is a relatively benign condition and all patients must be advised to stop smoking and to exercise regularly. However, severe claudication may have major implications for the social independence of the patient and cost implications for society if the patient is unable to work or to look after himself without help. Balanced against this is the variable evidence for the long-term efficacy of intervention, particularly when the risks and costs are taken into account.

Probably more important to the patient is the risk from generalized vascular disease. Patients with claudication have a risk of death >3-fold that of age-matched controls. This is almost exclusively due to ischaemic heart disease (50%), cerebrovascular disease (15%) and intra-abdominal vascular disease (10%). When treating patients with claudication, attention should therefore be directed to their general cardiovascular condition as well as their presenting problem.

Figure 15.2 is an algorithm for the treatment of claudication and the factors influencing the decision to intervene are outlined in Table 15.2.

Medical management

Having established the diagnosis and counselled the patient, many sufferers will be reassured and no further treatment is required. Identification of risk factors, including hyperlipidaemia, and correction when possible is important (see Chapter 6). Cessation of smoking and exercise are probably the most beneficial actions the patient can take and are likely to improve the claudication as well as reduce the general cardiovascular risk.

Structured exercise programmes

Telling patients to walk more is probably of little value, but structured exercise training is useful. A recent meta-analysis of 21 exercise training

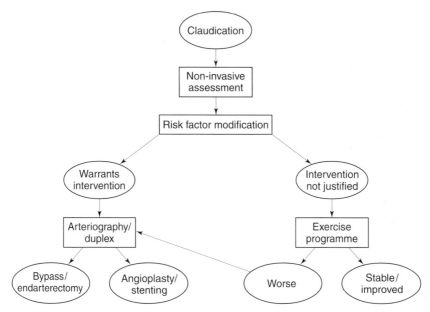

Fig. 15.2. Algorithm for the treatment of claudication.

Table 15.2. Factors influencing the decision to intervene in claudication.

For	Against
Severe symptoms	Short history
Job affected	Still smoking
No better after exercise	Severe angina/COAD
Aortoiliac disease	Femorodistal disease
Stenosis/short occlusion	Long occlusion
Unilateral symptoms	Multilevel disease

programmes showed that training for at least 6 months, by walking to near maximum pain tolerance, produced significant improvements in pain-free and maximum walking distances. Several randomized studies have shown the benefits of exercise programmes on maximum walking distance and the only controlled trial comparing exercise with translumi-nal angioplasty found exercise to be better than angioplasty. Exercise programmes are relatively cheap compared with surgery and angioplasty and certainly are safer, although compliance may be a problem.

Endovascular intervention

Since the first transluminal arterial dilation in 1964 and sub-sequent development of balloon dilatation catheters, the number of percutaneous transluminal angioplasties (PTA) performed has escalated dramatically. In some situations, such as aortoiliac disease, endovascular techniques have virtually replaced conventional surgery.

The optimum lesions for PTA are short stenoses or occlusions of the iliac and the proximal superficial femoral vessels, with good run-off (Fig. 15.3). The patency rates at 1 year are excellent (approximately 90% and 80%, respectively).

Although the morbidity of PTA is low, it does carry a 3–4% risk of complications such as groin haematoma and acute thrombosis of the dilated segment. The mortality rate is very low in most series (around 0.2%) but there is a small, but definite, risk of limb loss. This must be borne in mind when treating patients who are not at any current risk of amputation.

Metallic stents provide a rigid endovascular support which holds back the atheroma to improve the initial lumen gain and reduce the risk of embolization. Stents may be deployed on a balloon (e.g. Palmaz) or be self-expanding (e.g. Wallstent, Memotherm) and are available in a range of diameters and lengths. Aortoiliac stents are indicated if there is a residual stenosis after angioplasty alone, when dilatation has resulted in a flow-limiting dissection or in occlusions where the risk of distal embolization is high (Fig. 15.4). The use of stents more distally has been disappointing due to high restenosis rates related to low flow.

The endovascular treatment of long occlusions and distal popliteal and tibial lesions is more complex and probably inappropriate in most claudicants. If intervention is required in these cases, then bypass surgery probably gives better results in terms of patency, although there have been few randomized trials. The short hospital stay (day case or overnight) and avoidance of a general anaesthetic add to the appeal of endovascular treatment. This is especially true if the alternative operation is a major undertaking such as aortobifemoral bypass.

Surgery

The treatment options for femoropopliteal disease are outlined in Fig. 15.5.

The role of surgical bypass in claudication remains poorly defined due to a lack of well designed trials. The results of *above-knee femoropopliteal bypass grafting* are relatively good and in the first 2 years the patency of prosthetic grafts is similar to vein (80%), although the long-term results are less good. The use of prosthetic grafts in this position has the advantage that the vein is preserved for later use if necessary and the operation is considerably quicker. The commonest prosthetic material used is ring-reinforced, 6 mm expanded polytetrafluoroethylene (ePTFE) which is relatively non-thrombogenic and kink resistant.

Bypass to below the knee is harder to justify as patency rates are lower (70%) and although vein gives better results, postoperative graft surveil-

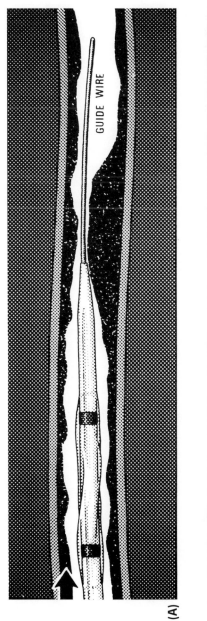

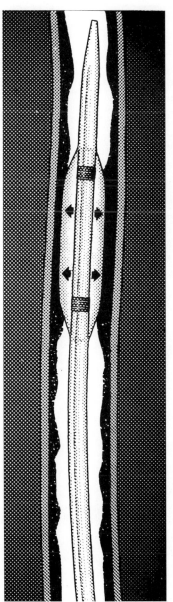

Fig. 15.3. Technique of percutaneous transluminal angioplasty. (A) Deflated balloon pushed along artery; (B) balloon inflated next to blockage.

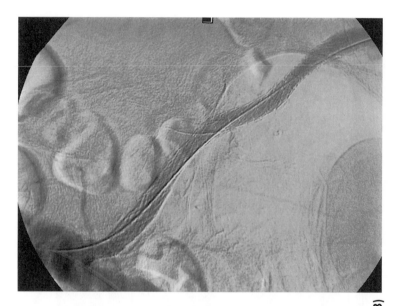

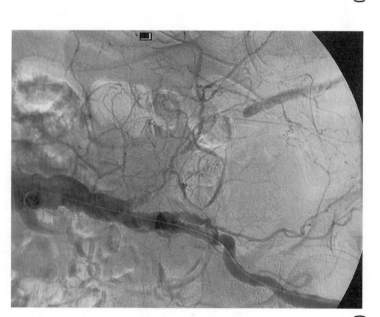

(A)

(B)

Fig. 15.4. (A) Long occlusion of the left common iliac artery; (B) treated by three Memotherm stents.

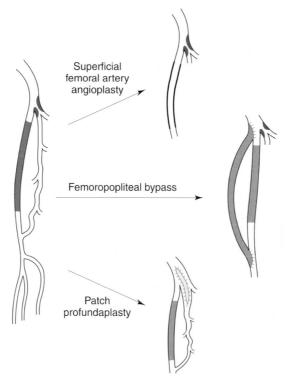

Superficial
femoral artery
angioplasty

Femoropopliteal bypass

Patch
profundaplasty

Fig. 15.5. **Treatment options for femoropopliteal disease causing claudication or ischaemic rest pain.**

lance is required with a 25–30% risk of a graft stenosis needing reintervention.

Bypass to a single calf vessel for claudication is rarely justified as the results and long-term patency, whilst highly acceptable for limb salvage, are not good enough for a claudicant.

The initial results of inflow procedures such as aortobifemoral bypass are excellent with a 5-year patency rate of >90% but are associated with a mortality of up to 5%. There is also a risk of prosthetic graft infection and postoperative impotence. Woven Dacron (polyester) is the standard prosthetic material. Collagen- or gelatin-sealed, knitted Dacron handles better, does not leak and can be pre-soaked in antibiotics, but is more expensive. Externally supported grafts should be used in extra-anatomic positions because of the risk of graft compression.

Cross-femoral and iliofemoral bypass provide technically satisfactory ways of dealing with unilateral iliac disease and in claudicants should give 90% 1-year patency rates. Axillobifemoral bypass is not justified for claudication because of lower patency rates (Fig. 15.6).

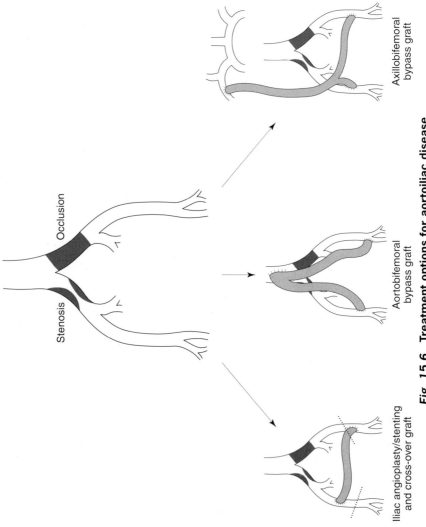

Stenosis

Occlusion

Axillobifemoral bypass graft

Aortobifemoral bypass graft

Iliac angioplasty/stenting and cross-over graft

Fig. 15.6. **Treatment options for aortoiliac disease.**

Critical Limb Ischaemia

Clinical features

The history is often clear with a gradual worsening of claudication progressing to nocturnal rest pain and ultimately ulceration and gangrene. The pain commonly occurs just after the patient has fallen asleep when the systemic blood pressure falls, so further reducing the perfusion pressure of the foot which is increased again by dependency. This produces the typical dusky red hue due to loss of capillary tone in the microcirculation. Elevation leads to pallor and venous guttering.

Approximately 20% of patients have a precipitous presentation due to an acute event superimposed on a chronic background. This may be due to thrombosis of a severely diseased arterial segment, embolization of atheroma distally or addition of another factor such as infection or injury that may occur during chiropody. As more interventions are carried out for PVD, it is quite common to see patients who, following successful initial treatment, re-present with further symptoms due to restenosis or graft occlusion (see Chapter 26).

As with claudication, careful clinical examination and pulse palpation can usually indicate the level of disease (see Chapter 3). The foot should be inspected carefully for ulceration of the heel and web spaces. Swelling may suggest deep infection. It helps to concentrate on determining whether the problem appears to be predominantly above the femoral artery (inflow) or infrainguinal. This is notoriously difficult, but a patient with a normal feeling femoral pulse is unlikely to have a haemodynamically significant lesion that will interfere with a distal bypass for limb salvage. This is quite different from the situation in a patient with claudication (see above).

Diagnosis

Identification of patients whose lower limb ischaemia is severe enough to place the leg at risk remains difficult and contentious. The European working group recommends that critical limb ischaemia (CLI) should be defined as:

- persistent rest pain of over 2 weeks duration requiring regular analgesia, with an ankle systolic blood pressure of <50 mmHg or a toe pressure of <30 mmHg; or
- patients with ulceration or gangrene of the feet, again with the same reduction of ankle blood pressure.

While this definition has improved the reporting of results of intervention, it is far from perfect. Even without treatment, many patients with

CLI do not end up with a major amputation. The measurement of ankle blood pressure may be falsely elevated, especially in diabetics where the vessels may be frankly calcified. The reasons for limb loss are often multi-factorial, and superimposed infection, the distribution of ulceration and other medical conditions all influence the outcome.

Investigation

Simple non-invasive assessment using a hand-held Doppler ultrasound probe to insonate the ankle arteries is useful to confirm the diagnosis and to establish a baseline prior to treatment. The ABPI is usually <0.5, and if it seems abnormally high should be checked by the elevation test or toe pressures.

Dependent Doppler and pulse-generated run-off (PGR) can help to determine the most suitable vessel for run-off in patients with distal disease if this cannot be demonstrated by angiography. Colour Doppler may localize the disease and help plan intervention, but currently nearly all patients with CLI proceed to angiography.

Biplanar views of the aortoiliac segment combined with measurement of pressure gradients at the time of angiography should determine the significance of any inflow disease. Distal imaging is used to confirm the non-invasive findings and to identify the most proximal segment of the vessel that can be used for run-off. If these cannot be identified pre-operatively, the situation can be clarified using per-operative angiography.

Management

Unlike claudication, CLI is usually caused by multi-segment disease and often the aortoiliac, superficial femoral and crural vessels are all affected. For these reasons it is very unusual to find a patient with truly limb-threatening ischaemia who can be salvaged with a simple above-knee femoropopliteal bypass or iliac angioplasty. If the preoperative investigations suggest a single level occlusion, then either the diagnosis should be questioned or distal or proximal disease has been missed, a common cause of graft failure.

A pragmatic definition of CLI is that the limb will be lost without revascularization. Therefore treatment focuses on limb salvage, although the need for risk factor modification must not be forgotten (Fig. 15.7).

Endovascular intervention

The same basic principles and techniques that apply to claudication also apply to CLI. However, more extensive revascularization of long occlusions and multiple stenoses may be attempted, whilst accepting higher complication and lower patency rates. Single level PTA and/or stenting

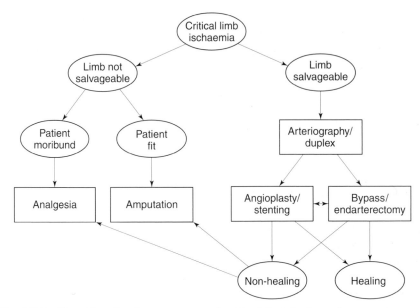

Fig. 15.7. **Algorithm for the treatment of critical limb ischaemia.**

may be sufficient to relieve ischaemic rest pain but healing of ulceration or gangrene usually requires vascular continuity to the foot. This may necessitate extensive dilatation of the superficial femoral, popliteal and tibial arteries. Limb salvage rates using endovascular techniques alone are reported to be 50–80% at 2 years.

Endovascular techniques can also reduce the magnitude of surgery. Dilation of an iliac lesion combined with a distal bypass is a better option than a multi-level operative procedure. Dilatation of a superficial femoral artery stenosis may allow the use of a popliteal–pedal bypass in a diabetic rather than a long femoropedal bypass. This reduces operation time and wound complications as the vein can be harvested from above the knee and transposed with the minimum number of incisions in the lower leg. Likewise dilation of a crural vessel stenosis may permit a femoropopliteal bypass rather than a femorocrural bypass (Fig. 15.8).

Surgery

If, after assessment, the pattern of arterial disease is not considered suitable for endovascular treatment, then surgery is required. Inflow disease can be dealt with in a conventional way. In younger patients who do not have significant cardiovascular problems, aortobifemoral bypass grafting should give excellent results. In those less fit, the options are cross-femoral or iliofemoral bypass for unilateral disease or axillobifemoral bypass for bilateral disease. If problems with the donor limb are

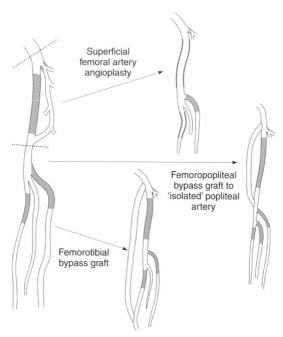

Superficial
femoral artery
angioplasty

Femoropopliteal
bypass graft to
'isolated' popliteal
artery

Femorotibial
bypass graft

Fig. 15.8. **Treatment options for femorodistal disease causing ulceration or gangrene.**

identified, then either pre- or per-operative PTA may correct the problem and allow a cross-femoral bypass to be undertaken (Fig. 15.6).

The main decision is whether to undertake concomitant distal bypass in the many patients with associated distal disease. If the profunda femoris artery is good and disease free and there is no frank tissue loss, then it is often better to carry out the inflow procedure alone, and only undertake distal bypass subsequently if correction of inflow alone proves insufficient. In patients with small or diseased profunda vessels or extensive pedal gangrene, it is usually expeditious to perform a combined procedure.

The majority of patients with distal disease require bypass to infrageniculate vessels and autologous vein should be used whenever possible because of better patency and reduced risk of infection. Preoperative duplex ultrasound mapping of the long saphenous vein has the advantage of making harvesting easier and allowing the use of discontinuous incisions as well as identifying small or diseased veins which are unsuitable for use. In these situations, vein can be harvested either from the arm, the opposite leg or the short saphenous vein. Autologous long saphenous vein can be used *in situ* or reversed with apparently equally good results (80% patency at 1 year). The merits of the reversed method

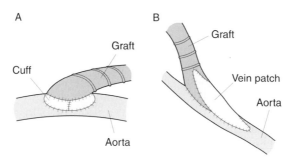

Fig. 15.9. **(A) Miller vein cuff and (B) Taylor vein patch.**

is that both proximal and distal anastomoses can be performed synchronously, reducing operation time, whereas the *in situ* technique allows the smaller distal end of the vein to be anastomosed to the smaller run-off artery. It is possible to prepare the *in situ* vein angioscopically, although this adds to the time the procedure takes. Side branches can be occluded with coils and the only incisions required are at the proximal and distal sites of anastomosis.

In the absence of autologous vein, polytetrafluoroethylene (PTFE) grafts to single calf vessels carry an unacceptably high failure rate. The use of either a vein patch or cuff at the distal anastomosis significantly improves the results with a 5-year patency rate of >50% (Fig. 15.9). The cuff makes it technically easier to perform a good quality anastomosis but there may also be an haemodynamic advantages. Many other prosthetic grafts are available, but none has been shown to be as good as vein or better than PTFE.

Other procedures such as profundaplasty have a limited role in CLI (Fig. 15.5). If there is no tissue loss, they may relieve rest pain, but the patient will often be left with claudication. Profundaplasty alone is usually inadequate to reverse distal ulceration or gangrene.

Postoperative anticoagulation is not undertaken routinely although all patients should receive aspirin 75 mg daily. All vein grafts must have a duplex scan at 6 weeks and then at 3-monthly intervals for at least the first year. Around 30% of vein grafts will develop a stenosis during this period and many will occlude if uncorrected. PTA should be attempted unless the lesion is long, although there is a high recurrence rate. If the stricture recurs or is >1 cm in length, vein patching or a jump graft is a better option (see Chapter 26).

Non-interventional management

In about 10% of patients, it will be technically impossible to revascularize the limb. Several pharmacological agents have been tried in these situations of which the most promising are prostanoids, particularly prostacyclin. A meta-analysis of 6 controlled studies of iloprost, a stable prostacyclin analogue, suggested a reduction of death and amputation in those patients receiving the drug.

In some patients the limb survives, but pain remains a problem. If simple analgesia is inadequate, then lumbar sympathectomy (surgical or chemical) or spinal cord stimulation may be helpful. It is unclear whether these procedures work by interruption of pain pathways or by improving microcirculatory perfusion.

If the general condition of the patient is very poor and the chances of survival are limited due to other co-existent pathology, it may be deemed reasonable to treat the patient with analgesia and palliative care alone. If the patient has a reasonable quality of life, and is likely to survive even for a few months, it is usually better to offer revascularization. It is a therapeutic failure for the patient to spend the remaining few months of his life struggling not only with his primary disease but also with an amputation (see Chapter 17).

Summary

- Claudication is a common condition and few patients progress to limb-threatening ischaemia.
- Non-invasive assessment confirms the diagnosis and gives some idea of the haemodynamic severity of the disease.
- An initial policy of non-intervention should be pursued in all but the most severely affected patients (stop smoking, keep walking, watch your cholesterol and take aspirin).
- Angioplasty and/or stenting is the first-line treatment for stenoses or short occlusions.
- Surgical bypass is only undertaken in patients with severe symptoms who are unsuitable for endovascular treatment.
- Critical leg ischaemia is an increasing problem, due to an aging population, and is caused by multi-level arterial occlusive disease.
- Diagnosis is confirmed by a Doppler ankle pressure of <50 mmHg. The elevation test or toe pressures are useful if arterial calcification is suspected.
- Most patients should undergo angiography with a view to endovascular treatment, if possible.
- Patent pedal arteries, not visualized by angiography, can be detected by dependent Doppler, duplex or pulse-generated run-off.
- Femorodistal bypass is technically demanding and time consuming. Autologous vein must be used if possible, with postoperative duplex surveillance.
- Primary amputation should be reserved for immobile patients and those with a non-viable foot.

Areas of controversy

- Is exercise therapy, angioplasty or surgery the most cost-effective treatment for claudication?
- Can colour Doppler completely replace angiography as the definitive investigation for lower limb ischaemia?
- Should complex intervention for limb-salvage be performed in specialist centres?

Further reading

- Housley E. Treating claudication in five words. *British Medical Journal* 1988;**296**: 1483–1484.
- Audit Committee of the Vascular Surgical Society of Great Britain and Ireland. Recommendations for the management of chronic critical lower limb ischaemia. *European Journal of Vascular and Endovascular Surgery* 1996;**12**:131–135.
- Ouriel K (ed). *Lower Extremity Vascular Disease.* Philadelphia: WB Saunders, 1996.
- Greenhalgh RM, Fowkes FGR (eds). *Trials and Tribulations of Vascular Surgery.* London: WB Saunders, 1996.

16
The Diabetic Foot

Jonathan E Shaw and Andrew JM Boulton

Introduction

Several different diabetes-related pathologies have their greatest impact on the foot, and so it is not surprising that foot ulceration is the commonest major end-point among diabetic complications. Diabetic neuropathy and peripheral vascular disease play major roles in foot ulceration and may act alone, together or in combination with other factors.

Previous or current ulceration is reported by up to 10% of diabetic patients, and lower limb amputation is performed 15 times more frequently amongst diabetic than non-diabetic patients. Following unilateral amputation, rates for both mortality and contralateral amputation are depressingly high.

Aetiology of foot ulceration

A number of risk factors play a role:

- previous ulceration;
- neuropathy;
- peripheral vascular disease;
- altered foot shape;
- high foot pressures;
- increasing age;
- visual impairment;
- living alone.

However, all diabetic foot ulcers can be attributed *primarily* to diabetic neuropathy and/or peripheral vascular disease.

Diabetic neuropathy

Although vascular disease and infection were once thought to be the main causes of foot ulceration, prospective studies have demonstrated the importance of neuropathy. Neuropathy leads to a 7–10 fold increase in ulceration and is responsible for up to 60% of foot ulcers.

The development of neuropathy is linked to poor glycaemic control over many years and thus increases in frequency with both age and duration of diabetes. Estimates of the prevalence of neuropathy vary because of different diagnostic criteria and populations studied, but it is probably about 30%.

There are numerous manifestations of diabetic neuropathy. As far as the diabetic foot is concerned, the *distal sensory neuropathy* is the most important type, although both motor and autonomic neuropathy also play a role.

Symptoms of neuropathy occur only in the minority of patients and most are completely unaware of their marked sensory loss, which can therefore only be detected by regular screening. As education about foot care is crucial to the prevention of neuropathic ulceration, all diabetic patients must be screened annually. When symptoms are present, they are usually easy to recognize, with patients typically describing burning, paraesthesiae and shooting pains. The features differentiating this from ischaemic pain are listed in Table 16.1.

Autonomic neuropathy reduces sweating in the skin and opens arteriovenous shunts leading to increased skin blood flow in the foot. Thus, the neuropathic foot is typically warm with bounding pulses and has dry, sometimes cracked, skin.

Motor neuropathy mainly affects the intrinsic muscles of the foot (as they are the most distal), with clinical evidence of wasting (guttering between the metatarsals) and an altered foot shape with clawed toes and prominent metatarsal heads.

Therefore, the insensitive neuropathic foot is at risk from:

- unperceived external trauma (e.g. ill-fitting shoes);
- repetitive injury to high pressure areas under the metatarsal heads;
- easy access of infection through cracked skin.

Table 16.1. Comparison of signs and symptoms of neuropathic and ischaemic pain.

	Neuropathic	Intermittent claudication	Ischaemic rest pain
Site	Foot/shin	Calf/thigh	Foot/calf
Nature	Tingling/burning/shooting	Aching	Aching
Exacerbating factors	Night time	Exercise	Exercise
Relieving factors	Exercise	Rest	Dependency of foot
Clinical signs	Warm, bounding pulses	Weak/absent pulses	Cold/pulseless

The diagnosis of neuropathy is usually simple and can be made by clinical examination which reveals a 'stocking' distribution of sensory loss and absent ankle reflexes.

Peripheral vascular disease

Atherosclerotic vascular disease is probably present (at least in a subclinical form) in all patients with diabetes of long duration. Vascular disease is responsible for up to 70% of deaths in non-insulin-dependent diabetes, and peripheral vascular disease may be 20-fold more common in diabetes.

Whereas in non-diabetic patients, peripheral vascular disease typically involves aortoiliac and femoral vessels, in diabetic patients, infrapopliteal

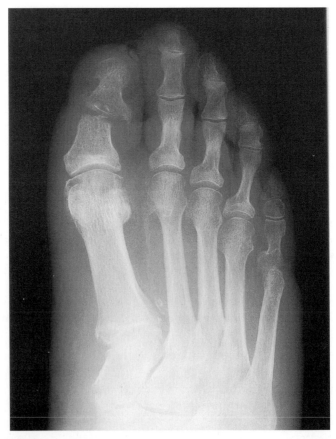

Fig. 16.1. Plain X-ray of diabetic foot demonstrating arterial wall calcification between 1st and 2nd metatarsals.

vessels are often diseased. Nevertheless, arteries in the ankle and foot are often patent and will allow a bypass with a distal anastomosis. The outcome of such surgery is good and may avoid amputation.

Despite significant disease, symptoms of intermittent claudication are often absent, especially if neuropathy co-exists, and the first clinical presentation may be ischaemic foot ulceration. Typically, this occurs at the ends of the toes, and in the absence of neuropathy is painful. The foot is usually cool with absent pulses and the most helpful non-invasive investigation is the measurement of the ankle brachial pressure index (ABPI). An ABPI below 0.9 is clearly indicative of ischaemia, but often it is falsely elevated due to medial calcification of vessel walls — a phenomenon frequently seen in diabetic neuropathy (Fig. 16.1). In this situation, the Doppler waveform is useful, as loss of the normal triphasic waveform indicates vascular disease. The elevation test or toe pressures can be used to assess the perfusion pressure.

Biomechanical aspects

Neuropathy alone does not lead to spontaneous ulceration. It is the combination of trauma and insensitivity that results in tissue damage. Usually this takes the form of repeated minor trauma, such as unperceived pressure from a shoe rubbing on the toes or increased pressure beneath the metatarsal heads during walking. It is now clear that elevated dynamic plantar pressures occur in neuropathy and predispose to ulceration. The presence of callus (produced in response to pressure) may exacerbate the problem, and its removal significantly reduces foot pressures.

The main cause of increased pressure is thought to be alteration in foot shape resulting in prominent metatarsal heads. Atrophy of the intrinsic muscles of the foot (predominantly plantar flexors of the toes) alters the flexor/extensor balance at the metatarsophalangeal joints and causes clawing of the toes, anterior displacement of the submetatarsal fat pads and reduced subcutaneous tissue thickness at the metatarsal heads.

The accurate measurement of foot pressure requires sophisticated and expensive systems. However, clinical examination, looking at foot shape and the presence of callus, provides invaluable information which can be used to select patients in need of pressure relief.

Abnormalities of the microcirculation

Thickening of capillary basement membranes can be found in most diabetic tissues, and although microvascular disease alone does not cause foot ulceration, it is almost certainly a contributory factor. The key abnormalities are:

- increased resting microvascular flow;
- impaired postural vasoconstriction;
- reduced hyperaemic response to nociceptive stimulation.

The loss of the nociceptive response, which is particularly marked in neuropathy, impairs the ability of the tissue to respond appropriately to trauma.

Other risk factors

Neutrophil function is impaired, and this may contribute to infection in the diabetic foot. Irreversible glycosylation of proteins leads to limited joint mobility and stiff tissues, which contribute to elevated foot pressures. Advancing age is frequently accompanied by impaired vision and immobility, both of which make foot inspection more difficult and delay help being sought for an ulcer.

Prevention of ulceration

The pathway to ulceration and amputation is often complex and two or more elements are nearly always required:

- Ulceration of the insensitive foot only occurs when it is subjected to trauma;
- the addition of peripheral vascular disease reduces the pressure at which ischaemia and tissue breakdown occur.

The corollary of this multifactorial aetiology is that the pathways can be interrupted at any point. Tight glycaemic control in the early years of diabetes will prevent the development of neuropathy and other complications, and the provision of good education about foot care to patients with high-risk feet may be equally successful at preventing ulceration (see below).

The 'at risk' foot

The identification of patients at risk of foot ulceration is most easily done by the annual screening of all patients with diabetes, as neuropathy, vascular disease and even ulceration are frequently asymptomatic. Peripheral neuropathy can be recognized with standard clinical methods. The peripheral vascular status is usually indicated by palpation of peripheral pulses. It should be remembered that absent foot pulses may be due to arterial wall calcification, not absent flow. The ABPI should be measured whenever there is any doubt. Foot inspection may reveal deformities of foot shape and areas of callus which indicate sites exposed to high pressure.

As most of the risk factors (apart from vascular disease) are not directly modifiable by treatment, the most important element of the management of high-risk patients is the provision of good education on foot care, as this can have a major impact on amputation and ulceration rates. The basic elements of foot care advice are:

- Target the level of information to the needs of the patient. Those patients not at risk require only general advice about foot hygiene and footwear.
- Make positive rather than negative recommendations:

  DO inspect the feet daily;
  DO report any problems immediately even if painless;
  DO buy shoes with a square toe box and laces;
  DO inspect the inside of shoes for foreign objects every day before putting them on;
  DO attend a fully trained podiatrist regularly;
  DO cut your nails straight across and not rounded;
  DO keep your feet away from heat (fires, radiators, hot water bottles) and check the bath water with your hand or elbow;
  DO always wear something on your feet to protect them and never walk barefoot.

- Repeat the advice at regular intervals and check for compliance.
- Disseminate the advice to other family members and health-care professionals involved in the care of the patient.

Management of ulcers

All diabetic patients presenting with foot ulcers need an examination of peripheral sensation and measurement of the ABPI in order to classify the ulcer as neuropathic, neuroischaemic or ischaemic. Any type of ulcer can be infected and the management of infection is considered separately.

Neuropathic ulcers

Typically, the foot is warm and well perfused with bounding pulses and distended veins. The ulcer is usually at the site of repetitive trauma and is most commonly due to a shoe rubbing on the dorsum of the toes or a high pressure area under the metatarsal heads.

The key to management is pressure relief. With shoe-induced ulcers, appropriate footwear must be provided. To relieve pressure from a plantar ulcer, a more aggressive approach is required. Bed rest is difficult to enforce in a patient who feels well and is free of pain. Specially

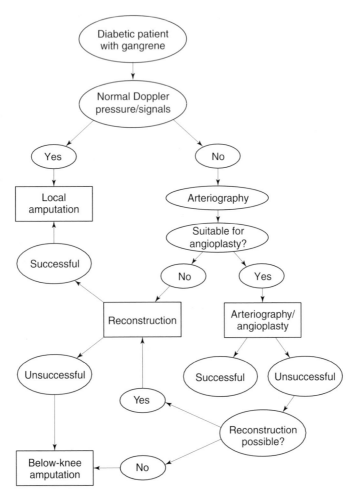

Fig. 16.2. Algorithm for the management of the diabetic patient with gangrene.

designed casts (total contact cast or Scotch cast boots) redistribute load away from high pressure areas, while allowing the patient to remain mobile.

Another important element of management of neuropathic ulcers is debridement of callus and necrotic tissue, which inhibit healing and encourage wound infection. This is usually required on a weekly basis and the continued presence of callus should prompt a review of pressure relief. Local amputation may be required for underlying osteomyelitis but should only be undertaken after vascular insufficiency has been excluded.

Ischaemic and neuroischaemic ulcers

The purely ischaemic ulcer is relatively rare and most are in fact neuro-ischaemic. Typical sites include the toes, heel and medial aspect of the first metatarsal head. Callus is usually absent and the ulcer is often surrounded by a rim of erythema and may have a necrotic centre. Pain only occurs in the absence of neuropathy. Ulceration is often precipitated by minor trauma and the commonest culprit is ill-fitting shoes. Prompt vascular assessment is crucial and angiography with a view to angioplasty is nearly always required. Revascularization should be performed whenever possible. If angioplasty is not possible, then a femorodistal vein bypass graft is usually required (see Chapter 15).

Although gangrene may complicate neuropathic ulceration (micro-organisms in infected digital ulcers may produce necrotizing toxins, which lead to thrombotic occlusion of digital arteries), it usually only occurs when significant vascular disease is present. Gangrenous tissue must be removed promptly (see Fig. 16.2), although a toe with dry gangrene may separate spontaneously. If arterial reconstruction is possible, then this can be combined with amputation to enable the healing of a distal amputation site (digit or ray amputation).

Infection

An infected diabetic foot ulcer can lead to limb loss in a matter of days, but by no means are all ulcers infected, although bacterial colonization is probably universal. The distinction between colonization and infection can be difficult and is not usually aided by microbiological investigations. Clinical signs are the most reliable indicators of infection. Evidence of systemic upset (e.g. fever, leucocytosis) is usually absent and signs of local inflammation and the presence of pus usually confirm the diagnosis.

Infections are usually polymicrobial and the most commonly isolated organisms include:

- staphylococci;
- streptococci;
- Gram negatives (e.g. proteus and pseudomonas);
- anaerobes (e.g. bacteroides).

In non-limb threatening infections, microbiological investigation is not essential, but when swabs are taken the method is important. Superficial swabs are likely to isolate colonizing rather pathogenic bacteria. Ideally, curettings from the ulcer base should be cultured aerobically and anaerobically.

Osteomyelitis should be suspected in any non-healing ulcer. Though sometimes obvious from plain radiographs (Fig. 16.3), bone scans or

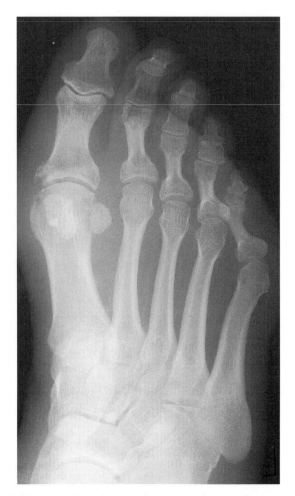

Fig. 16.3. **Plain X-ray of diabetic foot demonstrating cortical erosion indicating osteomyelitis, deep to an ulcer over the 1st metatarsophalangeal joint.**

MRI may be needed. The ability to probe the bone with a blunt instrument at the base of an ulcer is strongly associated with osteomyelitis.

The threshold for initiating antibiotic treatment should be low, and the agents used should have a broad spectrum of activity. Clindamycin or the combination of amoxycillin and clavulanic acid are suitable oral treatments. Aminoglycosides should be used with caution because of their potential nephrotoxicity, and quinolones should not usually be used alone because of their limited activity against Gram-positive cocci. Limb-threatening infections require urgent hospitalization, bed rest, surgical debridement and broad-spectrum antibiotics.

Charcot neuroarthropathy

Charcot neuroarthropathy affects 9% of patients with neuropathy. It can be one of the most devastating foot complications and is characterized by bone and joint destruction, fragmentation and remodelling. Weight bearing on an injured foot and a localized osteoporosis are both thought to be involved in the pathogenesis.

Typically, patients present with a warm, swollen foot. There is frequently discomfort, although not enough to prevent walking. Plain radiography is usually adequate to make the diagnosis, but isotope scans and MRI are sometimes necessary to exclude osteomyelitis.

The mainstay of treatment is rest and immobilization, usually in a plaster cast, which may need to be continued for many months, until disease activity and bone resorption have subsided. Surgery to the foot is contraindicated in the early stages, due to the gross hyperaemia of involved bone and the risk that it (like trauma) will trigger further bone resorption. Corrective surgery may, however, be useful at a later stage to remove bony prominences and appropriate (usually custom-made) footwear is required.

Summary

- Diabetic foot ulceration and amputation are common, but often preventable.
- Annual screening is vital to identify 'at risk' patients with neuropathy and peripheral vascular disease.
- Foot care education should be provided for all 'at risk' patients.
- Aggressive treatment of foot ulcers requires debridement, pressure relief, control of infection and often revascularization.

Areas of controversy

- Management of infection (indications for treatment, choice of antibiotic).
- Ideal methods of education on foot care.
- The pathogenic mechanisms of Charcot neuroarthropathy.
- The long-term benefit of femorodistal reconstruction versus below-knee amputation for neuroischaemic ulceration.

Further reading

- Malone JM, Snyder M, Anderson G, Bernhard VM, Holloway GA Jr, Bunt TJ. Prevention of amputation by diabetic education. *American Journal of Surgery* 1989;**158**: 520–523.
- Rith-Najarian SJ, Stolusky T, Ghodes DM. Identifying diabetic patients at high risk for lower-extremity amputation in a primary care setting. *Diabetes Care* 1992;**15**: 1386–1389.
- Veves A, Murray HJ, Young MJ, Boulton AJM. The risk of foot ulceration in diabetic patients with high foot pressure: a prospective study. *Diabetologia* 1992;**35**:660–663.
- Shaw JE, Boulton AJM. The Charcot foot. *The Foot* 1995;**5**:65–70.
- Shaw JE, Boulton AJM. The diabetic foot. In: Beard JD, Gaines PA (eds). *A Companion to Specialist Surgical Practice, vol VI. Vascular and Endovascular Surgery.* London: Saunders 1998:131–150.

17

Amputation and Rehabilitation

Neil CM Fyfe

Introduction

In patients presenting with intermittent claudication, the risk of an eventual amputation is <2%. However, in critical ischaemia, the probability of amputation being required is around 20% over 10 years. Amputation may be required following unsuccessful previous attempts at arterial reconstruction, because clinical conditions preclude such attempts or, with diminishing frequency, as a consequence of local non-availability of vascular surgical services.

Whatever the circumstances, clinicians and, most importantly, patients, should not look upon amputation as representing, in any sense, a 'failure'. Amputation is a perfectly valid management option following which the majority of patients do, with appropriate rehabilitation, learn to walk again and re-establish themselves in the community. The precise outcome for any individual depends on a range of factors relating both to surgical aspects of the amputation and to the general constitution (including co-existent disease) of the amputee; it is relative to the latter that goals should be set and outcomes judged. There are no absolutes in rehabilitation.

Aetiology

Peripheral vascular disease (PVD) is by far the commonest reason for lower limb amputation in Westernized societies. In the UK it accounts for >80% of all amputations and of these, 20–30% occur in patients with diabetes mellitus. In non-insulin-dependent diabetics the overall risk of amputation is 2% compared with 12% in insulin dependency. However, the risk can be substantially reduced with adequate foot care and footwear provision (see Chapter 16).

There is uncertainty regarding the total number of PVD amputations which are carried out annually in the UK due to the limitations of centralized NHS statistical records. In Denmark, the National Amputation Register has demonstrated a 27% fall in the number of major amputations due to PVD in the decade 1980 to 1990. This decline was attributed to the increased use of (distal) bypass operations. Similarly, a UK study published in 1994 showed a 32% reduction in the amputation rate was associated with an 11-fold increase in the 'volume' of arterial surgery over 8 years. However, in both studies the basal level of vascular surgical activity at the outset was extremely low.

By contrast, data from Maryland, USA, where vascular surgery had been well established, showed no change in the amputation rate when the volume of vascular surgery increased with the introduction of transluminal angioplasty. Thus, it seems that there is a point beyond which increased vascular surgical activity fails to exert any further downward pressure on amputation rates.

The progressive nature of arteriosclerosis is all too evident in PVD amputees: 30% may be expected to lose the contralateral limb within 3 years and half die within 5 years. At 4 years, only 20% are still alive without any further amputation having been performed.

The decision to amputate

Where there is extensive necrosis or ulceration such that even if surgical reconstructive possibilities do exist there is little or no likelihood of tissue viability, the decision that a primary amputation is required does not usually present difficulties provided that the situation is explained clearly to patient and relatives.

The role of amputation in the management of critical ischaemia remains controversial. There is little doubt that in such cases the ideal is for a revascularization procedure to be carried out with consequent recovery of ischaemic tissue, loss of pain and full restoration of function. Unfortunately, it is impossible to predict with certainty which patients will fail to respond to revascularization. However, most surgeons would agree that if the procedure does not result in a functioning limb for at least a year, primary amputation would, in retrospect, have been the appropriate management option.

Where a patient with critical ischaemia demonstrates co-existent disabilities which would render him unable to make use of a salvaged limb, the case for primary amputation is strengthened. Such patients include those previously immobile with, for example, a dense hemiplegia or other paralytic condition or severe arthritis. Marked cardiopulmonary disease may, of itself, contraindicate arterial surgery.

In summary, the decision on amputation in PVD may not be clear-cut but it should always be borne in mind that the fundamental aim of whatever treatment modality is adopted is restoration of maximum independence over the *medium to long term*, and that short-term limb salvage may not be consistent with this goal.

Amputation surgery

Level selection

The fundamental requirement for amputation is that healing should be expected at the level chosen. However, it must also be considered that in general the more distal the amputation site, the better the rehabilitation result in terms of walking ability (Fig. 17.1).

Starting with the most distal levels, individual or multiple toe amputations generally fail to heal unless the foot can be revascularized, except in the case of diabetics with good foot pulses. Transmetatarsal amputation using a long plantar flap gives excellent functional results in the few cases in which the local circulation will support it. Other partial foot amputations (Chopart) and Symes (through ankle) amputation are not recommended even if feasible as their long-term viability is poor and they present considerable prosthetic difficulties. Thus, the major levels in PVD are trans-tibial (TT, below knee), knee disarticulation (KD) or Gritti-Stokes (GS) and trans-femoral (TF, above knee) (Fig. 17.2).

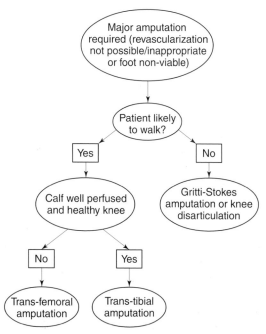

Fig. 17.1. Algorithm for the selection of amputation level.

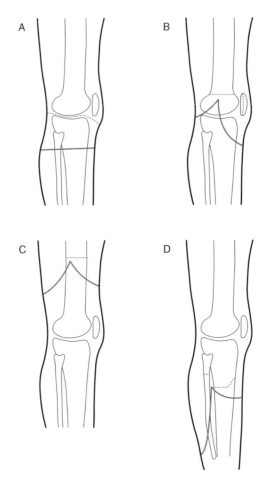

Fig. 17.2. Skin incisions (——) and level of bone section (- - - -) for (A) knee disarticulation (KD), (B) Gritti-Stokes (GS), (C) transfemoral (TF) and (D) transtibial (TT) amputations. The commonly used equal anterior and posterior flaps (TF) and the long posterior flap (TT) are used for illustrative purposes.

The following principles may be used as a guide to level selection:

- When a prosthetic limb is likely to be fitted, the TT level should always be attempted whenever there is a reasonable chance of healing. This results in superior rehabilitation.
- When there is a *severe* (i.e. >45°) knee flexion deformity, there is little point in preserving the knee joint and a higher amputation level is appropriate.
- If the patient is definitely unsuitable for prosthetic rehabilitation, a long stump such as a KD or GS can be very valuable as a 'lever'. This is especially true for double amputees.

Surgical techniques

Amputations must be carried out with an appreciation that a new organ of locomotion is under construction. This requires specific knowledge of the important principles and the procedure should never be delegated to unsupervised junior staff who lack experience of the procedure.

Important general points include:

- Flaps should be over sized initially, then shaped as required.
- Bone edges should be smoothed off and bevelled as appropriate.
- Muscles should not be dissected from deep facia or skin or the latter may be devitalized. Excess muscle should be filleted to avoid producing a bulky or bulbous stump.
- Nerves should be pulled down, divided cleanly and allowed to retract with, usually, no attempt at haemostasis required.
- Skin edges should be handled atraumatically. Subcuticular closures supplemented by adhesive strips are recommended.

Specific points are given below for each level of amputation.

Transfemoral

- Adequate myoplastic cover of the femoral end to avoid pain and discomfort caused by upward traction of tissues against the bone by the prosthetic socket and to allow balanced action of opposing muscle groups.
- Sufficient clearance above the knee joint centre (at least 12 cm) to allow room for the prosthetic knee joint without knee centre lowering and knee protrusion when sitting.

Knee disarticulation

- Mediolateral flaps so that the scar retracts into the intercondylar notch, away from the end-bearing area.

Gritti-Stokes

- Adequate fixation of the patellar remnant. Non-union thwarts the intention of end bearing.

Transtibial

- The long posterior myoplastic flap (Burgess) procedure gives excellent long-term compatibility with prosthetic wearing. The 'skew' flap utilizes the same posterior muscle flap but the skin flaps are 'skewed' with the aim of improving early skin healing.
- Bone section should be 15 cm below the joint line. Muscle wasting causes a longer stump to develop into a pointed bony 'strut' which

causes discomfort in the prosthetic socket. If necessary, stumps as short as 8 cm can be fitted using supracondylar sockets.

- Adequate myoplastic cover and bevelling of the tibial end.
- Avoidance of an excessively bulbous distal end by reducing flap muscle bulk.

The rehabilitation process

Organization

The rehabilitation of the elderly vascular amputee is a complex, multi-faceted process which demands a multidisciplinary approach. To this end the concept of the *team* approach has gained currency. The core members of an amputee rehabilitation team should include a vascular surgeon, specialist in rehabilitation medicine, physiotherapist and occupational therapist with specific training in this area, and a prosthetist. Others whose ready availability is invaluable are a social worker, community nurse, housing officer and general practitioner.

The problem with the team approach is that since most hospitals perform <10 amputations per year, it may not be feasible to constitute a team as described. In this event, it is still essential to have one or two named individuals who will accept responsibility for co-ordinating the rehabilitation process for every amputee. A suitably knowledgeable 'key therapist' is generally capable of co-ordinating the care of all amputees in an average district hospital.

Early assessment

If conditions allow, a preamputation consultation by the rehabilitation specialist (or key therapist) will prepare the patient for the likely programme to come, and realistic expectations may be implanted. A further assessment should be carried out 1 week postoperatively. At this time, it may be evident that certain patients are extremely unlikely to benefit from a prosthesis and, if so, early training in the independent use of a wheelchair should be initiated. Absolute contraindications to prosthetic rehabilitation are:

- extreme frailty;
- severe dementia;
- contralateral hemiplegia;
- severe cardiorespiratory disease;
- gross flexion deformities;
- severe arthritis of upper or lower limb joints;
- non-healing stumps.

In many cases it will not be apparent for some time whether or not a prosthesis is appropriate and postamputation mobility aids, which should be used in all prospective limb wearers, will often help in this decision. These devices are the pneumatic post-amputation mobility aid (PPAM aid) for TT stumps and the ischial bearing 'Femurett' for TF stumps. Apart from their use as assessment tools, these devices also allow strengthening of the remaining leg and upper limbs and are of considerable psychological benefit.

Other important preprosthetic measures are:

- elevation and active and passive movement of the stump to avoid contractures and to promote resolution of oedema;
- application of graduated compression stump socks designed to 'shape' the stump for prosthetic fitting.

Prostheses

Recent technological advances in prosthetic design have followed the strict application of biomechanical principles which have been derived from extensive studies in gait analysis. Furthermore, application of materials such as plastics (thermoplastic and thermosetting), carbon fibre and lightweight alloys have allowed the development of the *modular* approach to prosthetic construction with only the socket being bespoke to the patient. It is now usual for prostheses to be available for fitting within 5 working days compared to the 3 months or more that were required before the introduction of modular systems 15 years ago.

Outcome

The prime determinants of functional achievement amongst patients who are fitted with prostheses are:

- mental attitude and approach;
- physical constitution;
- level of amputation;
- condition of remaining limb;
- ability to put on and take off the limb;
- intensity of the rehabilitation programme.

Age and preamputation mobility are not good predictors. However, walking with the aid of a prosthesis involves a considerably increased energy cost — up to 33% in the case of a single TF amputation. Where energy reserves are restricted, as in the case of co-existent cardio-respiratory disease, prosthetic walking ability will be necessarily limited. Likewise, grossly impaired cognitive ability reliably augurs a poor mobility outcome.

The influence of *amputation level* on walking ability is all important. The outcome after TT amputation is approximately twice as good as after TF. However, this difference becomes less marked with the passage of time.

Overall, if amputees are correctly selected for prosthetic fitting, around 90% will have some useful function from their prostheses. However, the extent of prosthetic use is very variable:

- 20% of amputees regain unlimited mobility;
- 30% have limited mobility outdoors;
- 40% are restricted to home and garden;
- 10% despite having prostheses, remain chairbound.

In general, it seems that long-term mobility is best preserved in those living with relatives. Those living alone fare less well, whilst of those living in residential care only 30% continue to walk.

Summary

- Peripheral vascular disease accounts for 80% of all amputations.
- Management decisions in critical ischaemia should not be constrained by the short-term view.
- Amputation level selection and techniques are prime determinants of prosthetic rehabilitation outcome.
- Although only two-thirds of vascular amputees are suitable for prosthetic fitting, modern prosthetic and rehabilitation techniques allow 90–95% of these to regain walking ability.

Areas of controversy

- Has vascular surgery now reached its limit of amputation prevention in the population?
- Should more primary amputations be performed?
- Should the rehabilitation of amputees involve greater or lesser use of prostheses?

Further reading

- Murdoch G, Wilson AB (eds) *Amputation Surgical Practice and Patient Management.* Oxford: Butterworth-Heineman, 1996.
- Murdoch G, Wilson AB. *A Primer on Amputations and Artificial Limbs.* Springfield: Thomas, 1998.

● Greenhalgh RM, Jamieson CW, Nicolaides AN (eds). *Limb Salvage and Amputation for Vascular Disease*. Philadelphia: WB Saunders, 1988.
● Vitali M, Robinson KP, Andrews BG, Harris EE, Redhead RG. *Amputations and Prostheses*, 2nd edn. London: Baillière Tindall, 1986.

18

Varicose Veins

Alun H Davies

Introduction

A varicose vein is a superficial vein, mainly in the lower limb, with incompetent valves. About 1 in 1000 people in Europe undergo surgery per annum for varicose veins.

Aetiology

Valve incompetence may be secondary to valvular damage following recanalization after thrombosis or may be related to a vein-wall deficiency defect which causes dilatation and hence renders the valves non-functional. The deep vein perforators and the main long or short saphenous trunks may also be incompetent. However, it is only the superficial vein tributaries that become visible or palpable under the skin.

The commonest source of reflux is the saphenofemoral junction which leads to reflux in the long saphenous vein and its tributaries (Fig. 18.1). Long saphenous reflux may occur secondary to incompetence of the isolated mid-thigh perforator.

Long saphenous reflux as determined by duplex occurs in approximately 65% of patients complaining of varicose veins. The anatomy in the popliteal fossa is very variable.

Only 60% of patients have true saphenopopliteal incompetence and the remainder may have incompetence in the gastrocnemius veins or the posterior perforator in the thigh, from a connection of the long saphenous vein.

Risk factors

Risk factors for varicose veins include:

- family history;
- pregnancy;
- past history of deep venous thrombosis or fracture.

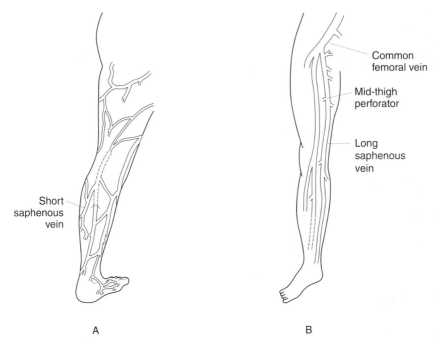

Fig. 18.1. (A) Posterior and (B) anterior views of the superficial venous system.

The precise family history with respect to the aetiology of varicose veins is uncertain but there does seem to be a strong association. Pregnancy is a well established risk factor due to impaired venous return caused by inferier vena cava or iliac vein compression compounded by the hormonal effects on the vein wall. Varicose veins may regress after pregnancy although significant reflux may remain. Similarly, in rare cases, pelvic or abdominal tumours causing more proximal vein pressure may give rise to distal vein symptoms.

Any person known to have had a deep venous thrombosis or long bone fracture should be regarded as having deep venous insufficiency unless proven otherwise by duplex.

Clinical features

Symptoms may relate to cosmesis, reflux or complications of varicose veins.

Most patients regard varicose veins as a cosmetic problem. Patients may complain of skin changes such as eczema or frank ulceration. Aching and heaviness in the lower limb with swelling classically towards the end of the day may well be due to reflux in the main long and short saphenous vein systems, although there is often little relationship between the size and extent of varicose veins and the symptoms. It should be noted also that symptoms, particularly those of venous reflux, may occur with little or no visible varicosities.

Diagnosis

Examination

The following questions are important:

- Does the patient have varicose veins?
- What is the distribution of the veins?
- Is there any skin damage?
- Are the foot pulses palpable?
- Is there any evidence of previous surgery?
- What is the likely source of the reflux?

A patient's own diagnosis of varicose veins may be variable and include dilated superficial venules, thread veins or visible veins that are not technically varicose.

Thread veins are a common cause for complaint in females due to their unsightly appearance. They often occur during pregnancy and may be related to hormonal change and have little relation to varicose veins, being more common in the thigh. Treatment is only justified for cosmetic reasons.

The visibility of *superficial veins* depends on the amount of sub-cutaneous fat and skin colour. Those with pale skin often have visible veins on their legs and arms which are normal. Veins may also become prominent in people who exercise regularly, hence the term 'athletic vein'. There are no symptoms and no indication for treatment.

Aching and swelling of the leg may be related to other causes such as osteoarthritis, immobility and lymphoedema.

Distribution of the veins

It is important to assess the extent and distribution of varicose veins as this will influence the form of treatment given (Fig. 18.1). Varicose veins of the thigh or medial calf are usually due to long saphenous vein reflux, whereas those in the popliteal fossa or posterior calf may be due to short saphenous reflux. However, it should be noted that distribution may be an unreliable guide to the source of reflux.

Skin damage

This may be present as small patches of eczema over prominent varices or more sinister changes of lipodermatosclerosis and/or ulceration of the gaiter region of the ankle, classically above the medial malleolus.

These changes are secondary to long-standing venous hypertension causing impaired tissue perfusion. Venous hypertension can arise purely due to isolated superficial venous reflux but is more commonly associated with deep venous insufficiency and perforator incompetence (see Chapter 19).

Foot pulses

The presence of foot pulses should be documented. This is important for two reasons: if there is ulceration present the problem may actually be a mixed arterial venous ulcer; and some surgeons regard varicose veins in a patient with claudication as being a contraindication for surgery as the vein may need to be used as a bypass conduit.

Previous surgery

A scar at the site of the saphenofemoral ligation or previous surgery in the lower limb may indicate that the long saphenous vein has been stripped. Previous surgery may be associated with evidence of saphenous neuralgia. Patients having undergone previous surgery are generally thought to require some formal imaging prior to treatment, such as a duplex scan.

Which system is refluxing?

This is an important question clinically because the optimal treatment depends on abolishing the source of the reflux. The clinical test of choice is the Trendelenburg test using either an elastic tourniquet or the hand to compress the saphenofemoral junction and then looking at the filling when the leg is put in the dependent position and the tourniquet or hand released (see Chapter 3). However, many feel that a more formal investigation may be required, the minimum being the use of a hand-held Doppler. Others believe a duplex examination should be performed (Fig. 18.2).

With respect to either deep vein occlusion or significant incompetence, the only clinical test available is Perthes' test. This involves placing a tourniquet around the thigh and then asking the patient to exercise his calf muscles for 3 min. A positive test is associated with marked pain in the lower limb.

Doppler examination

With the patient standing, the long saphenous vein in the thigh is located with the hand-held Doppler by squeezing and releasing the calf.

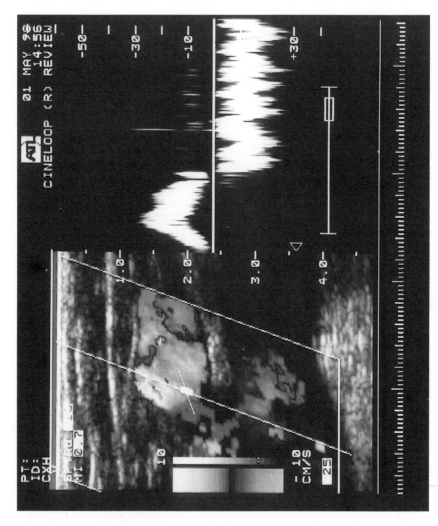

Fig. 18.2. Duplex scan showing saphenofemoral vein junction incompetence.

A classical venous sound is heard in the normal long saphenous vein on compression of the calf. However, in the presence of incompetence, when the calf is released there is a classic 'whooshing' sound. This can be further elaborated by getting the patient to lie flat, elevating the legs to 45° and performing a Trendelenburg test with the Doppler rather than by hand. If the reflux is still present when the tourniquet occludes the upper region, this may be suggestive of some mid-thigh perforator incompetence. Short saphenous vein incompetence can also be excluded by performing the Doppler test with the probe at the lower part of the popliteal fossa. However, at this point it should be noted that there is variable anatomy and any positive test should be confirmed using duplex ultrasound.

The exact role of duplex ultrasound in the assessment of primary varicose veins is uncertain. Certainly, it is more sensitive than hand-held Doppler in the evaluation of veins and in any patient with suspected short saphenous vein incompetence it is the investigation of choice.

The following are guidelines for which patients should undergo colour Doppler ultrasound:

- reflux in the popliteal fossa on hand-held Doppler examination;
- varicose veins in the popliteal fossa;
- reflux not controlled by an above-knee tourniquet;
- recurrent varicose veins (particularly in patients who have had previous surgery);
- past history of deep venous thrombosis or fracture;
- presence of lipodermatosclerosis and/or ulceration.

The aim of the duplex scan is to confirm and locate the source of the reflux when short saphenous reflux or recurrent saphenofemoral incompetence is suspected. Deep venous insufficiency should be excluded if there is a past history of deep vein thrombosis, fracture or evidence of skin damage at the ankle.

Venography

This has the major disadvantage of being invasive with a small risk of inducing phlebitis but is an acceptable alternative to duplex. There are undoubtedly those who still advocate conventional ascending venography to confirm deep venous occlusion and that deep venous reflux requires descending venography for confirmatory diagnosis (see Chapter 5).

Management

The presence of varicose veins is not necessarily an indication for treatment. Patients with symptoms due to or secondary to varicose veins should be treated. Any patient undergoing treatment for varicose veins should be reminded that treatment is not necessarily curative but palliative.

Treatment can be divided into:

- Medical;
- Sclerotherapy;
- Surgery.

Medical treatment

Many patients can be managed non-operatively, including those who have deep venous incompetence or are unfit for surgery. The patient with marked varicose veins may benefit from the use of class II support hosiery stockings below the knee. Full-length stockings are useful in those patients who have symptomatic varicose veins but compliance can be poor and they are difficult to apply. Other measures include elevation of the legs, and regular walking to improve the calf muscle pump.

In patients with eczematous or ulcerative disease there is a role for four-layer bandaging. Superficial thrombophlebitis is also often treated by support hosiery, non-steroidal anti-inflammatory agents and antibiotics.

Sclerotherapy

This can involve the injection of either a sclerosant or the use of laser treatment. The former aims to damage the endothelium and hence by thrombosis obtain occlusion of that segment. A sclerosant can be used for thread veins and minor varicose veins without evidence of significant reflux. However, patients should be warned of two possible risks: skin staining and exudation of sclerosant resulting in local ulceration.

Laser sclerotherapy is available for thread veins. The success of this technique is dependent on the wavelength used. Patients should be warned that there is a risk of hypo/hyper skin pigmentation over the area of treatment.

Surgery

The aims of surgery are:

- correction of reflux;
- removal of varicosities.

Correction of reflux

Reflux is corrected by ligation of either the saphenofemoral or saphenopopliteal junctions. With respect to the long saphenous vein, in the case of reflux, there is increasing evidence that stripping should be performed to the knee. This adds to postoperative discomfort but reduces recurrence rates; stripping to the knee level has not been shown to increase the risk of saphenous nerve stripping, unlike stripping the vein to the ankle. Furthermore, as a rule, the short saphenous vein is not stripped and is just ligated to avoid the potential risk of damage to the sural nerve.

Varicose veins due to isolated perforator incompetence without underlying deep venous thrombosis are uncommon other than in the case of mid-thigh perforator incompetence when they are usually dealt with by stripping the long saphenous vein.

Removal of varicosities

This is usually performed in conjunction with the procedure for correction of reflux. However, for cosmetic reasons, it may be performed as an isolated procedure and if there are very few avulsions/phlebectomies can be performed under local anaesthetic. This often gives better cosmetic results than sclerotherapy.

Treatment of the complications of varicose veins

Bleeding

Initial treatment is with compression and then surgical correction of the varicose vein.

Superficial thrombophlebitis

Initially this is treated conservatively with non-steroidal anti-inflammatory agents, antibiotics and support hosiery. Then, suitable investigations should be arranged and once the phlebitis has settled, appropriate venous surgery offered.

With respect to eczema and ulcers, venous surgery should be offered once sufficient evidence exists to suggest that there is reflux in the superficial system that needs correcting.

In pregnancy, no treatment should be offered if possible and management is with support hosiery; however, surgery can be performed under local anaesthetic if necessary.

Outcome

The results of surgery are variable with a recurrence rate of 5–30%. There may be a return of symptoms or varicosities. Overall, patient satisfaction with varicose vein surgery is in the region of 80–85% with a substantial number of patients being dissatisfied with the overall outcome.

Recurrent varicose veins

These are a very difficult problem to treat; a surgical treatment should not be offered until the patient has been adequately assessed. Treatment is obviously dependent on the cause of the recurrence and the severity of the symptoms. Initially, the patient, as a minimum, should have a duplex examination and may even need to have venography. The patient should be told that his revision surgery is associated with a higher risk of complications.

In the presence of deep venous reflux, conservative management with support hosiery is probably the ideal choice. Persistent or recurrent saphenofemoral reflux should be treated by redo saphenous vein surgery. It is imperative that these patients are told, as previously, that venous surgery is not curative and only palliative.

Summary

- Varicose veins may cause aching, cosmetic problems, eczema or ulceration of the limb.
- Treatment may be medical with support hosiery or sclerotherapy, or surgical.
- Indications for duplex are recurrent varicose veins and preoperative assessment of the saphinopopliteal junction.
- The standard operation is saphenous vein flush ligation, stripping and avulsions.

Areas of controversy

- Role of duplex scanning in the assessment of primary varicose veins.
- Relative benefits of stripping the long saphenous vein and superficial flush ligation.

Further reading

- Negus D. *Leg Ulcers*. Oxford: Butterworth-Heinemann, 1991.
- Browse NL, Burnand KG, Lea Thomas M. *Diseases of the Veins: Pathology, Diagnosis and Treatment*. London: Edward Arnold, 1988.
- Tibbs DJ. Venous disorders, vascular malformations and chronic ulceration in lower limbs. In: Morris PJ, Malt RA (eds) *Oxford Textbook of Surgery*. Oxford: Oxford University Press, 1994, pp 503–596.
- Tibbs DJ. *Varicose Veins and Related Disorders*. Oxford: Butterworth-Heinemann, 1992.

19
Venous Ulceration

Alun H Davies

Introduction

Between 1.5 and 3 per 1000 of the population have active leg ulcers and the prevalence increases with age up to 20 per 1000 in those over 80 years. Leg ulceration is mainly associated with venous disease; however, arterial disease is present in approximately 20% of cases.

Aetiology

The underlying cause of venous ulceration is venous hypertension. This derives from two mechanisms:

- 'adynamic' — hydrostatic pressure due to valve failure and the weight of the blood pressing distally (gravitational/immobility);
- 'dynamic' — the muscles contract and blood travels from the superficial to the deep system. However, when these valves are incompetent blood is transmitted superficially and the intra-compartmental forces are transmitted directly to the subcutaneous veins and dermal capillaries.

The above would suggest that perforator veins have an important role in the development of venous ulcers, but the stage at which a perforator vein becomes of critical importance in the development of a venous ulcer is controversial. The exact cellular changes that occur are again a matter for speculation.
  The two main theories are:

- white blood cell become trapped and cause increased peripheral resistance and ultimately tissue ischaemia;
- the development of fibrin plugs leads to tissue ischaemia.

Clinical features

The patient will often have obvious varicosities with evidence of varicose eczema, skin pigmentation and frank ulceration. Clinical examination is as for primary varicose veins (see Chapter 18).

The key clinical test is the Perthes test which involves occluding the superficial venous outflow of the limb with a tourniquet or compressing it with an elastic bandage, and then getting the patient to exercise. Severe pain on exercise suggests that there is deep venous occlusion as the superficial veins are collapsed and unable to empty the blood.

Investigation

The investigations for a patient potentially presenting with a new leg ulcer include:

- venous duplex;
- ankle brachial pressure index (ABPI), if ABPI is <0.8, the patient needs arterial duplex or angiography;
- biopsy;
- blood tests, full blood count, Zn, Mg, vasculitic screen and glucose level.

Although hand-held Doppler is easily performed, it has been superceded by colour Doppler which allows full evaluation of the veins and identification of all sites of valvular insufficiency, venous thrombosis and venous occlusion.

Photoplethysmography, light reflective rheography, mercury strain gauge plethysmography and air plethysmography have all been used to elucidate venous pathology. None has gained widespread clinical use and they are mainly used as research tools.

Differential diagnosis

The differential diagnosis of a venous ulcer is listed in Table 19.1 and the classic sites of various ulcers in Table 19.2.

Management

Conservative treatment of venous ulceration always precedes any thought of surgical intervention (see Fig. 19.1).

The main form of non-operative treatment is compression therapy. In the UK the four-layer bandaging (orthopaedic wool, crepe, Elset, Coban) technique is very popular, in Europe short stretch bandaging is used and in the USA the Unna boot is the chosen method. In the trials to date there is no evidence that any of these methods is superior with respect to healing rates. Antibiotics are only indicated in the treatment of specific infections which are identified following microbiological testing.

The role of one-stop clinics in confirming diagnosis and therefore commencing appropriate treatment is becoming more important with a subsequent move to management in the community.

Table 19.1. Differential diagnosis of leg ulcers.

Venous	Gravitational, phlebitis
Arterial	Atherosclerosis (Martorell's ulcer of shin, arteriovenous fistula)
Lymphatic	Infection, trauma, ischaemia
Vasopastic	Raynaud's phenomenon, pernio, paralysed limb, erythrocyanosis frigida (Brazin's disease)
Traumatic	Pressure (e.g. POP casts) self-inflicted, burns, injections, sclerosant, cortisone, drug addict
Infective	Chronic bacterial, tuberculous, treponemal, progressive synergistic bacterial gangrene (Meleney), tropical, osteomyelitis (Brodie's abscess), yaws, leprosy, anthrax
Neoplastic	Epithelioma, rodent ulcer, Marjolin's wound cancer, basal cell carcinoma, leukaemia, squamous cell carcinoma, lymphoma
Malnutrition	Scurvy, pellagra, senility, diabetes mellitus, necrobiosis lipoidica, acholuria familial jaundice, ulcerative colitis, pyoderma gangrenosum
Neuropathic	Diabetes mellitus, spina bifida, syringomyelia, stroke
Rheumatoid	
Vasculitic	Scleroderma, polyarteritis nodosa

Table 19.2. Differential diagnosis by 'classical' location of ulcer.

Gaiter area	Venous
Sole of foot	Arterial
	Nerve — tabes, neuropathy, lower motor neuron
Toes	Vasospastic
	Fungal
	Trauma
	Osteomyelitis

Drugs

There is no evidence to support the systemic use of any pharmacological agent to increase ulcer healing rates.

Surgical treatment

Surgical intervention is thought to be indicated if conservative measures are failing or in the prevention of recurrence. Straightforward venous surgery involves long saphenous vein ligation, stripping and short saphenous vein ligation.

Methods of dealing with the incompetent communicating and perforator veins have gained increasing popularity with the development of subfascial endoscopic perforator surgery (SEPS). The main advantage of this technique is that surgery can be offered from a distance and does not require division of poor skin to allow access to the veins (Fig. 19.2).

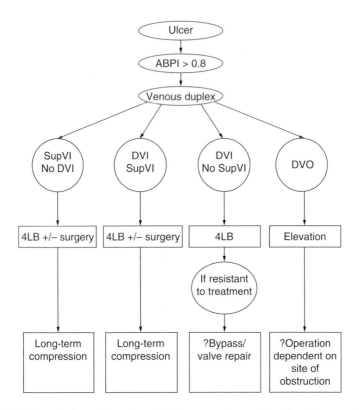

Fig. 19.1. **Diagnosis and treatment of venous ulceration. SupVI, superficial vein incompetence; DVI, deep vein incompetence; 4LB, 4-layer bandaging; DVO, deep vein obstruction.**

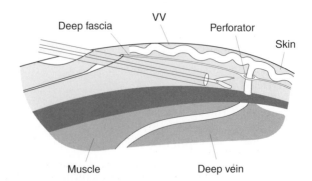

Fig. 19.2. **Subfascial endoscopic surgery involves placing a telescope beneath the fascia of the calf. Perforating veins traversing the subfascial space are interrupted under direct vision.**

The role of deep venous reconstruction is still unproven. Various procedures have been described such as a bypass procedure using competent vein or direct valve repair.

Surgery also has a role in ulcer excision and primary skin grafting can give good initial results. In the case of significant arterial disease, appropriate revascularization treatment by angioplasty or bypass may be indicated.

Outcome

Using standard medical treatment, healing rates of 70% at 12 weeks are often found but rates >80% are hard to achieve. The overall rate of recurrence is influenced by subsequent treatment following healing. Undoubtedly the use of compression stockings reduces the rate of recurrence. Class III compression stockings have a lower recurrence rate than Class II but patient compliance is not as great and hence there is a certain trade-off when deciding which to use. To date there is no pharmacological medication that improves outcome.

Summary

- Venous ulcers are a major cause of morbidity worldwide.
- Compression therapy can significantly improve healing rates.
- Compression stockings prevent the recurrence of venous leg ulcers.
- Patients with untreated arterial disease are unsuitable for compression therapy.

Areas of controversy

- Best method of compression for optimum treatment.
- Role of surgery in the treatment of venous ulcers.
- Best way to prevent ulcer recurrence.

Further reading

- Compression therapy for venous leg ulcers. *Effective Health Care* 1997;**3**:4.
- Negus D. *Leg Ulcers*. Oxford: Butterworth-Heinemann, 1991.
- Browse NL, Burnand KG, Lea Thomas M. *Diseases of the Veins: Pathology, Diagnosis and Treatment*. London: Edward Arnold, 1988.
- Tibbs DJ. Venous disorders, vascular malformations and chronic ulceration in lower limbs. In: Morris PJ, Malt RA (eds) *Oxford Textbook of Surgery*. Oxford: Oxford University Press, 1994, pp 503–596.
- Tibbs DJ. *Varicose Veins and Related Disorders*. Oxford: Butterworth-Heinemann, 1992.

20
Deep Venous Thrombosis and Pulmonary Embolism

Alun H Davies

Introduction

The true incidence of deep venous thrombosis (DVT) and pulmonary embolism in patients admitted to hospital is uncertain. The overall incidence, of DVT is thought to be 50 per 100 000 patients with the incidence of pulmonary embolism being about half this. It has been estimated that up to 30% of patients undergoing general surgical procedures and 50% of those undergoing major orthopaedic procedures may have a DVT.

Deep venous thrombosis

Aetiology

The classic causes were laid down by Virchow who emphasized the need for there to be stasis, potential injury to the wall vessel and/or increased coagulability. DVT occurs most commonly in the calf veins, especially those within the soleal plexus. Moving up the leg, they become rarer from the calf femoral common iliac and inferior vena cava.

There is evidence to suggest that thrombosis is more common in the left limb. This may be related to the relationship with the left and right common iliac arteries.

Thrombosis mostly remains confined to the calf vessels and the majority undergo spontaneous resolution. In about 20% of patients the calf vessel thrombosis propagates into the popliteal, femoral and iliac vessels. The overall consensus is that 10% of patients who have proximal DVT, if not treated, will go on to develop a pulmonary embolism.

Risk factors

There are numerous risk factors for DVT.

- age over 40;
- pregnancy/oestrogens;
- heart disease;

- malignancy;
- trauma;
- sepsis;
- hypercoagulable states;
- previous DVT/pulmonary embolism;
- cryofibrinogenaemia;
- Behçet's syndrome;
- varicose veins.

The identification of high-risk patients preoperatively should allow suitable prophylactic treatment.

Clinical features

The majority of patients presenting with a DVT do not have any symptoms; however, if present, the commonest is pain followed by swelling of the limb. Distension of the superficial veins with some erythema may be present. The patient may present with a pyrexia. On examination Homans' test may be positive, i.e. this is pain experienced in the calf with forced dorsal flexion of the foot.

There are two extreme types of DVT:

- *phlegmasia alba dolens* in which the limb is oedematous, painful but not ischaemic and function is normal;
- *phlegmasia caerula dolens* in which the extremity is blue, very oedematous, has bullae and there may be a risk of arterial insufficiency and nerve damage. There is clinical evidence of sensory and motor deficits.

In these cases it is certainly possible for venous gangrene to occur.

Table 20.1 summarizes the criteria and a method for assessing the clinical probability of a DVT.

Investigation

A potential investigation protocol is given in Figure 20.2.

D-dimers are unique fragments derived from fibrin by the hydrolytic action of plasma. Thrombus is associated with an increase in the plasma level of D-dimer and there is increasing evidence that normal levels of D-dimer can 'rule out' a diagnosis of DVT.

The non-invasive investigation of choice is colour Doppler imaging which allows B-mode imaging to be combined with Doppler signalling (Fig. 20.1). Thrombosis is diagnosed from occlusion of the vein, lack of compressibility of the vein or direct visualization of the thrombus. The specificity for duplex and venography has been as good as 98% and 95%, respectively. It should, however, be noted that duplex scanning is operator dependent.

Table 20.1. **Clinical diagnosis of deep venous thrombosis.**

Major criteria	Active cancer
	Paralysis or recent plaster immobilization of leg
	Recently bedridden (>3 days) or major surgery (<4 weeks)
	Past history of DVT or strong family history
	Thigh and calf swelling
	Calf swelling 3 cm > asymptomatic side
Minor criteria	History of recent leg trauma (<60 days)
	Hospitalization within the last 6 months
	Unilateral pitting oedema
	Unilateral erythema or dilated superficial veins
Clinical probability	*High*
	>3 major points and no alternative diagnosis
	>2 major points and >2 minor points + no alternative diagnosis
	Low
	1 major point + >2 minor points + alternative diagnosis
	1 major point + >1 minor point + no alternative diagnosis
	0 major points + >3 minor points + alternative diagnosis
	0 major points + >2 minor points + no alternative diagnosis
	Moderate
	All other combinations

Ascending venography may be regarded as the gold standard investigation. However, it is an invasive procedure which requires contrast to be injected into veins in the dorsum of the foot. The criteria required to make the diagnosis of DVT are constant filling defects, cut-off of a contrast column, opacification of part of the vein, lateral flow and presence of torturous collaterals. This technique is not widely used because of the development of more reliable non-invasive techniques.

Impedance plethysmography allows non-invasive assessesment of volume changes in the limb. However, it is not as sensitive as duplex and cannot detect calf veins or non-occluding thrombi.

Using hand-held Doppler, thrombosis is indicated by an absence of flow or the absence of augmentation of flow with respiration and compression. This again is not as reliable as Duplex imaging.

Management

The commonly-held opinion is that the incidence of DVT and pulmonary embolism can be reduced by the limitation of venous stasis. Therefore, much emphasis is being put on prophylactic measures that

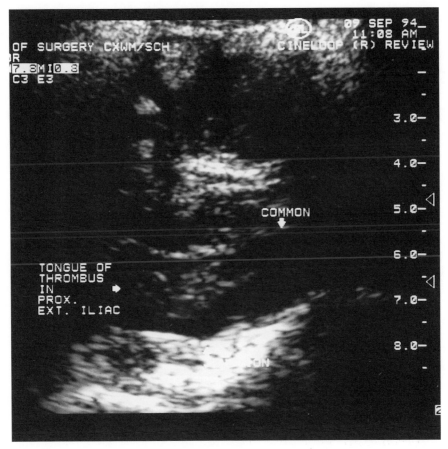

Fig. 20.1(A). **Duplex scan showing thrombus in the external iliac vein.**

can be used to prevent venous thrombosis. These can be divided into physical and pharmacological measures.

Physical measures

Early mobilization with leg exercises following surgery has been shown to decrease the incidence of DVT.

There are two forms of compression:

- thromboembolic (TED) stockings are used to improve venous return and minimize the effects of the post-phlebitic syndrome. Support hosiery is recommended for a variable time depending on the patients symptomatology with respect to swelling and other changes.
- pneumatic compression devices in the operating theatre stimulate emptying of the deep venous plexus, especially in the foot and calf, and increase venous return and fibrinolytic activity.

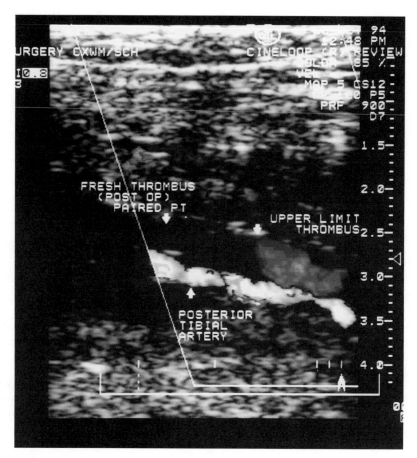

Fig. 20.1(B). Duplex scan showing thrombus in a calf vein.

Pharmacological measures (see also Chapter 6)

The administration of low-dose *subcutaneous heparin* has been shown to reduce the incidence of DVT and also to decrease the number of fatal pulmonary emboli. The usual regimen for administration is 5000 units subcutaneously preoperatively and 5000 units either 8 or 12 hourly post-operatively. Complications include thrombocytopenia and haemorrhage. The benefits of using low-molecular-weight heparin are in the process of being evaluated.

Warfarin is undoubtedly effective at preventing venous thrombosis and is used in orthopaedic surgery. However, it needs to be used with great care and careful monitoring of the prothrombin times because of a risk of haemorrhage. Other side-effects include dermatitis, hypersensitive

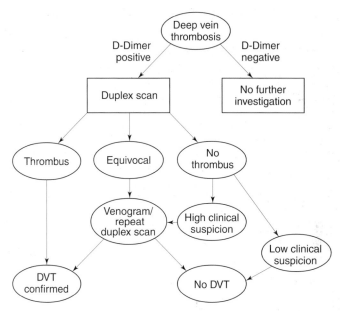

Fig. 20.2. **Protocol for investigation of a patient with a deep vein thrombosis.**

reactions and nausea and vomiting. Furthermore, it should not be used during pregnancy as it has the potential to cross the placenta and is teratogenic. Other potential problems with warfarin administration are patient compliance and interactions with other drugs and disease states (Table 20.2).

Dextran (70 and 40) functions by decreasing platelet adhesion and reduces the plasma concentration of Factor VIII. This used to be popular prior to the introduction of subcutaneous heparin. The dosage is 500 ml of a 6% solution and 1000 ml of a 10% solution over 24 h for up to 72 h. It is now regarded as a second-line agent in the prevention of thromboembolic disease.

Intravenous heparin is effective in preventing the progression of thromboembolic complications in patients who have a DVT. Initially the patient is given a low dose of 5000 units of IV heparin followed by an infusion which normally commences at about 1000–2000 units/h, the aim being to run an APPT of about double the control value. IV heparin is usually continued until oral anticoagulation using warfarin has been evaluated and is sufficient. However, there is evidence that high-dose low-molecular-weight subcutaneous heparin may be as effective in the outpatient setting, although this has resource implications for primary health-care services. Long-term oral anticoagulation with warfarin is usually recommended for 3–6 months.

Table 20.2 **Interactions of warfarin with other medications and disease states.**

Potentiates effect (prolongs PT)	Inhibits effect (shortens PT)
Medications	Medications
Alcohol	Barbiturates
Allopurinol	Cholestyramine
Amiodarone	Corticosteroids
Anabolic steroids	Diuretics
Aspirin	Glutethimide
Cimetidine	Griseofulvin
Clofibrate	Oral contraceptives
Disulfiram	Rifampin
Erythromycin	
Metronidazole	Disease states
NSAIDs	Uraemia
Phenylbutazone	High vitamin K diet
Phenytoin	High vitamin C diet
Quinidine	Hypermetabolic states
Thyroxine	Low vitamin K diet
Trimethoprim-sulphamethoxazole	Hepatic insufficiency

PT = prothrombin time.

A major dilemma with respect to the treatment of DVT is whether patients with calf vein thrombosis should receive anticoagulation since only 20% will go on to develop a more proximal thrombus. One suggestion is that patients should not receive treatment unless on subsequent, either duplex or venography, investigation, they have developed a proximal propagation.

Contraindications to the administration of heparin are:

• active bleeding;
• recent neurosurgery;
• an intracerebral bleed.

Gastrointestinal bleeding and a recent stroke may be considered to be relative contraindications. Indeed, thrombolysis can be used to bring about the dissolution of DVT. There is some evidence to suggest that there is a lower incidence of postphlebitic syndrome in patients who have had thrombolytic therapy. However, this advantage has to be weighed against the potential complications of thrombolysis administration: haemorrhage, allergic response to the thrombolytic agent, and risk of small clots embolizing and resulting in pulmonary emboli.

Surgery

Patients who have a major long-term contraindication to anticoagulation and have had recurrent pulmonary emboli may be suitable for the insertion of a device, either by direct operative procedure or by placing of an intraluminal device such as a Greenfield filter, to interrupt flow in the inferior vena cava. The main aim of this is to prevent a fatal pulmonary embolism. The role of iliofemoral thrombectomy has not been well established and may well be superseded by catheter-directed thrombolysis.

In patients with long-standing iliofemoral disease limb swelling is a major problem and reconstructive venous procedures may be appropriate, e.g. a Palma operation in a patient with an occlusion of the iliofemoral venous system which involves mobilizing the contralateral long saphenous vein and performing an anastomosis to the common femoral vein in a similar manner to a femorofemoral cross-over.

Pulmonary embolism

Pulmonary emboli occur mainly when thrombi are dislodged from lower limb vessels, particularly the iliofemoral vessels. They occur in about 10–20% of patients who have confirmed proximal DVT. The overall mortality rate for pulmonary emboli in hospital is 5–9%.

Clinical features

Patients may present with:

- dyspnoea;
- haemoptysis;
- pleuritic pain;
- tachypnoea;
- tachycardia;
- clinical thrombophlebitis.

In view of the diversity of clinical presentation, a high index of suspicion must be kept.

Investigation

A potential investigation protocol is given in Figure 20.3.

The initial investigation is a chest X-ray: the abnormalities to look for are an hyperlucent area or the presence of an effusion, but its main benefit is the exclusion of other causes or diagnoses. An ECG is often performed but again may not be diagnostic.

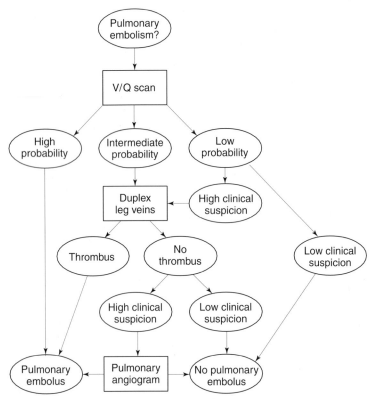

Fig. 20.3. Protocol for investigation of a patient with a pulmonary embolism.

In the immediate situation, arterial gases may suggest a problem with oxygen transfer and may support the diagnosis of a pulmonary embolism.

The commonest investigation for the confirmation of pulmonary embolism is a ventilation perfusion (V/Q) scan. The diagnosis of a pulmonary embolism is suggested if the ventilation scan is normal but abnormalities can be seen on the perfusion scan. However, again this is not 100% diagnostic.

The gold standard investigation for confirming the diagnosis of pulmonary embolism is pulmonary angiography (Fig. 20.4). However, this is an invasive procedure and should only be performed in those patients in whom it is anticipated that thrombolysis or surgery may be indicated.

Management

The aims of treatment are to:

- prevent propagation of further thromboembolic episodes;
- aid the natural fibrinolytic activity;
- prevent recurrence.

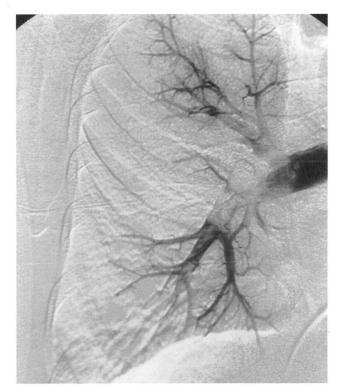

Fig. 20.4. **Pulmonary angiography showing a large pulmonary embolus.**

Initially, respiratory support may be required in the form of administration of oxygen by mask or tracheal intubation. Any evidence of hypertension or heart failure may suggest the need for inotropic support. There is evidence to suggest that aggressive fluid management by improving left atrial filling may be important. It is important that those patients who have had a major pulmonary embolism are nursed in an appropriate environment.

Anticoagulation

The patient is given a loading dose of 5000–10 000 u of heparin, and then 1000 unit/h. The aim is to keep the APPT about twice the normal range. Heparin is then administered for between 5 and 10 days and the patient is then put routinely on oral anticoagulation for a minimum of 3 months. Patients who are confirmed to have a DVT are given thromboembolic stockings (see above).

The incidence of recurrent pulmonary emboli on adequate heparinization is approximately 10–15%, but without it the risk is up to 40%.

Thrombolysis

The major cause of death following a massive pulmonary emboli is that of right-sided cardiac failure due to the marked pulmonary vessel resistance. The advantage of thrombolysis is that it may be able to dissolve this clot more quickly and help lower hypertension and thereby reduce cardiac output. However, there is no long-term evidence to suggest that thrombolytic therapy is beneficial except in patients who have had a massive embolus.

Surgery

Operative embolectomy again is only of benefit in patients who have had a massive pulmonary emboli. Preoperative angiography is required to confirm the diagnosis and the procedure is associated with up to 50% mortality. With the development of endovascular techniques, there is evidence to suggest that directed suction embolectomy may be a future alternative.

Outcome

Up to 10% of patients presenting with a clinical DVT may develop a pulmonary emboli. The use of prophylactic measures has reduced the number of postoperative DVT and the number of fatal pulmonary emboli.

Summary

- Deep venous thrombosis is common after surgery.
- D-dimer has a role as a screening test for DVT.
- The initial investigation of choice is duplex examination.
- The use of prophylactic measures is important to prevent deep venous thrombosis and pulmonary embolism.
- Drug interactions with warfarin should be considered.
- A postphlebitic limb can be a major cause of morbidity.
- Pulmonary angiography is the gold standard for confirming the diagnosis of pulmonary embolism.

Area of controversy

- Which patients should receive perioperative thromboprophylaxis?
- Should patients presenting with deep venous thrombosis be treated with intravenous or subcutaneous high-dose heparin?
- Should isolated calf deep venous thrombosis be treated?
- Role of thrombolysis in the treatment of deep venous thrombosis or pulmonary embolism remains undefined.

Further reading

- Tibbs DJ. *Varicose Veins and Related Disorders.* Oxford: Butterworth-Heinemann, 1992.
- Kim Lyerly H, Sabiston DC. Deep vein thrombosis and pulmonary embolism. Morris PJ, Malt RA (eds) *Oxford Textbook of Surgery.* Oxford: Oxford University Press, 1994, pp 597–607.
- Corris P, Ellis D, Foley N, Miller A. Suspected acute pulmonary embolism: a practical approach. *Thorax* 1997;**52**:S1–S24
- Sissons GRJ. Investigation of suspected lower limb venous thrombosis. *Roy Coll Surg Engl* 1998;**80**:49–54.
- Khaira HS, Mann J. Plasma D-dimer measurement in patients with suspected DVT — a means of avoiding unnecessary venography. *European Journal of Vascular and Endovascular Surgery* 1998;**15**:235–238.
- Wells PS, Hirsch J, Andersen DR *et al.* Accuracy of clinical assessment of deep vein thrombosis. *Lancet* 1996;**348**:983–987.

21
Lymphoedema

Catharine L McGuinness and Kevin G Burnand

Introduction

Lymphoedema is an accumulation of tissue fluid in the extracellular compartment as a result of defective lymphatic function. It is associated with an increased pool of extravasated plasma proteins and recirculating lymphocytes, monocytes and Langerhans cells. There is an additional impairment of transport of autologous and foreign proteins. The production of cytokines by the parenchymal and immune cells may be responsible for the proliferation of fibroblasts and epithelial cells, which cause subsequent sclerotic changes of the skin and subcutaneous tissues.

Lymphoedema may be primary (of unknown cause) or secondary to other diseases which damage the lymphatics. The incidence of primary lymphoedema is difficult to ascertain but in 1985 it was estimated that 1 in 6000 births will develop primary lymphoedema with a female:male ratio of 3:1.

Aetiology

Primary lymphoedema

Of patients with primary lymphoedema 30% have a family history, suggesting that there is a genetic defect. Primary lymphoedema affects the lower limb with a far greater frequency than the upper limb. The scrotum, genitalia and face are occasionally affected.

Congenital lymphoedema

True congenital lymphoedema (Milroy's disease) is hereditary and presents within 1 year of birth. It affects boys more often than girls and is a result of hypoplasia or aplasia of the lymphatics. It is rare (1 in 33 000), accounting for <5% of cases of primary lymphoedema. In 90% of congenital lymphoedemas the lower limb is affected (Fig. 21.1). Congenital lymphoedema is associated with other abnormalities or syndromes, e.g. Pierre Robin or Turner's.

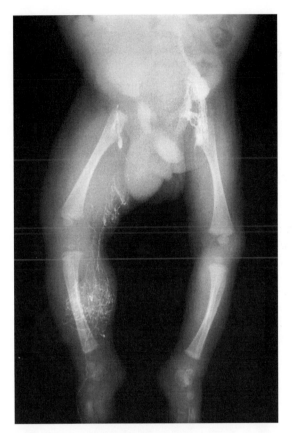

Fig. 21.1. Lymphangiogram showing congenital lymphoedema of the right lower limb as a result of proximal hypoplasia causing distal distension of the lymphatics. Contrast on the right is halted at the groin.

Lymphatic hyperplasia also affects boys more frequently than girls and may be associated with an absent thoracic duct. Lymphangiograms show increased numbers of lymphatics that do not function effectively and are often associated with increased numbers of small nodes.

Megalymphatics usually cause unilateral swelling and affect boys and girls equally. They are often associated with lymphatic abnormalities and leak into the abdominal cavity (chylous ascites), pleural space (chylothorax), genitalia (chylometrorrhoea) and urinary tract (chyluria). The primary abnormality is an absence of lymphatic valves causing reflux of lymph fluid under the influence of gravity. The skin in the area drained by the affected lymphatics commonly develops vesicles that leak chyle as the absorbed mesenteric lymph refluxes down the lower limbs (Fig. 21.2).

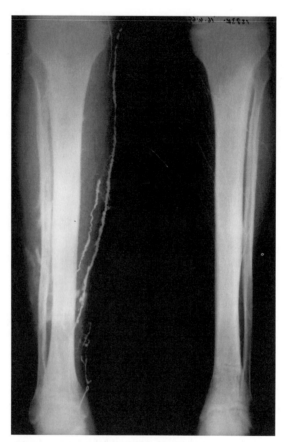

Fig. 21.2. **Megalymphatics of the right lower leg.**

Acquired or 'late-onset' primary lymphoedema

The majority of patients with primary lymphoedema fall into this category. Subdivisions can be made on the lymphangiographic appearance of the lymphatics. The reason for a delayed onset of an apparently congenital abnormality is still unexplained.

Distal obliterative lymphoedema usually affects women at or around puberty. It often affects both legs with the swelling confined to below the knee. The lymphatics are usually reduced in number but may be absent. The inguinal and iliolumbar nodes are normal, as are all the proximal lymph channels.

Proximal obliterative lymphoedema may present at any age. The ratio of men : women is 1:2 and half the cases are bilateral. At the onset, the swelling affects the thigh, but eventually progresses to involve the whole limb. Initially, the lymphatics in the distal part of the limb are dilated and increased in number. The inguinal and pelvic nodes are often fibrosed and the lymphatics in the limb eventually become reduced in number by 'die-back'. Die-back is the phenomenon that occurs after prolonged lymphatic obstruction such that the site of obstruction moves more distally. These patients may be considered for enteromesenteric bridge operation provided that some channels are present and suitable nodes are demonstrated at groin exploration.

Secondary lymphoedema

Causes include:

- filariasis;
- non-filarial elephantiasis;
- other chronic infection, e.g. tuberculosis, lymphogranuloma venereum, hidradenitis suppurativa;
- acute infection, e.g. cellulitis, toxocariasis;
- trauma, including node dissection or clearance;
- malignancy (primary or secondary infiltration of nodes or by mass effect);
- rheumatoid arthritis (cause unknown);
- ionizing radiation;
- artefactual, e.g. tourniquet.

Worldwide by far the most important cause is infection. Filariasis can be caused by several species of filarial parasites including *Wuchereria bancrofti*, *Brugia malayi* and *Brugia timori*. Various arthropod vectors transmit the parasites. The worms enter the lymphatics and produce a fibrotic inflammatory reaction, particularly in the nodes. Non-filarial elephantiasis has been reported in certain parts of East Africa and Ethiopia where filariasis does not exist. It is thought that the condition is a result of an obstructive lymphopathy caused by aluminosilicate and silica absorbed from soil through the soles of the feet. The silica causes a dense fibrotic reaction in the inguinal nodes of the barefoot tribesmen.

In Europe and North America the majority of cases of lymphoedema occur as a result of radiotherapy and/or surgical excision of regional lymph nodes as part of the treatment for carcinoma, especially of the breast. The incidence of lymphoedema following surgical excision of lymph nodes largely depends upon the primary pathology for which the excision is being performed and also whether adjuvant radiotherapy is given. For example, lymphoedema following lymphadenectomy for penile and vulval carcinoma occurs in 15% of patients, whereas following a block dissection for cutaneous cancer it affects more than half. The incidence following a further groin exploration for recurrent varicose veins is about 0.5%.

The level of axillary clearance affects the incidence of secondary lymphoedema of the arm, but overall it is of the order of 5%. The incidence is much higher when radiotherapy is also given and is greater when infection complicates surgical excision.

Clinical features

Most patients present with swelling of one or both lower limbs. The patient may attribute the onset to an insect bite, infection or local injury such as a twisted ankle. It is possible that in a predisposed individual such an episode may further damage a previously 'coping' lymphatic drainage, thus initiating a now irreversible lymph overload.

The oedema at early presentation usually pits easily on digital pressure. Later in the disease process after subcutaneous fibrosis has begun, the greater tissue resistance makes pitting more difficult to demonstrate. The oedema of long-standing lymphoedema used to be described as 'non-pitting', but this is not so, as even in the most chronic cases, pitting can always be seen after prolonged firm pressure.

Verrucous skin changes may develop and lymphocutaneous fistulae may be present in patients with megalymphatics. The fistulae usually leak clear lymph or white chyle and often result in the surrounding skin becoming macerated and secondarily infected with yeasts and fungi. Ulceration is rare.

Complications

Infection

The normal lymphatic system is 99% effective in protecting the bloodstream from particulate matter, malignant cells and bacteria. The most efficient points of filtration are the initial lymphatics and the first node. Bacteria are trapped at all points of the lymphatic tree and their localization in trunks between the initial lymphatic entry point and first node may explain the rapid appearance of lymphatic streaks observed in lymphangitis. Nevertheless, some authors have suggested that the lymphatic clearance of bacteria from soft tissues is unimportant as a host defence mechanism as less than a third of experimentally injected bacteria are cleared within 24 h. This may explain why the soft tissue in lymphoedematous patients is so susceptible to infection.

Observations in developing bacterial infections reveal that there is a dramatic reduction in flow within the draining lymphatics. This phenomenon must increase the oedema further. 'Open junctions' have been shown to develop in lymphatics within inflamed tissue. These enlarged junctions allow proteins and fluid to leak more, which again increases the oedema. Histological examination of tissue taken from areas of recurrent erysipelas demonstrates degeneration and in some cases, obliteration of lymphatic channels. Despite these observations, infections more commonly complicate lymphoedema than act as a cause. Breaches in the skin of patients with concomitant dermatological conditions allow the ingress of bacteria. Lymphangitis may result, which in turn may cause permanent damage to the lymphatics. Lymphoedema, with its stagnant protein-rich extracellular fluid, is prone to infection and inflammation and so the condition tends to be self-perpetuating.

In patients with skin vesicles and constant lymph leak from fistulae, maceration of the skin may occur and this predisposes to fungal and secondary bacterial infection. A similar problem is seen in patients with deep clefts in verrucous lymphoedema, particularly in the foot and lower leg. These clefts may also be colonized by anaerobic bacteria and an offensive leakage may then develop. When failure of conservative treatment with antiseptic baths, systemic antifungals and antibiotics fails, the problem may be best remedied by 'shaving of verrucae' and application of split-skin grafts.

Tinea pedis and other fungal infections of the interdigital spaces, particularly of the toes, are very common in patients with lower limb lymphoedema. Patients are therefore advised to use antifungal topical agents after bathing.

Cellulitis spreads along the subcutaneous or subfascial planes, often as a result of infection with *Streptococcus pyogenes*, which has entered the tissue via a wound or accidental minor trauma. Because cellulitis within lymphoedematous tissue can progress so quickly, patients are given antibiotics to keep available to start immediately if any symptoms occur. Recurrent attacks in which no cause is found can be treated with long-term continuous low-dose antibiotic prophylaxis.

Malignancy

Lymphangiosarcoma is an uncommon complication of chronic lymphoedema. It is most often seen in the arms of lymphoedema patients with previous breast cancer who have been treated by axillary clearances and radiotherapy. An endovascular papillary angioendothelioma-like tumour has also been reported.

Diagnosis

The absence of stigmata of chronic venous insufficiency or the presence of obvious unilateral elephantiasis usually indicates the correct clinical diagnosis. Isotope lymphography should, however, be performed to confirm the diagnosis and to identify the level of obstruction. In some patients with a proximal block, bypass surgery is possible but in the majority the problem is distal and conservative management is the mainstay of treatment.

In the UK, technetium-99m(^{99m}Tc)-labelled rhenium sulphide or ^{99m}Tc antimony sulphide colloid is used for isotope lymphography. The micro-colloid is taken up by the lymphatics after injection of a calculated weight-dependent dose into the web-space of the affected limb. The colloid should normally be concentrated by the nodes. The percentage uptake of the original dose present in the regional nodes at 30 and 60 min can be calculated. An ilioinguinal uptake of <0.6–3% is typical of lymphoedema (Plate 5). Patients with proximal obstructions have normal uptake in the nodes, but clearance of colloid from the nodes is delayed. Patients with venous oedema have an increased isotopic clearance and are easily differentiated from those with lymphoedema.

Lymphoscintography is minimally invasive, reasonably reliable and can be performed on an outpatient basis. False negatives occur with poor injection technique and false positives with proximal blocks. The investigation cannot distinguish between the various types of primary lymphoedema or between primary and secondary causes but it is a good screening test as further investigations are usually not required.

Contrast lymphangiography is reserved for patients in whom the results of isotope lymphography are equivocal, or when an isotope scan has confirmed lymphoedema and bypass surgery is being contemplated. In cases of reflux when lymphatic ligation is required, a formal lymphangiogram is helpful in order to define precisely the region of concern.

A short transverse incision is made on the dorsum of the foot (or hand) and a lymphatic is dissected out using an operating microscope. Fine instruments are required. The lymphatic is cannulated and an oily contrast medium (Lipiodol) is injected using a slow-speed infusion pump. Lipiodol, which is made from poppy seed oil and contains 38% iodine, remains within the lymphatics and is therefore ideal for lymphography. The contrast moves proximally and the lymph nodes remain filled for many weeks. Delayed films give good pictures of the nodes. Some patients are allergic to iodine or poppy seed and oil embolism to the lungs is a possible complication if excessive amounts of contrast are administered (>20 ml).

Differential diagnosis

The differential diagnosis of lymphoedema is:

- cardiac failure;
- renal failure;
- hepatic failure;

- malabsorption, malnutrition;
- lipodystrophic disorders;
- voluntary and involuntary dependency or disuse;
- idiopathic cyclic oedema;
- venous oedema;
- erythrocyanosis frigida crurum puellarum;
- arteriovenous fistulae;
- gigantism;
- abnormalities in antidiuretic hormone production/response;
- allergies;
- Klippel–Trenaunay syndrome;
- arterial reperfusion.

Attempts should be made to exclude other causes of oedema before lymphography is requested.

Cardiac failure is an important cause of bilateral lower limb oedema. It should be suspected from finding an elevated central venous pressure. Chest auscultation and radiographs should confirm the diagnosis. Chronic renal failure will be apparent on renal function tests. Low albumin is found in cases of malnutrition and malabsorption in association with weight loss. Abnormal liver function tests, clotting studies and a low serum albumin are found in patients with hepatic cirrhosis and oedema.

Allergic conditions are usually diagnosed from the history. Hereditary angio-oedema, a dominantly inherited autosomal condition, results from a deficiency (true or functional) of C1 esterase inhibitor. It causes recurrent attacks of facial swelling which may be associated with peripheral oedema. It resolves spontaneously within 48–72 h but mortality from asphyxia in untreated cases is as high as 30%. It can be confirmed by finding low blood levels of C1 esterase inhibitor, or low C4 levels during an attack.

Idiopathic cyclic oedema occurs in women of childbearing age and typically causes mild swelling of both lower limbs in the premenstrual week. The diagnosis should be obvious from the history.

Unilateral ankle oedema most commonly results from chronic venous insufficiency. Other features of venous disease, including ulceration, venous flares, eczema, lipodermatosclerosis or varicose veins are usually present (see Chapters 18–20). Occasionally, iliac vein compression or caval occlusion may not cause much in the way of signs, although an abdominal mass, abnormal pelvic examination or dilated abdominal wall collateral veins may give a clue to the underlying pathology. An ascending venogram or duplex scan confirms the diagnosis. Venous occlusion cannot cause lymphoedema unless there is a pre-existing subclinical abnormality of the lymphatics when the increase in extravasated fluid and protein caused by the venous occlusion may overload the lymphatics.

Klippel–Trenaunay syndrome, which is associated with varicose veins, bony and soft tissue anomalies, increased limb length, capillary naevi and abnormal or absent deep veins, also causes oedema. In more than half of these patients, a primary abnormality of the lymphatics co-exists.

Oedema can be observed in patients with long-standing paralysis but occasionally is produced by patients with psychological problems by deliberate limb disuse.

Lipodystrophy occurs most frequently in women and is associated with obesity. The fat distribution is abnormal and when confined to the lower legs may appear similar to lymphoedema. The fat never pits and isotope lymphography is normal.

Erythrocyanosis frigida is a condition of young, often heavily built women who have cold and blotchy reddish shins. It is the result of slow cutaneous circulation and is almost always symmetrical.

Gigantism may be associated with hypertrophy of the underlying bone and soft tissue but lymphatic drainage is normal. Similarly, patients with Parkes Weber syndrome (multiple arteriovenous fistulae) also have limb lengthening and oedema but their lymphatics are normal. The limb is warm, a thrill may be palpable and a machinery murmur may be audible on auscultation. The Branham sign of pulse slowing in response to occlusion of the arterial inflow to the fistula confirms the diagnosis.

Metabolic causes of oedema include abnormalities of the production of antidiuretic hormone (ADH) and reperfusion of an ischaemic limb. The osmolality of the blood in patients with ADH abnormalities and oedema is very low and is associated with other electrolyte effects depending on the severity of the dilution. Reperfusion oedema should not cause a diagnostic problem. It is frequently seen in the early postoperative course whereas postoperative lymphoedema occurs after many days or weeks and when the patient is mobile.

Management

Conservative and prophylactic treatment

Achieving *compression* with hosiery may be difficult in patients with oddly shaped limbs and severe lymphoedema. Compression bandaging is sometimes the best option under these circumstances. Fitted below- or above-knee graduated compression hosiery is otherwise prescribed. Lymphoedema of the arm can also be treated by application of a gauntlet. Pneumatic compression devices (e.g. ®Lymphapress) can be used at home or on the hospital ward preoperatively. These use sequential inflation to 'massage' the lymphoedema up the limb.

Elevation is always effective, if impracticable. It should be used at night and whenever the patient is not actively exercising.

Massage has a measurable but poorly sustained effect. Patients like this expensive form of therapy.

Antibiotics may be necessary for cellulitis, which usually complicates a breach of the integument. The skin pathology of recent attacks should be treated and eventually long-term low-dose antibiotics may be required.

Foot care is important. Interdigital infection is difficult to cure unless the patient bathes daily, dries his skin thoroughly and wears well-fitting footwear. Many patients need specially fitted shoes. Several drugs are effective topically against dermatophytes (clotrimazole, tolnaftate and miconazole). Lamisil (terbinafine) 250 mg once daily orally is effective systemically. Cutaneous candidiasis may be problematic in moist areas and in patients with cutaneous lymph leakage. Nystaform HC ointment (nystatin with Vioform and Hydrocortisone) is a very effective treatment.

General hygiene can be promoted with ®Hibiscrub baths in patients with repeated infections and in preoperative cases.

Benzopyrones are reported to reduce lymphoedema by increasing proteolysis by tissue macrophages. The benzopyrone, 5,6-benzo-α-pyrone, has been used orally in randomized double blind trials in patients with filarial lymphoedema, primary lymphoedema and other causes of secondary lymphoedema with success gauged on statistical criteria. The clinical improvement in affected legs has been small.

Surgical procedures

Only a small percentage of patients with lymphoedema require surgery. Many operations have been described but they almost all fall into the categories of debulking, bypass or ligation procedures.

Reducing operations

The number of infective episodes may be reduced by the removal of excess bulk, although this is not always the case.

Homans' operation is named after a Boston surgeon, John Homans, although Auchincloss first described the procedure in 1930. Flaps of skin are raised and a wedge of skin and subcutaneous tissue is excised down to the fascia (Fig. 21.3). The principle can be applied to reduce the thigh, lower leg and foot but only if the skin quality is good. A medial Homans' procedure is usually performed initially, but can be followed by a lateral reduction at a later date if required.

Dermal flap procedures, where a flap of de-epithelialized skin is buried in the subfascial space in an attempt to allow skin lymphatics to drain directly into deep channels, have been abandoned. The complications of pilonidal sinus formation combined with the poor scar gave worse results than the standard Homans'. There was no evidence that the lymphatics ever joined.

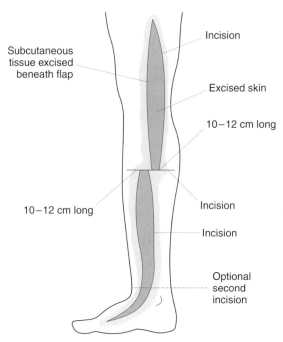

Subcutaneous
tissue excised
beneath flap

Incision

Excised skin

10–12 cm long

10–12 cm long

Incision

Incision

Optional
second
incision

Fig. 21.3. **Homans' procedure.**

Charles' operation was originally described by Sir Havelock Charles for the treatment of tropical elephantiasis. It is often now used for large lower limbs with warty excrescences, deep clefts or lymph leakage from poor quality skin. The procedure involves circumferential excision of the skin and subcutaneous tissue from the calf and application of split-skin grafts onto the exposed fascia. 'Darts' are fashioned at the knee and ankle to produce a well-shaped limb without a pantaloon appearance. Charles' reductions can be complicated by excessive warty skin and hypertrophic scars, which can be shaved off with a skin-graft knife.

Bypass procedures

Many bypass operations have been described and abandoned. Two which remain in use today are *lymphovenous anastomosis* and the *mesenteric bridge bypass*.

Lymphovenous fistulae

In this operation lymphatics are directly anastomosed to veins and the results appear to depend on the number of anastomoses created. The results are disappointing in patients with primary lymphoedema but good results have been reported in the treatment of filariasis. Preoperative identification and confirmation of the presence of lymphatics is required, as it is not possible to perform the bypass when there is lymphatic aplasia. A suitable lymphatic cannot be identified intra-operatively in some patients and the procedure then has to be abandoned.

Bridging operations

Many types of bridging operations have failed. Pedicled omental grafts are no longer popular. The poor results obtained have been attributed to insufficient lymphatics within the omentum. In 1994, however, optimistic results were reported after combined free omental autotransplants and lymph nodal-venous anastomosis to omental veins.

The enteromesenteric bridge is still used in a few patients with obstruction at the pelvic level (Fig. 21.4). The submucosal lymphatics of the ileum are profuse. A small length of ileum is prepared as a pedicle on the mesentery, which must be able to reach the groin of the affected side. The small bowel continuity is restored by an end-to-end anastomosis. The isolated pedicle is laid open along the antimesenteric border and the mucosa is stripped after it has been raised from the submucosa by injection of adrenaline and saline. The rectangular graft is laid onto one or more bivalved nodes in the groin or pelvis. Good results can be obtained in at least half of a group of well-selected patients. The procedure may be complicated by bowel obstruction and the other complications of lower midline laparotomies and groin incisions.

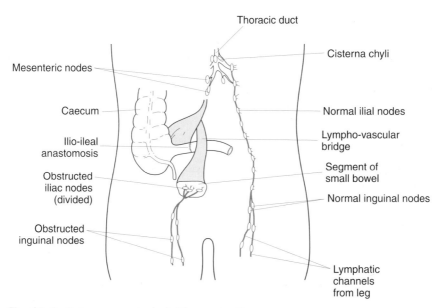

Fig. 21.4. Enteromesenteric bridge operation.

Ligations

Massive lymphatic ectasia with valvular incompetence encourages chyle to leak back into vesicles, peritoneum or pleural cavity. A contrast lymphangiogram can often define the site of leakage with sufficient accuracy to allow local lymphatic ligation to be performed. Chylothorax is best treated by pleurectomy unless there has been trauma to the thoracic duct, which is then best ligated at the level of T10 through a left thoractomy. Chylous ascites may be treated by local ligation, underrunning of the fistula or by the insertion of a peritoneal-venous shunt (Denver or LeVeen), although replacement due to blockage is frequently necessary.

Outcome

This seems to be determined early in the natural history. For example, it is unusual for oedema to spread up the leg if only the lower leg has been affected for sometime. If oedema develops in the contralateral limb it is often less severe. The distal lymphatics are obliterated in most patients (90%) with primary lymphoedema.

The condition can usually be contained by correctly fitting compression hosiery or pneumatic compression, which may be combined with regular massage or tight bandaging. Reduction surgery is required for <5% of patients but can give very satisfactory results and return limb function in a few patients with massive limb swelling.

Summary

- Other causes of oedema should be excluded.
- Isotope lymphography should be used to confirm the diagnosis.
- Contrast lymphography should still be performed when the diagnosis is in doubt, when bypass is contemplated or if ligation of megalymphatics is being undertaken.
- Most cases of lymphoedema are best managed by conservative measures using limb compression therapy.
- Operations should be reserved for patients with impaired mobility because of massive limb size, proximal obstruction with functioning distal lymphatics or refluxing megalymphatics.

Areas of controversy

- Can lymphoedema be managed with expansive massage, bandaging and support programmes alone?
- Place of lymphovenous anastomosis and mesenteric bridging.

Further reading

- Kinmonth JB. *The Lymphatics. Disease, Lymphography and Surgery,* 2nd edn. London: Edward Arnold, 1982.
- O'Brien BMcC. *Microvascular Reconstructive Surgery.* Edinburgh: Churchill Livingstone, 1977.
- Browse NL. *A Colour Atlas of Reducing Operations for Lymphoedema of Lower Limb.* London: Wolfe Medical Publications, 1986.
- Reed RK, McHale NG, Bert JL, Winlove CP, Laine GA. *Interstitium, Connective Tissue and Lymphatics.* London: Portland Press Proceedings, 1995.

22
Vasospastic and Sympathetic Disorders

Bruce Campbell

Introduction

Raynaud's phenomenon (RP) is by far the commonest of the vasospastic disorders affecting up to 30% of women in cool climates to some degree. Others include erythromelalgia, acrocyanosis, chilblains, livido reticularis and reflex sympathetic dystrophy. Only a minority of patients who experience frequent and troublesome symptoms present to hospital and they are seen by a variety of specialists, including rheumatologists, general physicians, vascular surgeons and angiologists.

Raynaud's Phenomenon

In 1862 Maurice Raynaud described a syndrome of episodic digital blanching, followed by cyanosis and rubor, with attacks precipitated by cold or emotion. The clinical features may, however, be atypical and there may be other precipitating factors. Patients can be subdivided into those with primary idiopathic Raynaud's disease and those with an associated underlying disorder.

The prevalence of RP in the population is about 10%. Ninety percent of sufferers are female, and among women of working age the incidence is about 20%. There is commonly a familial predisposition in cases developing before the age of about 30 years: many women who develop symptoms in their teens experience gradual improvement about the time of the menopause. About 5–10% of patients with RP eventually develop a connective tissue disease (CTD).

Aetiology

Raynaud's phenomenon is classified as:

- primary (idiopathic), with no identifiable cause or associated disorder — usually called Raynaud's disease (RD); or

- secondary to an aetiological agent or associated with another disorder — usually called Raynaud's syndrome (RS) in the European literature.

Raynaud's syndrome may be associated with a wide variety of underlying disorders or causative agents (Table 22.1).

Vasospasm is the excessive and inappropriate contraction of small blood vessels (in contrast to normal vasoconstriction). Factors which may contribute to the vasospasm seen in RP are:

Table 22.1. Causes of Raynaud's syndrome.

Connective tissue diseases	Systemic sclerosis (scleroderma; RS in 90% of cases)
	Mixed connective tissue disease (RS in 85% of cases)
	Systemic lupus erythematosus
	Sjögren's syndrome
	Dermatomyositis and polymyositis
	Rheumatoid arthritis
Arterial occlusive diseases	Atherosclerosis
	Buerger's disease
	Thoracic outlet syndrome
	Peripheral embolism
Occupational and trauma	Vibration white finger
	Frozen food packers
	Frostbite, trench foot
	Injury by heat, electric shock, percussion
Neurological disorders	Reflex sympathetic dystrophy
	Carpal tunnel syndrome
	Paralysis of a limb
Blood dyscrasias	Hyperviscosity syndromes
	Cold agglutinin disease
	Cryoglobulinaemia
	Myeloproliferative diseases
Drugs and toxins	Ergotamine and other migraine therapies
	β-Blockers (even when cardioselective)
	Cytotoxics — bleomycin, vinblastine
	Bromocryptine
	Sulphasalazine
	Vinylchloride
Miscellaneous diseases	Hypothyroidism
	Malignancy
	Arteriovenous fistula
	Hepatitis B, pulmonary hypertension, uraemia

- *Sympathetic nervous activity and reactivity.* An altered and increased sensitivity of both α and β receptors has been demonstrated in RP. Local vibration of one hand produces vasoconstriction in the other in RP patients, and body cooling (without cooling the hands) also causes digital blanching. These findings suggest some kind of involvement of the central nervous system.
- *Endothelial function.* Abnormal levels of chemicals derived from vascular endothelium have been identified in patients with RS, with reduced generation of the vasodilators nitric oxide and prostacyclin and excessive production of the vasoconstrictor endothelin. Elevated levels of von Willebrand factor (generated by the endothelium) may signal endothelial damage, and a deficiency of fibrinolysis has also been observed.
- *Blood constituents.* Increased platelet aggregation occurs in RP, with increased release of thromboxane A_2. Erythrocytes are less deformable and are therefore more likely to obstruct flow in small vessels when vasospasm occurs. Increased leucocyte activation has also been demonstrated.

It is important to note that blood and endothelial abnormalites have been found largely in patients with RS, rather than those with primary RD. How many of them have a causal role and how many are epiphenomena remains uncertain.

Clinical features

The diagnosis of RP is usually obvious from a clinical history of episodic digital blanching on exposure to cold. Subsequent cyanosis or rubor on rewarming is common and patients often complain of paraesthesiae or numbness during attacks, but these symptoms are not fundamental to the diagnosis. Patients who develop cyanosis only, without blanching, have acrocyanosis.

Although digital colour change is the cardinal feature of RP, vasospasm may occur in other parts of the body:

- tip of the nose;
- ear lobes;
- cerebral arteries (producing headaches);
- pulmonary arteries;
- coronary arteries (possibly producing myocardial contraction band necrosis in CTDs);
- oesophagus (possibly producing symptoms in the absence of stricture or achalasia).

Cold is the classic stimulus precipitating attacks, but emotion is also an important factor in many patients; others include tobacco smoke and trauma (e.g. pressure on the metatarsal heads).

An attempt to differentiate between RD and RS is vital, and the history should always include questions which might elucidate an underlying cause:

- occupation (vibrating tools, exposure to chemicals or cold temperatures);
- drugs (commonly β-blockers or migraine therapies);
- features of CTD (especially arthralgia, dry mouth or eyes, dysphagia, ulcers or rashes).

In addition to symptoms suggesting the presence of a CTD, other clinical features associated with progression to RS include:

- onset in childhood or old age;
- recurrence of chilblains in adult life;
- vasospasm all year round;
- asymmetrical attacks;
- digital ulceration.

Examination should include:

- digits — colour, digital pitting, sclerodactyly, ulceration, presence of obvious nailfold megacapillaries;
- arteries — pulses, blood pressure (both arms), auscultation above and below clavicle, provocation manoeuvres for thoracic outlet syndrome;
- search for features of CTD or carpal tunnel syndrome.

Investigations

The particular investigations required in each case will be guided by the clinical findings. Some tests should be done routinely, but more complex investigations (e.g. cold challenge tests and measurements of digital blood flow) are only necessary in selected cases.

Blood tests

Routine tests are:

- full blood count and erythrocyte sedimentation ratio (ESR):
- thyroid function;
- antinuclear antibody;
- rheumatoid factor;
- blood glucose.

Tests for selected cases are:

- serum protein electrophoresis (if ESR is elevated);
- cryoglobulins (rare and require special handling of blood samples).

Radiology

The routine test is a chest X-ray for pulmonary fibrosis in CTD or cervical rib. Special views may be needed and it should be remembered that thoracic outlet compression may be caused by fibrous bands.

Tests for selected cases are:

- arteriography;
- duplex ultrasound scanning (for suspected thoracic outlet syndrome);
- hand X-rays (for digital calcification).

Vascular laboratory tests

The routine test is capillary nailfold microscopy. Abnormally dilated capillary loops develop in the nailfolds of patients likely to progress to a CTD. These are best demonstrated using a specially designed microscope, which allows photography of the nailfold vessels, but the changes can also be seen using an ophthalmoscope (Fig. 22.1).

Tests in selected cases measure digital systolic pressure or flow before and after a cold challenge and, traditionally, form part of the investigation of RP, but in practice there is seldom a need for their use.

Management

All treatment is palliative and the methods used depend on the severity of symptoms. Certain general measures are applicable to all patients, but for those with troublesome symptoms a wide range of therapeutic agents has been used none of which is predictably or thoroughly successful (Fig. 22.2).

General measures

These include:

- *Counselling.* A clear explanation of the nature of the problem is essential for all patients.
- *Withdraw possible causative agents.* Drugs known to cause or exacerbate RP should be stopped. Occasionally, there appears to be a link

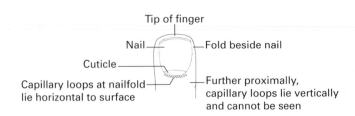

Fig. 22.1. Nailfold vessels.

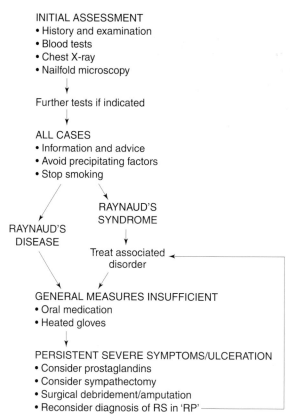

INITIAL ASSESSMENT
- History and examination
- Blood tests
- Chest X-ray
- Nailfold microscopy

Further tests if indicated

ALL CASES
- Information and advice
- Avoid precipitating factors
- Stop smoking

RAYNAUD'S SYNDROME

RAYNAUD'S DISEASE

Treat associated disorder

GENERAL MEASURES INSUFFICIENT
- Oral medication
- Heated gloves

PERSISTENT SEVERE SYMPTOMS/ULCERATION
- Consider prostaglandins
- Consider sympathectomy
- Surgical debridement/amputation
- Reconsider diagnosis of RS in 'RP'

***Fig. 22.2.* Algorithm for the management of Raynaud's phenomenon.**

between the contraceptive pill or hormone replacement therapy (HRT) and development of RP, in which case a trial of stopping therapy is worthwhile. There is, however, no good evidence for stopping the pill or HRT as a routine. Patients whose occupation is linked with RS should consider a change of job.

- *Stop smoking* (because it causes vasoconstriction).
- *Avoid cold.* Apart from commonsense measures to avoid cold environments, this may simply mean wearing warm gloves and thick socks for patients with mild symptoms. Well insulated shoes or boots keep the feet warm and padded insoles also militate against vasospasm precipitated by pressure. Disposable or reusable hand warmers are available for occasional use, but for patients with troublesome symptoms, electrically heated gloves and socks can be very helpful.

Drug treatment

Drug treatment should be reserved for patients who still suffer distressing symptoms despite the general measures described above. The most commonly used drugs include calcium channel blockers and inhibitors of the sympathetic nervous system:

- nifedipine (initially 10 mg bd — maximum 20 mg tds)
- inositol nicotinate (initially 500 mg tds — maximum 750 mg bd of inositol nicotinate forte)
- naftidrofuryl (initially 100 mg tds — maximum 200 mg tds)
- thymoxamine (initially 40 mg qds — maximum 80 mg qds)
- oxpentifylline (initially 400 mg tds — maximum 800 mg tds).

The calcium channel blocker nifedipine is particularly popular. Its dosage is limited by side-effects such as headache, dizziness, palpitations and flushing: these can be kept to a minimum by starting with 10 mg bd and increasing the dose every 1–2 weeks.

Prostaglandin E_1 (PGE_1) and I_2 (Prostacyclin, or a synthetic analogue — Iloprost) have both been used quite extensively in the treatment of severe RP, although neither is yet fully licensed for this purpose. Both drugs are potent vasodilators and inhibitors of platelet aggregation.

Some benefit has been demonstrated with a variety of other agents:

- evening primrose oil preparations (need at least 3 months' trial);
- stanozolol (important side-effects — virilization, liver dysfunction and dyspepsia);
- ketanserin (a serotonin antagonist, which is no longer readily available).

None has yet gained widespread acceptance, nor is any currently licensed specifically for the treatment of RP. They are best considered only for refractory cases.

Sympathectomy

Upper limb

This requires ablation of the second and third thoracic ganglia and intervening sympathetic chain. The stellate ganglion should be studiously avoided, because Horner's syndrome will result if it is damaged. Some descriptions have advocated removal of the lower part of the stellate ganglion, but there is no good evidence that this improves results. The fourth and fifth thoracic ganglia may also be ablated when denervation of the axilla is required (e.g. in combined palmar and axillary hyperhidrosis).

A number of surgical approaches have been described for upper thoracic sympathectomy, of which the transaxillary and supraclavicular approaches have been by far the most popular. Nowadays, the operation is usually done endoscopically by the transaxillary route. Complications of the procedure must be discussed with the patient preoperatively. These include:

- pneumothorax;
- Horner's syndrome (see above);
- compensatory sweating;
- arm/thoracic pain.

Upper limb sympathectomy was traditionally used in the treatment of RP until proper evaluation of results during the last 30 years demonstrated a very high relapse rate. Poor results are the rule in RS and even in RD the majority of patients relapse within a year. These disappointing results have led many surgeons to abandon upper limb sympathectomy altogether in RP. However, it may still have a limited yet useful place in patients with very severe trophic changes, threatened loss of digits and poor response to medical therapy. In such advanced cases, sympathectomy may offer a chance of improvement and healing. Deterioration within a few months is common, but often ulcers do not then recur.

There have been reports of worthwhile improvement from digital artery sympathectomy, with healing of ulcers in severe RP, but the place of this technique is not yet clear. It is done under the operating microscope (usually by plastic surgeons).

Lower limb

Lumbar sympathectomy involves ablation of the second and third (ideally also the fourth) lumbar sympathetic ganglia and the intervening sympathetic chain. Classically, this was done as a surgical procedure, by an anterior retroperitoneal approach, splitting or cutting the abdominal muscles just lateral to the rectus sheath at about the level of the umbilicus. There is little evidence that this works any better than lumbar phenol sympathectomy, during which an injection is done under radiological control using a long needle inserted by a translumbar route. This is commonly done under local anaesthesia.

Problems after lumbar sympathectomy are uncommon. Some patients complain of dysaesthetic aching in the anterior part of the thigh, but this almost always resolves after a few weeks. Postural hypotension and impotence are said to be risks of bilateral lumbar sympathectomy, but their incidence is unknown and they seem to be rare.

In complete contrast to upper limb sympathectomy, lumbar sympathectomy for lower extremity RP generally works well (particularly when done for RD rather than RS).

Plasma exchange

Plasma exchange removes immune complexes, lowers blood viscosity and affects the activity of blood cells. It has been shown to have possible benefit in RP patients with refractory ulceration, but is rarely used.

Behavioural methods

Methods such as biofeedback and Pavlovian conditioning have been investigated in RP and seem to offer benefit in a small proportion of well motivated patients.

Vibration white finger syndrome

This has assumed particular importance since being declared an industrial injury, for which compensation may be due to sufferers, and vascular surgeons are among those approached for medical reports on suspected cases.

The diagnosis rests on a history of exposure to vibration, with subsequent onset of RP symptoms. The nature of the machinery used, the number of years of exposure and the duration of exposure during the working day or week are all important elements of the history. Symptoms and disability can be graded by the Stockholm Workshop Scale or the scale described by Taylor and Pelmear.

Regular use of vibrating tools should be stopped and most employers remove sufferers from this kind of employment permanently. If patients need to use vibrating machinery, then intermittent prolonged periods of use are less damaging than more frequent use of such tools. Gripping machinery more loosely and using vibrating tools of lighter weight are other helpful measures. It is particularly important for sufferers to stop smoking.

Erythromelalgia

Erythromelalgia (occasionally referred to as erythermalgia) is a distressing condition characterized by redness, increased skin temperature and burning pain of the extremities. Like RP, there are primary and secondary forms and treatment is often difficult. Erythromelalgia is generally less well recognized and understood by clinicians than RP: the literature is contaminated by dubious cases and the true incidence is obscure.

Acrocyanosis

Acrocyanosis is characterized by persistent blue discolouration of the fingers, which sometimes also affects the toes, face and ears. The discolouration may worsen on exposure to cold and hyperaemia may be seen on rewarming. The affected extremities are cool, often sweaty, and there may be slight swelling of the digits.

The aetiology and pathogenesis of acrocyanosis remain rather obscure. As a rule it is not progressive or associated with underlying disorders and the general measures described for treatment of RP are usually adequate.

Chilblains (Pernio)

Chilblains are raised red or blue patches, a few millimetres in diameter, which develop on the extremities as a response to cold. They appear on the feet, hands or shins, usually as a result of repeated cold exposure. Several lesions often appear at once and generally resolve over 1–2 weeks. They may itch and can ulcerate, sometimes leaving pigmented areas on healing. Acute and chronic forms of pernio have been described.

Chilblains most often affect young women and are then intermittently troublesome throughout life. Sufferers tend to find cold exposure in general quite distressing. The underlying pathology is a form of vasculitis.

The most important aspects of treatment are avoidance of cold exposure and putting warm clothes on the extremities. Nifedipine has been claimed to hasten resolution of chilblains.

Livedo reticularis

In this condition the skin develops a mottled red and blue appearance, which is most marked on exposure to cold and which recovers on rewarming. The legs are most often affected, the upper extremities less commonly, and the trunk rarely. Livedo reticularis is quite common. It is usually mild and of cosmetic significance only. Treatment is by reassurance and advice to avoid exposure to cold and to dress warmly.

A more severe form of primary livedo reticularis has been described, associated with vasculitis, vascular thromboses and ulceration. In addition, livido reticularis may occasionally be seen in association with conditions such as CTDs (particularly systemic lupus erythematosus), atheroemboli and hyperviscosity syndromes.

Reflex sympathetic dystrophy

This is a clinical syndrome of pain, hyperaesthesia, discolouration, swelling and trophic changes affecting a limb, which usually follows trauma. It is poorly understood and difficult to treat. Reflex sympathetic dystrophy is sometimes also called algodystrophy, Sudeck's atrophy or shoulder hand syndrome.

Hyperhidrosis

Although not strictly a vasospastic condition or a sympathetic disorder, hyperhidrosis is mentioned here because it responds predictably and well to sympathectomy (see above). Sympathectomy is used most commonly for patients with disabling hyperhidrosis of the hands. There is often excessive axillary sweating as well (although axillary hyperhidrosis alone can usually be dealt with by topical means).

Summary

- The true mechanisms underlying most vasospastic and sympathetic disorders remains elusive.
- Unilateral Raynaud's phenomenon usually has a local rather than a systemic or idiopathic cause.
- Idiopathic (primary) Raynaud's phenomenon is usually a benign condition.
- A proportion of patients with primary Raynaud's phenomenon subsequently develop connective tissue disease.
- There are few predictable or well proven treatment modalities.

Areas of controversy

- Role of drug therapy.
- Indications for sympathectomy.

Acknowledgement

The author thanks John Tooke, Professor of Vascular Medicine in Exeter, for his advice and comments during the preparation of this chapter.

Further reading

- Belch J. Temperature-associated vascular disorders: Raynaud's phenomenon and ery-thromelalgia. In: Tooke JE, Lowe GDO (eds). *A Textbook of Vascular Medicine*. London: Edward Arnold 1996, pp 329–352.
- Byrne J, Walsh TN, Hederman WP. Endoscopic transthoracic electrocautery of the sympathetic chain for palmar and axillary hyperhidrosis. *British Journal of Surgery* 1990;**77**:1046–1049.
- Isenberg DA, Black C. Raynaud's phenomenon, scleroderma, and overlap syndromes. *British Medical Journal* 1995;**310**:795–798.

- Landry GJ, Edwards JM, McLafferty RB, Taylor LM, Porter JM. Long-term outcome of Raynaud's syndrome in a prospectively analyzed patient cohort. *Journal of Vascular Surgery* 1996;**23**:76–86.
- Paice E. Reflex sympathetic dystrophy. *British Medical Journal* 1995;**310**:1645–1648.
- Palmer RA, Collin J. Vibration white finger. *British Journal of Surgery* 1993;**80**:705–709.

23
Vascular Trauma

Alasdair J Walker

Introduction

Injury to the major blood vessels is uncommon, but the combined problems of arrest of haemorrhage and restoration of vessel continuity can be most challenging to the admitting surgeon. Trauma is the commonest cause of death in young persons, and major vascular trauma is often the primary cause of death or an important contributory factor.

Aetiology

In the UK, blunt trauma from road accidents is the commonest cause of vascular trauma. Elsewhere, penetrating trauma is common due to high levels of urban violence (Table 23.1).

Blunt injury

Deceleration and shearing forces act to disrupt the central vessels tearing the less elastic intima and media, raising flaps and causing thrombosis or aneurysm. More commonly, fractures and dislocations are associated with damage to limb vessels, particularly those around joints where the vessels are more vulnerable. The extent of soft tissue and vascular damage is often underestimated and needs most careful evaluation.

Table 23.1. **Causes of vascular trauma.**

Blunt injury	Road traffic accident
Penetrating injury	Stabbings
	Domestic and industrial accidents
	Gunshot wounds
Iatrogenic injury	Radiological procedures
	Drug abuse

Penetrating injury

Stabbing injuries and lacerations with broken glass due to domestic or industrial accidents usually cause direct vessel puncture or transection. The extent of gunshot wounds depends on energy transfer to the tissues from the bullet or missile. A high-energy transfer projectile causes considerable tissue damage, with secondary damage resulting from fragmentation of the projectile and splintering of bone. Vessel contusion or transection can occur distant from the entry point due to cavitation effects. Missile embolism is a rare complication.

Iatrogenic injury

Diagnostic interventional radiological techniques are using larger catheters to deploy stents and endovascular prostheses. False aneurysm of the femoral artery is a recognized complication of transfemoral catheterization. Cardiac catheterization procedures via the brachial or radial artery can disrupt these vessels. Inappropriate intra-arterial injection by IV drug abusers can lead to distal microembolization of the hand or foot, which seldom requires operative treatment but does need systemic heparinization.

Clinical features

Severe haemorrhage is an obvious feature of large vessel injury, but is not always present. Signs and symptoms of arterial damage are variable:

- reduced or absent distal pulse;
- major haemorrhage (class II — loss of >15–30% of blood volume);
- ischaemia;
- enlarging haematoma;
- bruit at or distal to the injury site;
- damage to anatomically related structures (nerves).

Complete transection of vessels such as the common femoral or popliteal arteries will lead to distal ischaemia with absent pulses. Bleeding may temporarily arrest due to contraction and haematoma formation, leading to a false sense of security. In partial transection, where part of the vessel wall remains intact, or where there is vessel contusion, limited distal flow reduces the signs of ischaemia. For this reason, distal pulses may be palpable and audible with Doppler, and the severity of the injury is missed initially or ignored.

Diagnosis

Clinical

A high index of clinical suspicion is essential in the diagnosis of vascular injury. The possibility of vessel injury must be entertained in all cases of long bone fracture (Fig. 23.1) or major joint dislocation and in all penetrating wounds to the neck. External blood loss is obvious, but occult blood loss into a body cavity or expanding haematoma should be considered when hypovolaemic shock fails to respond to adequate resuscitation. Clinical reassessment at regular intervals is mandatory as some vascular injuries do not become apparent for some time. Pulses initially observed may be absent on reappraisal. Palpable thrills, audible bruits and distal ischaemia are all highly suggestive of vessel damage.

Hand-held Doppler

Doppler assessment of peripheral pulses may be helpful in the initial assessment. However, it lacks specificity as apparently normal values can be seen despite vascular injury.

Duplex

Duplex is a useful technique for assessing the flow in and patency of most vessels and is highly specific.

Plain Film Radiography

Plain X-rays cannot be relied upon to demonstrate vascular injuries. They do demonstrate fractures and dislocations or displacement of soft tissues by large haematomas, adding to the 'index of suspicion'.

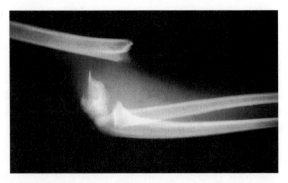

Fig. 23.1. X-ray showing supracondylar fracture of the humerus.

Computerized axial tomography

This modality may be useful in examining the multiply injured patient who has been resuscitated and is stable. It allows evaluation of the thoracic and abdominal viscera and the great vessels, especially when contrast is administered. It is not sensitive enough to allow examination of the peripheral arteries and veins.

Magnetic resonance imaging

This may be of greater value than CT scanning being both non-invasive and safe. It should be able to detect even minor abnormalities and clearly delineate tissue planes. However, there is little published experience as yet of the use of MRI in vascular trauma.

Arteriography

Arteriograms are used preoperatively to establish the need for surgery, demonstrate suspected but otherwise undetectable injuries and help plan the operation. If the patient fails to respond to initial resuscitation, an emergency arteriogram should not be delayed and may be performed in the operating room.

Indications for emergency angiography are:

- penetrating injuries to the base of the skull;
- thoracic outlet injuries (first rib fracture, clavicular fracture with signs of distal ischaemia);
- penetrating chest injuries;
- widening mediastinum on chest X-ray;
- extremity injuries with extensive soft tissue injury;
- shotgun injuries (multiple pellets).

It should be remembered that arteriograms are not infallible and the apparent absence of angiographic abnormalities should not detract from the clinical impression. They do aid the planning of surgery by demonstrating the location and extent of the injury. Intimal flaps, extensive thrombosis, false aneurysm and arteriovenous fistula can all be demonstrated.

Management

Initial management

The basic principles of trauma management must not be neglected because of the dramatic appearances of haemorrhage or ischaemia.

Priority is given to the establishment of an airway and the maintenance of adequate tissue oxygenation. Haemorrhage can then be controlled by direct pressure or tourniquet while the circulating blood volume is replaced through large-bore IV cannulae. Blind clamping of vessels is to be avoided.

A primary survey of the patient at this stage should identify treatment priorities. Head, chest and cardiac injuries may take precedence, but prolonged ischaemia should be avoided whenever possible. Regular repeat assessments should be made once baseline studies are recorded as the appearance of vascular injuries can be delayed or masked by initial hypovolaemia. Broad-spectrum antibiotics and tetanus toxoid should be given to minimize the risk of subsequent infection.

Careful liaison between the vascular and orthopaedic surgeons is important at this stage in limb trauma. Rapid reduction of dislocations or straightening of fractures may result in return of distal pulses (supracondylar fracture of the humerus or ankle dislocation). However, in most cases vascular repair should take precedence over orthopaedic or plastic surgical interventions, especially when there is damage to the popliteal artery and vein. Where there is concern that subsequent orthopaedic manipulations to achieve internal or external fixation may disrupt an anastomosis, temporary intraluminal shunts have been used to bypass the damaged artery and vein, preventing prolonged ischaemia and permitting vascular reconstruction after manipulation (Fig. 23.2).

The assessment of limb survivability can be very difficult and requires a senior opinion. Extensive crush injuries, associated major nerve damage and fixed plantar flexion of the foot are all poor prognostic signs. In these cases, a primary amputation may lead to more rapid recovery avoiding the complications of myoglobinuria and acute tubular necrosis.

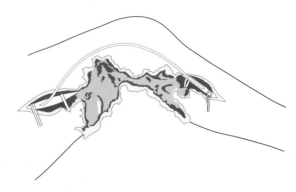

Fig. 23.2. Extraluminal shunt.

Surgery

Basic principles

Generally, patients are positioned supine allowing access to the chest, abdomen, neck and all four extremities. Wide exposure is essential to allow control of the affected vessels both proximally and distally. An uninvolved leg should be exposed also to allow harvesting of the long saphenous vein. Vertical incisions are preferred as they can be easily extended and run parallel to the major neurovascular bundles in the extremities. Access is particularly difficult at the base of the skull, root of the neck and superior mediastinum. Incisions along the anterior border of sternocleidomastoid can be extended into a median sternotomy if necessary. Penetrating wounds should not be extended as they seldom offer ideal access and control, especially in the root of the neck.

Vascular sloops, atraumatic clamps and intraluminal balloon occluders (e.g. Fogarty catheters) are used to gain control, the latter being particularly useful in controlling haemorrhage from major veins. Once control is achieved, operative blood loss is minimized and careful haematoma evacuation is possible to demonstrate the extent of the injury.

Minor veins can be ligated without complication, but the great veins and those at or proximal to the popliteal and axillary veins are best repaired.

Arterial repair

Methods of arterial repair are:

- lateral suture;
- patch angioplasty;
- end-to-end anastomosis;
- interposition graft (reversed vein, ?PTFE).

Shredded and damaged vessels should be trimmed back to viable undamaged intima. Proximal clot can be removed by milking the vessel, but restoration of distal patency may require gentle passage of a Fogarty catheter.

Ligation is only appropriate in 'non-essential' vessels, e.g. branches of the external carotid and abdominal and chest wall vessels.

Lateral suture with continuous or interrupted monofilament sutures is appropriate where there will be no significant vessel narrowing, i.e. lacerations to larger vessels. Smaller vessels can rarely be repaired by this technique without venous patch angioplasty.

Where there is loss of vessel length of <1– 2 cm, direct end-to-end anastomosis can be performed as long as there is no tension on the suture line. Larger gaps need an interposition graft, preferably of reversed long

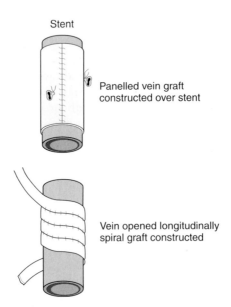

Stent

Panelled vein graft
constructed over stent

Vein opened longitudinally
spiral graft constructed

Fig. 23.3. (A) Panel and (B) spiral graft.

saphenous vein. Should a large artery require repair, and there is considerable size mismatch between it and the native long saphenous vein, a
'panel' or 'spiral' graft may be constructed from the long saphenous
vein. This technique adds time to the operation as either two pieces
of vein are opened longitudinally and then anastomosed, or after
longitudinal opening the vein is reconstructed in a spiral about a stent
(Fig. 23.3).

The use of artificial graft material in potentially infected wounds is
controversial. Most vascular surgeons would prefer autogenous material,
but some recent studies suggest that infection is not as great a problem
in the presence of artificial plastic prostheses, especially polytetrafluoroethylene (PTFE). These grafts have potential where size mismatch is a
problem (iliac vessels). Extra-anatomical routes with anastomoses away
from the site of injury may also be appropriate with such grafts. All grafts
must have adequate soft tissue cover.

Venous repair

Proximal ligation can lead to acute venous gangrene and postphlebitic
syndromes. In combined popliteal artery and vein trauma, failure to
repair the vein leads to unacceptably high amputation rates.

Methods are similar to arterial repair with lateral suture, vein patch,
end-to-end anastomosis and interposition grafting all possible. Anastomoses should be under no tension and carried out using fine mono-

filament sutures. Prosthetic grafts tend to thrombose and have no place in venous reconstruction. Some surgeons insert a distal arteriovenous fistula to improve venous flow and long-term patency. They are associated with potential haemodynamic complications if too great in diameter and may have to be closed after several weeks. Postoperative heparinization may be used to improve patency if the other injuries allow, but if this is contra-indicated low-molecular-weight dextrans might be more appropriate.

Specific injuries

The extremities

Injury to the femoral vessels is more common than that to vessels of the upper limbs. Acute ligation of the common femoral artery is associated with a 49% amputation rate which is only surpassed by ligation of the popliteal artery (73%). Injuries to these vessels require urgent surgical repair. Popliteal venous injury must be repaired at the same time as arterial, otherwise venous hypertension may impede graft patency. Superficial femoral injuries rarely cause severe ischaemia on their own, and repair may be temporarily delayed until orthopaedic procedures are performed. All injuries to the tibioperoneal trunk need repair. Severe ischaemia of the distal limb is only seen where two of the three calf arteries are damaged, allowing ligation in single vessel injury.

Four-compartment fasciotomy is mandatory when there is prolonged ischaemia, extensive soft tissue injury or any evidence of neurological deficit.

Axillary artery damage is uncommon and brachial artery injury is most frequently seen in the upper limb due to penetrating trauma or in associ-ation with fracture (supracondylar). Iatrogenic injuries at cardiac catheterization can cause brachial thrombosis. Few patients will require upper limb amputation due to the excellent upper extremity collateral circulation, but some will exhibit exercise-induced ischaemic symptoms. Isolated radial or ulnar artery injuries, but not both, can be safely ligated if repair is not possible. Associated nerve injuries, especially to the brachial plexus, most often determine the outcome in upper limb vascular trauma.

The neck

In the UK, stabbing is the commonest cause of wounds to the cervical vessels. Gunshot wounds are more common in the USA. The common carotid is most often involved on the left side. Associated pharyngeal, tra-cheal and oesophageal injuries may contaminate the wound. The pres-ence of severe neurological deficit (coma or dense hemiplegia) leads to difficult management decisions where revascularization of a carotid occlusion may lead to fatal haemorrhage into an ischaemic infarct.

Preoperative angiography is essential in stable patients with thoracic outflow wounds (proximal common carotid) and wounds above the angle of the mandible (distal internal carotid) where clinical examination is difficult. Patients with mid-cervical wounds and no neurological deficit may be operated on without angiography if urgent. In future, MRI scanning may have a place to play in more accurately identifying vessel patency than angiography, as all patent vessels should be repaired. Most surgeons would agree that wounds penetrating the platysma must be explored, but some would adopt a selective exploratory policy to mid-cervical wounds.

Carotid injuries may be repaired primarily or may require interposition grafting. A temporary intraluminal bypass shunt may maintain cerebral blood flow while repair is effected.

Vertebral arterial injuries are less common and may be identified only at angiography. If there is good contralateral flow, primary ligation is acceptable, but where there is a single or dominant vessel, repair is necessary.

Venous injuries to the neck can mostly be ligated except where there is bilateral internal jugular damage.

The thorax

Blunt injury is most often seen to the proximal descending thoracic aorta and the proximal innominate artery. The enormous shearing and deceleration forces in high-speed road traffic accidents (RTAs) cause tearing of the relatively fixed descending thoracic aorta, which is frequently fatal. Penetrating wounds are commoner in all other great vessel injuries. Clavicular and first rib fractures can be seen in association with subclavian injuries.

A history of a high-speed RTA, the death of another occupant in the same car or penetration of the mid thorax should alert the admitting surgeon to the possibility of great vessel damage in an otherwise apparently stable patient. Chest radiography may show a widening superior mediastinum, deviation of a nasogastric tube or trachea from the midline. However, X-rays in the acute trauma situation can be notoriously difficult to interpret. Although CT and MRI may be useful modes of evaluation, aortography is still preferred clearly to delineate great vessel damage in the stable patient.

Surgical approaches may be via a median sternotomy or left fourth intercostal incision. Limited median sternotomy with 'trap door' extensions may be sufficient to expose subclavian injuries.

Partial or complete cardiopulmonary bypass is recommended by some surgeons to limit potential spinal cord ischaemia while thoracic aortic injuries are being repaired. Primary repair, interposition Dacron grafting or extra-anatomical bypass grafting may all be appropriate in injuries to the innominate and subclavian vessels.

Injuries to the superior vena cava (SVC) and azygos vein are usually penetrating ones, leading to high blood loss and difficult exposure. Ligation of the azygos vein with lateral repair of the SVC is indicated.

The abdomen

Most abdominal vascular injuries (80%) are penetrating. Blunt trauma is often seen in association with other serious injuries to the abdominal viscera and pelvis which prove fatal. However, deceleration may occasionally avulse mesenteric or renal branches of the aorta or cause intimal tears, and seat-belt compression may cause aortic thrombosis. Resulting haemorrhage may be free intraperitoneal with hypovolaemic shock or contained within the retroperitoneum.

The need for rapid surgical exploration is usually obvious from the history and clinical signs. However, when there is contained haemorrhage in a stable patient, plain X-rays, CT scanning and aortography all may be helpful. All reasonably stable patients with penetrating abdominal trauma should have an excretion urogram to evaluate the renal blood supply, delineate the ureters and exclude urinary extravasation. If necessary this may be done in the operating theatre. Diagnostic peritoneal lavage usually adds little to the clinical picture and false positive results can occur.

The availability of autotransfusion equipment in theatre is desirable. A midline incision allows good exposure and can be extended into the thorax. Major haemorrhage can be controlled by cross-clamping the supracoeliac aorta or the thoracic aorta via a left thoracotomy. Packing of the abdomen can then be performed and the small bowel swung to the right to allow inspection of the abdominal cavity and identification of the source of bleeding. Suprarenal injuries can only be adequately exposed by mobilizing the spleen, left colon, left kidney and tail of the pancreas to the right. The method of repair is determined by the nature of the wound, with lateral suture and patch angioplasty being usually sufficient for stab wounds. Where there is tissue loss, interposition grafting is appropriate, unless there is also gross faecal soiling when oversew of the infrarenal aortic stump with extra-anatomical bypass grafting should be considered. Alternatively, some surgeons advocate PTFE as a conduit when there is faecal soiling.

Single injuries to the coeliac, superior mesenteric and inferior mesenteric arteries can be safely ligated at their origins in the young trauma victim due to the excellent marginal blood supply to the gut. Injuries to the superior mesenteric artery distal to the inferior border of the pancreas require repair. Injuries to the renal arteries should be repaired, if necessary by reimplantation, to revascularize the kidney. The iliac vessels can be approached directly and repaired. Where there is iliac vein injury, control may only be achieved by dividing the overlying artery first, and then repairing the vein and artery in sequence.

There is a high mortality associated with wounds of the inferior vena cava (IVC). Anterior wounds to the IVC can be controlled with a partial occlusion clamp (Satinsky) to allow lateral suture. The posterior wall should be carefully examined for injury before the cava is closed. More extensive wounds may necessitate caval ligation. Injury to the retro-hepatic IVC is difficult to expose and may require temporary atriocaval bypass shunting.

Postoperative management

An intraoperative Doppler assessment may give evidence of distal patency. However, completion angiography should be performed when-ever possible to allow assessment of anastomoses and certainly if there is any doubt about the adequacy of flow. It can demonstrate hitherto un-recognized intimal flaps, false aneurysms and arteriovenous fistulae. These complications should be treated immediately as they will jeo-pardize the preceding repair — both false aneurysms and arteriovenous fistulae will increase in size and complexity, making delayed surgery more difficult. Ideally, they should be identified preoperatively allowing planning of the initial operation. Regrettably, they can be missed in the haste of preoperative assessment and only reveal themselves after repair re-establishes flow.

Broad-spectrum antibiotics should be given to all patients in the post-operative period. Systemic anticoagulation may help in isolated vascular injuries, but may complicate the recovery of patients with multiple injuries.

Summary

- Vascular injuries are associated with a high level of mortality and morbidity.
- Most wounds are due to road traffic accidents in the UK, but urban violence leads to high levels of penetrating injury.
- Assessment can be difficult unless there is obvious blood loss.
- Angiography is important in the assessment of the stable patient, but should not delay surgery in those failing to respond to resuscitation.
- Good access, proximal and distal control and careful surgical technique are essential to ensure successful management.
- Concomitant venous repair is important in popliteal injuries.

Areas of controversy

- Role of MRI angiography in assessment of vascular trauma.
- Order of surgical precedence when there is combined orthopaedic and vascular trauma to the limbs.
- Place of temporary arterial and venous bypass shunting in limb vascular trauma.
- Use of artificial (PTFE) grafts in potentially contaminated wounds.
- A selective operative policy in penetrating mid-cervical wounds.
- Role of delayed primary lavage in abdominal vascular trauma.

Further reading

- Perry MO. Vascular trauma. In: Moore WS (ed) *Vascular Surgery.* Philadelphia: WB Saunders, 1993, pp 630–647.
- Franklin DP, Cambria RP. Arterial and venous injuries. In: Morris PJ, Malt RA (eds) *Oxford Textbook of Surgery.* Oxford: Oxford University Press, 1994, pp 454–460.
- McCroskey BL, Moore EE, Rutherford RB (eds). Vascular trauma. *Surgical Clinics of North America* 1988;**68**(4).

24
Renal Artery Stenosis

George Hamilton

Introduction

Renal artery stenosis (RAS), an increasing problem in the ageing populations of the Western world, is the commonest cause of severe hypertension, renal failure and their morbidity and mortality. Unfortunately, because of its slowly progressive and largely asymptomatic nature, this condition goes unrecognized until it is well advanced.

Aetiology

Causes of renal artery disease are:

- atherosclerosis;
- fibromuscular dysplasia;
- middle aortic syndrome;
- neurofibromatosis;
- Marfan's syndrome;
- Takayasu's disease;
- systemic vasculitis;
- idiopathic hypercalcaemia;
- renal artery aneurysm.

of which the two major causes are fibromuscular dysplasia in the young and arteriosclerosis in the elderly.

Renal artery fibromuscular dysplasia

This is an heterogeneous group of diseases which are not due to arteriosclerosis or inflammatory vascular disease. It is rare, occurring in only 0.5% of the general population, most commonly in caucasians. This condition is the commonest cause of correctable renal hypertension in the young. The dysplastic process mainly involves the media and the adventitia of the artery but with intimal dysplasia alone accounting for only 5% of all dysplastic renal artery lesions. This latter condition usually presents

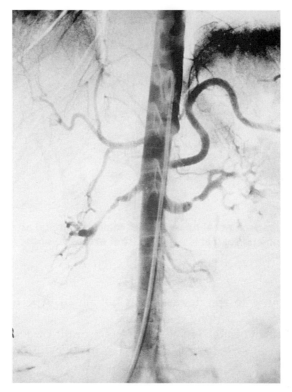

Fig. 24.1. Typical angiographic appearance of fibromuscular dysplasia of the renal artery.

as a smooth focal stenosis of the main renal artery itself. The commoner medial muscular dysplasia gives a classical appearance of 'a string of beads' and occurs most often in females (Fig. 24.1).

Atherosclerotic renal artery stenosis

In the majority of patients the atherosclerotic process does not arise in the renal artery but is a continuation of severe widespread aortic wall disease which involves the origin or ostium of the renal arteries. Arteriosclerotic disease of the main stem renal artery is much less common. Thus, atherosclerotic renal artery disease is classified into either osteal or non-osteal (Fig. 24.2).

Atherosclerotic RAS is most commonly a progressive lesion, particularly in stenoses >60%. Thus, the severity of the stenosis is predictive of the eventual outcome. Duplex studies of the natural history of stenoses >60% have revealed occlusion rates of 5% at 1 year and 10% at 2 years. Because of the development of a collateral circulation, progression is

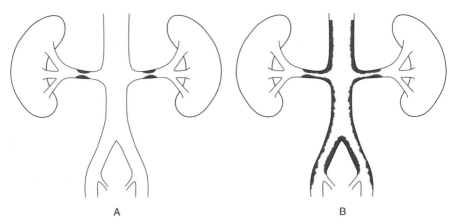

Fig. 24.2. Comparison of (A) non-osteal or main stem renal artery stenosis with (B) the commoner osteal lesion as part of extensive aortic atherosclerosis and calcification.

always silent but with the development initially of hypertension and in the later stages renal atrophy and failure.

Renovascular hypertension develops as a result of activation of the renin–angiotensin system as a response to hypoperfusion of the juxta-glomerular apparatus. This is further compounded by the development of fibrotic change and glomerulosclerosis secondary to long-standing hypertension. This insidious development of renal failure results from ischaemic atrophy of the renal cortex manifest by shrinkage of the kidney. Once the serum creatinine has increased above 200 mmol/l, approximately 50% of renal parenchyma and function has been lost.

Renal artery stenosis secondary to Takayasu's arteritis

Takayasu's arteritis is probably the commonest cause of RAS presenting in young adults in the East and Africa. It is associated with multiple arterial occlusions, typically with complete occlusion of the proximal renal artery.

Clinical features

Clinical presentations of renovascular disease are:

- severe hypertension;
- acute renal failure (often with ACE inhibitors);
- chronic renal failure;
- flash pulmonary oedema;
- asymptomatic finding at angiography.

Severe hypertension

Fibromuscular dysplasia, Takayasu's arteritis and congenital causes of RAS all present as severe hypertension developing in childhood or early adulthood. These syndromes are rarely associated with progression to severe renal failure. These are rare syndromes and the bulk of reno-vascular disease presenting to the vascular specialist is secondary to atherosclerosis.

Atherosclerotic renovascular disease increases markedly with age with an incidence of over 70% in the over 70s having been reported in post-mortem studies. Clearly the majority of these patients are asymptomatic but this high incidence underlines the frequency of the condition. The true incidence of hypertension in patients with atherosclerotic renovascular disease remains unclear.

Renal failure

Acute renal failure in the elderly often develops in severe atherosclerotic renal artery disease particularly during treatment for associated hyper-tension with angiotensin converting enzyme (ACE) inhibitors. Approx-imately 15% of patients over the age of 50 presenting with acute renal failure will have renal artery stenosis as the sole underlying precipitating condition. Because of inhibition of the mechanism described above, the use of ACE inhibitors is causing a greater proportion of previously asymptomatic patients to present with renal failure.

Patients with atherosclerotic RAS requiring dialysis have a very poor outcome, due to associated conditions such as myocardial ischaemia, left ventricular dysfunction, peripheral vascular disease and cerebral vas-cular disease. The median survival of 25 months with only 18% surviving at 5 years and 5% at 10 years compares with median survival of 52 months for all dialysis patients with 44% surviving 5 years and 23% 10 years.

Flash pulmonary oedema

This is a condition specific to RAS occurring in patients who do not have severe left ventricular dysfunction but who frequently develop severe life-threatening and often refractory pulmonary oedema. It occurs mostly in patients with poorly controlled hypertension and renal failure with bilateral renal artery stenosis; over half have a completely occluded renal artery. Again, the situation is often aggravated by the use of ACE inhibitors for the treatment of the presumed left ventricular failure.

Asymptomatic renal stenoses

Since RAS occurs as part of widespread arteriosclerosis it is not surprising that there is a high prevalence of this condition noted at angiography for other conditions:

- peripheral vascular disease (22–59%);
- aortic aneurysmal and occlusive disease (28–38%);
- coronary artery disease of >50% stenosis (15%).

Diagnosis

Hypertension occurring in childhood or in the young carries a very high likelihood of RAS and this diagnosis must be excluded by angiography. At the other end of the age spectrum, any patient over the age of 50 who has risk factors for arteriosclerotic disease and has resistant hypertension or any degree of renal failure should be considered as having atherosclerotic RAS until proven otherwise.

Renal vein renin measurement

This is an old diagnostic methodology which is now of value only in the assessment of renovascular hypertension where there are bilateral renal artery lesions. The demonstration of a high renal vein/inferior vena cava ratio (>1.5) indicates the presence of a significant RAS meriting intervention.

Ultrasound assessment

Ultrasound assessment of the size of the kidneys is an extremely valuable first investigation. The length of the kidneys is a good predictor of outcome after revascularization. Kidneys <8–9 cm in length are unlikely to yield significant renal function after revascularization. The demonstration of asymmetrical kidneys is highly predictive of significant RAS.

Duplex scanning

Because of the anatomical disposition of the origin of the renal arteries and their posterolateral course, duplex scanning of the hilar arteries is a technically very demanding procedure. This difficulty is further compounded by overlying intestinal gas and in most hands this is not a reliable investigative modality. Further improvements in the diagnostic accuracy of duplex scanning may come with the advent of ultrasonic contrast media.

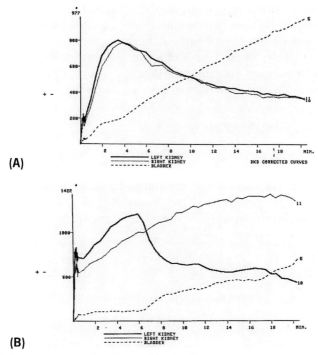

Fig. 24.3. Renogram of patient with a unilateral renal artery stenosis (A) before and (B) after captopril.

Captopril renography

Captopril renography is based on the physiological response to glomerular hypoperfusion of renin release and eventual conversion to angiotensin II. If significant change to a DTPA or MAG III scan is found after the administration of captopril in comparison to the pre-administration study, then it is likely that a significant RAS is present (Fig. 24.3). Studies have confirmed good sensitivity and specificity for this test but only for stenoses of >50%. The best results have been obtained in young patients with hypertension, with more difficulty in the assessment of older patients with bilateral renal artery disease.

Contrast angiography

Intra-arterial digital subtraction angiography with anterior and oblique views of the renal artery origin remains the gold standard in the investigation of RAS. It is obviously associated with risks because of its invasive nature and the nephrotoxicity of the contrast load. Thus this investigation should be performed only where there is a high clinical suspicion and need for intervention. Intravenous hydration and monitoring of urine output is mandatory before, during and after angiography, particularly in patients with a degree of renal failure. Because of the high prevalence of involvement of the coeliac and superior mesenteric arteries, lateral views of these vessels are valuable, particularly where an extra-anatomic reconstruction of the renal circulation is being considered.

Carbon dioxide angiography

Reasonable imaging can be obtained with this technique using a high volume injection of carbon dioxide which is extremely soluble and is very quickly absorbed and excreted by the lungs. Because of its low viscosity, carbon dioxide can be given through smaller delivery systems but requires a special injector pump. However, imaging of the segmental and small vessel arteries is poor.

Spiral CT angiography

Spiral CT scanning with 3D-reconstruction gives good imaging of the renal vessels in expert hands. Sensitivity of 90% with a specificity of 80% has been reported when compared to arterial angiography. Intra-arterial injection is not needed but a major contrast load is still required.

Magnetic resonance angiography

This technique carries much promise since there is no need for arterial cannulation or use of contrast agents. With present technology good images can be obtained but the severity of the stenotic lesions typically is over-estimated.

Management

Medical management

Hypertension, often severe and difficult to control, is a frequent feature of renovascular disease whatever the cause. Management in conjunction with a nephrologist or relevant physician will be required, particularly in atherosclerotic disease. Postural hypotension is common and the standing blood pressure should be used as a guide for treatment. Triple or quadruple antihypertensive therapy is often required.

Modulation of hyperlipidaemia and other cardiovascular risk factors such as fibrinogen and lipoprotein (a) is important in reducing long-term risk of death from myocardial disease.

Optimization of function in the presence of renal failure is worthwhile and to this end the use of ACE inhibitors and non-steroidal anti-inflammatory drugs must be avoided.

Intervention

The indications for renal revascularization are:

● difficult to control hypertension;
● flash pulmonary oedema;
● progressive renal failure;
● to halt progression of renal artery stenosis.

Endovascular renal revascularization

Angioplasty is the treatment of choice for fibromuscular dysplasia in the vast majority of cases. Repeat angioplasty of recurrent stenoses is usually successful but in rare cases, particularly those involving distal segmental arteries, surgical reconstruction will be required (see below).

In atherosclerotic RAS the results of angioplasty are not as good as in fibromuscular dysplasia, particularly where the lesion is osteal, with best results achieved in main stem renal artery lesions. Angioplasty of osteal lesions remains controversial but good technical and clinical success rates have been reported recently (Fig. 24.4). Improved technical success rates have been reported with stent angioplasty which has the theoretical advantage of resisting the high tendency to restenosis from aortic recoil at the site of the renal ostium.

Renal artery angioplasty carries with it a small but real risk of major complications such as renal artery rupture, complete occlusion at the angioplasty site and major renal ischaemia. This procedure must not be performed without the backup of appropriate renovascular expertise in the event of such a catastrophe.

Because of the tendency to restenosis, careful follow-up post renal angioplasty is essential. To obtain good results, redo angioplasty, or if necessary surgical revascularization is required in up to 20% of patients. Restenosis, due to myointimal hyperplasia, may make reintervention extremely difficult.

Surgical renal revascularization

The surgical options for renal revascularization include:

● aortorenal bypass (saphenous vein, PTFE, Dacron);
● aortic replacement and renal bypass;
● endarterectomy of renal artery stenosis;
● extra-anatomical bypass (hepato- and spleno-renal, iliac, supracoeliac);
● bench reconstruction/autotransplantation.

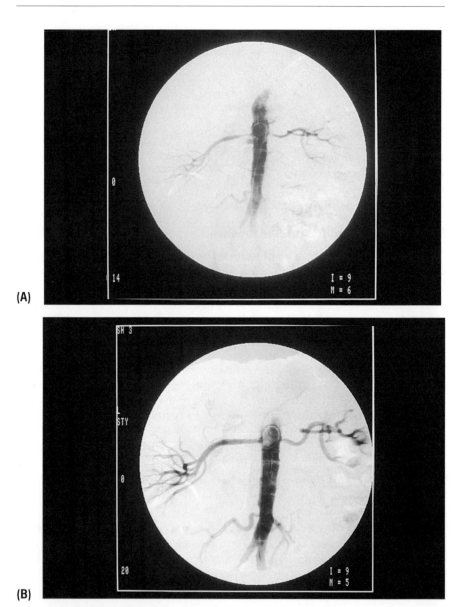

Fig. 24.4. Balloon angioplasty of osteal right renal artery stenosis. (A) Before and (B); after angioplasty.

Aortorenal bypass

Simple bypass grafting from the aorta to the renal artery is the most straightforward approach to surgical renal revascularization. This is the treatment of choice where the aorta is not severely diseased and is the

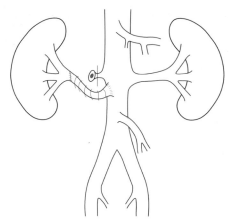

Fig. 24.5. Aortorenal bypass grafting with spatulated end-to-end anastomosis.

commonest procedure used in younger patients. The origin of the bypass graft is most commonly taken from the anterolateral aspect of the infra-renal aorta (Fig. 24.5). The graft material can either be saphenous vein or prosthetic, either polytetrafluoroethylene (PTFE) or Dacron, 6–8 mm in diameter. There are no prospective comparisons of these materials but the literature does not indicate any difference in performance. However, saphenous vein has a tendency with time to dilate.

Aortic replacement and renal reconstruction

Aortic replacement is most often indicated where there is a significant infrarenal abdominal aortic aneurysm. A 6–8 mm limb of prosthetic

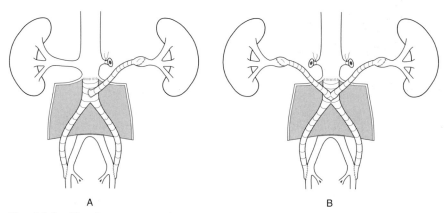

A   B

Fig. 24.6. Simultaneous aortic replacement and (A) unilateral and (B) bilateral renal revascularization.

material is sutured onto the trunk of the aortic graft and then anastomosed onto the appropriate renal artery. Bilateral renal revascularization
can be best obtained by suturing a small reversed bifurcated prosthetic
graft onto the front of the *in situ* aortic graft and then anastomosis of
each limb made to the renal arteries (Fig. 24.6).

Endarterectomy of renal artery stenosis

Endarterectomy requires extensive exposure of the juxtarenal aorta, left
renal vein and inferior vena cava. After partial aortic clamping across the
renal artery origin, an incision is made from the aorta across the stenosis
onto the main stem renal artery. Under direct vision, an endarterectomy
is performed and the arteriotomy closed with a patch of prosthetic material (Fig. 24.7). Excellent results with this approach are reported in those
few centres which regularly use it.

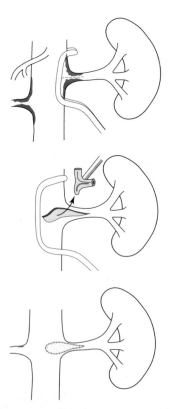

Fig. 24.7. Unilateral aortorenal endarterectomy with patch angioplasty.

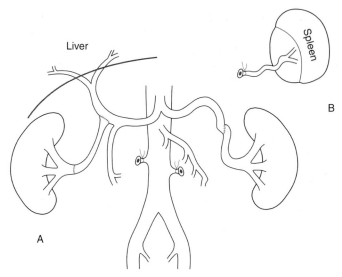

Fig. 24.8. Extra-anatomical renal revascularization; (A) Hepatorenal and (B) splenorenal bypass.

Extra-anatomical renal revascularization

This approach has considerable advantages, particularly in patients in whom the aorta does not require resection. The procedure can be achieved through a subcostal incision and there is no need to dissect or clamp the aorta. Most commonly, the hepatic artery on the right and the splenic artery on the left are used as the inflow sites (Fig. 24.8). In an hepatorenal bypass the gastroduodenal artery is of sufficient calibre in up to 50% of patients to allow anastomosis of this artery end-to-end onto the renal artery. In other cases, either saphenous vein or a 6 mm prosthetic graft is used as an inter-position graft. In a splenorenal bypass the splenic artery is divided after careful mobilization at its mid point and anastamosed end-to-end onto the left renal artery. The spleen remains viable on its collateral circulation and the short gastric blood supply.

Bench reconstruction/autotransplantation

In the presence of segmental stenosis of the renal artery, particularly where these are multiple or where there has been previous surgery to the main stem renal artery, bench reconstruction is an attractive option. The kidney is removed after division of the main stem renal artery and the renal vein, cooled and perfused in exactly the same way as a harvested kidney for renal transplantation. Bench reconstruction of multiple stenosis can be undertaken with either multiple saphenous vein patches or the internal iliac artery with its branches, if this is healthy. Using this approach there are no time constraints to the reconstruction. Once complete the kidney can be autotransplanted either into its native bed or onto the iliac circulation.

Nephrectomy

Where a kidney is too small for revascariztion (<8 cm in length) and is shown to produce excessive quantities of renin, nephrectomy may help to aneliorate severe hypertension. In the situation of successful revascularization of a solidarity functioning kidney with the contralateral kidney producing renin, 'a chemical' nephrectomy can be induced by the administration of an ACE inhibitor.

Outcome

Successful renal revascularization can be defined in terms of the effect on hypertension and renal function.

Hypertension

- Cure is defined as diastolic pressure ≤90 mmHg without medication.
- Improvement is defined as 50% decrease in diastolic pressure or diastolic pressure <90 mmHg with decrease in quantity of antihypertensive medication.

Renal function

- Improvement is defined as a fall in serum creatinine >15%.
- Renal function is stabilized if no increase in serum creatinine on follow-up; renal function is worse if >15% rise in serum creatinine.

Cure of renovascular hypertension will occur in only 15% of patients with improvement occurring in 70% and deterioration in the remainder. Similar results can be expected for preservation of renal function.

Endovascular renal revascularization

There is only one prospective randomized trial comparing angioplasty (non-stent) with surgery and this documents a primary patency rate for angioplasty of 70% with a secondary patency rate of 90% at 2-year follow-up. However, 17% of patients required surgical revascularization to obtain clinical success. The conclusion from this trial was that angioplasty is the primary treatment of choice, certainly for renovascular hypertension provided there was careful follow-up with prompt reintervention either by redo angioplasty or surgical reconstruction.

Complications of angioplasty are greater in the elderly patient, in particular in those with a solitary functioning kidney. Major haemorrhage or acute thrombotic occlusion may lead to emergency surgery, a scenario which carries a high mortality approaching 40%.

There has been a recent explosive increase in the use of renal stents because of the extremely high technical success rates of 90–100%. However, there is a significant restenosis rate at 6 months of 12–40%. Until the long-term results of ongoing trials are available, the use of stent angioplasty should be limited to that of a secondary procedure. This is because of the technical problem of reintervention.

Surgical renal revascularization

Results of surgical intervention for RAS in the young are good with excellent long-term clinical success rates and low mortality being reported. However, the atherosclerotic patient being older with multiorgan involvement has a much higher risk from surgery.

Combined renal revascularization and aortic resection carries a significant morbidity and the highest mortality rate of all the procedures. The experience of several centres, including the author's, documents a mortality rate in the region of 15%. Renal revascularization without aortic reconstruction carries significantly lower mortality rates of between 3% and 6%. Risk factors associated with elevated mortality include:

- advanced renal failure (serum creatinine >250 mmol);
- aneurysmal rather than occlusive aortic disease;
- complex renal and visceral renal reconstructions;
- significant coronary artery disease.

Summary

- Renal artery stenosis is endemic in today's atherosclerotic population.
- A high index of clinical suspicion for the presence of this condition in elderly arteriopaths is important.
- Intervention is indicated in the presence of severe, intractable hypertension and progressive renal failure (serum creatinine >150 mmol) and in renal artery stenoses >60%.
- Best results are obtained by a multidisciplinary approach involving the nephrologist, interventional radiologist and vascular surgeon.

Areas of controversy

- Should an asymptomatic renal artery stenosis be treated?
- Is the use of primary stent angioplasty for osteal renal artery lesions indicated or justified?
- Is angioplasty of a high-grade stenosis in a solitary kidney better than surgical revascularization?
- Which has the better long-term results — angioplasty or surgical revascularization?

Further reading

- Zierler RE, Bergelin IO, Isaacson JA, Strandness BE. Natural history of atherosclerotic renal artery stenosis; a prospective study with a duplex ultrasonography. *Journal of Vascular Surgery* 1994;**19**:250–258.
- Connolly JO, Higgins RM, Walters HL *et al.* Presentation, clinical features and outcome and different patterns of atherosclerotic renovascular disease. *Quarterly Journal of Medicine* 1994;**87**:413–421.
- Kidney DD, Deutsch L-S. The indications and results of percutaneous transluminal angioplasty and stenting in renal artery stenosis. In: Wilson SE (ed) *Renal Disease and the Vascular Surgeon. Seminars in Vascular Surgery* 1996;**9**:188–197.
- Weibull H, Bergqvist D, Bergentz S-E *et al.* Percutaneous transluminal renal angioplasty versus surgical reconstruction of atherosclerotic renal artery stenosis; A prospective randomised study. *Journal of Vascular Surgery* 1993;**18**:841–852.
- Novick A, Scoble JE, Hamilton G (eds). *Renal Vascular Disease.* London: WB Saunders, 1996.

25

Mesenteric Ischaemia

Ian M Williams and John HN Wolfe

Introduction

Mesenteric ischaemia is a relatively uncommon vascular emergency and accounts for fewer than 4000 emergency abdominal operations in the UK. Since the other effects of vascular disease are now being managed more effectively and patients are living longer, the incidence of mesenteric ischaemia is likely to increase. The clinical presentation may be misleading with vague symptoms. Indeed, once signs are obvious mesenteric infarction has usually occurred and the situation has become irremediable. The diagnosis should be considered in any patient with pre-existing cardiovascular disease who has a sudden onset of abdominal pain which is out of proportion to the physical signs.

The typical presentation of chronic mesenteric ischaemia is that of extreme weight loss and abdominal pain on ingestion of food which prevents the patient eating. Unlike most other causes of abdominal pain the patient is hungry but is frightened to eat. Many patients present with a much vaguer history. They do, however, usually have evidence of widespread vascular disease.

Acute mesenteric ischaemia

Aetiology and diagnosis

Superior mesenteric artery embolus

One-third of cases of acute mesenteric ischaemia are due to arterial embolism. The embolus originates in the left atrium and atrial fibrillation or a history of peripheral embolism are particularly relevant. Fifteen percent of the emboli lodge at the ostium of the superior mesenteric artery, 50% distal to the proximal jejunal and middle colic branches and the remainder travel distally.

Physical signs may be subtle but a catastrophic clinical course of rapid development of peritonitis and hypovolaemic shock may ensue (if the condition is not diagnosed and treated promptly and aggressively). If the proximal jejunum is viable, embolus is more likely than thrombosis; this sparing occurs because the embolus has lodged beyond the proximal jejunal branches (85% of patients). The development of peritonitis usually indicates irreversible bowel infarction and almost invariably has a fatal outcome.

Superior mesenteric artery thrombosis

The pain in this condition may develop more insidiously (since the pre-existing arterial disease may have led to the development of collaterals) and signs of shock and peritonitis can be delayed. Approximately 50% of patients describe symptoms related to mesenteric ischaemia prior to the acute episode. Similarly, there may be evidence of arterial disease in the peripheral, coronary and extracranial arteries. The extent of the infarction is usually greater than for embolism and may extend from the duodenum to the transverse colon. The thrombotic process tends to involve the superior mesenteric artery at its origin which is proximal to the jejunal and middle colic arteries. Due to the necessity for complicated revascularization, the long-term outcome is worse than for embolism.

Mesenteric venous thrombosis

This condition can be classified as primary or secondary. The number of mesenteric venous thromboses classified as primary has decreased as increasing numbers of causative factors have been identified. Secondary mesenteric venous thrombosis is usually associated with:

- protein C and S deficiency;
- antithrombin III deficiency;
- Leiden antibody;
- polycythaemia;
- thrombocytosis;
- other rarer causes, such as following blunt abdominal trauma and portal pyaemia.

Mesenteric venous thrombosis can be classified into either acute or chronic depending upon whether symptoms have been present for 4 weeks or more. In this condition, the prodromal period is usually prolonged with an average duration of pain of up to 2 weeks prior to admission. Reports indicate that it may be responsible for up to 30% of cases of acute mesenteric ischaemia. The fact that mesenteric thrombosis is secondary to a procoagulant state in many patients is supported by a history of deep vein thrombosis or pulmonary embolism in 50% of patients.

Diagnosis is usually difficult although patients with a prior history of hyperthrombotic states presenting with abdominal pain with no obvious cause should raise suspicion.

Non-occlusive mesenteric ischaemia

This affects the superior mesenteric artery almost exclusively and appears to be a multifactorial process. Those affected invariably have a stenosis at the origin of the superior mesenteric artery and abnormal cardiac function. Factors which contribute to this presentation include dehydration, sepsis and recent cardiac surgery. The cause is a drop in perfusion pressure which secondarily causes microcapillary sludging. On arteriography, all the major mesenteric branches appear patent, but the secondary and tertiary branches of the superior mesenteric artery show narrowings and irregularities.

Investigations

Mesenteric ischaemia should be carefully considered in the differential diagnosis of sudden onset abdominal pain, especially in the elderly.

There is no specific laboratory investigation that reliably indicates the presence of ischaemic bowel. Common biochemical findings in ischaemic bowel may be leucocytosis, hyperamylasaemia and abnormal liver function tests. Evidence has been presented that elevated serum phosphate was diagnostic but other studies have not substantiated this.

A plain abdominal X-ray may exclude other causes of abdominal pain but signs specific to mesenteric ischaemia are rare and most patients have a normal film.

The most accurate method of demonstrating mesenteric ischaemia is angiography. As no reliable screening test is available the use of angiography has to be based upon clinical suspicion. Unfortunately, in some reports, false negatives are as high as 50%.

The investigation of choice for suspected mesenteric venous thrombosis is CT, providing there is no peritonitis, although this is being superceded by MRI. The recognized radiological features are thrombus in the superior mesenteric vein, thickened bowel wall and pneumatosis. If this investigation is inconclusive, then angiography with a delayed venous phase may reveal the diagnosis. Once the diagnosis is made, intravenous heparinization is the current treatment.

Management

Medical management

Three major factors are involved in the pathophysiology of acute mesenteric ischaemia and each has important therapeutic implications:

- fluid sequestration;
- reperfusion injury;
- splanchnic vasoconstriction.

Fluid loss

The amount of fluid lost in mesenteric ischaemia is considerable and must not be underestimated. Animal experiments have suggested that one-third of the circulating fluid may be lost after superior mesenteric artery occlusion. This is primarily plasma and a rise in haematocrit is common. When the arterial flow is restored and the gut revascularized, there is marked reactionary haemorrhage into the bowel lumen.

The initial replacement in these patients should commence with 2–3 litres of colloid infusion. Blood transfusion may then be necessary. Many patients with acute mesenteric ischaemia are frail and elderly and have associated cardiorespiratory problems; therefore, careful fluid replacement with central venous pressure monitoring on an intensive care unit should be arranged. Regular measurements of arterial blood pressure, pulse, heart rate and urinary output are obviously mandatory.

Reperfusion injury

When the gut is reperfused following a period of ischaemia, acidosis and anaerobic metabolism trigger the cascade that results in reperfusion injury. The main detrimental effects of reperfusion are manifest in the production of free radicals [superoxide (O_2), peroxide (H_2O_2) and hydroxyl (OH)]. Their release is associated with a systemic inflammatory response resulting from the release of cytokines and platelet activating factor. Release of these factors into the systemic circulation activates monocyte, neutrophil and endothelial cell activity and may result in renal dysfunction, adult respiratory distress syndrome and bone marrow suppression. The end result may be disseminated intravascular coagulation with widespread vascular permeability resulting in extensive fluid loss from the circulation.

Mannitol is useful as it is not only a diuretic but also a free radical scavenger. Allopurinol (a xanthine oxidase inhibitor) has the same effects but although shown to be effective in animal models, evidence in patients is currently tenuous.

Splanchnic vasoconstriction

Even after successful revascularization of the gut, vasoconstriction may persist, rendering the perfusion inadequate. The selective injection of papaverine into the superior mesenteric artery may improve survival rates and appears to be an attractive prospect in patients with a generally poor medical outlook.

Surgical management

All patients require full resuscitation with central lines, urinary catheter and continuous cardiopulmonary monitoring. A full laparotomy is indicated and a long midline incision is required. On opening the abdomen and discovering mesenteric ischaemia, the question is whether the bowel is viable or not. If the bowel is clearly infarcted, then a considered decision must be made at a senior level as to whether resection is appropriate. Elderly patients requiring resection of the entire small bowel should probably not be subjected to such a procedure.

The difficulty arises when the surgeon is confronted with bowel of doubtful though probably reversible viability. Under these circumstances full intraoperative resuscitation may alter the appearance; patience and warm packs while the anaesthetist optimizes the circulation can be rewarding. Clinical assessment of the arteries can be supplemented with a hand-held Doppler in a sterile glove and sleeve.

The cause of the ischaemia is fundamental to the operative approach and the clinical presentations discussed above assist the surgeon in making the decision. The segment of dead gut should be removed before revascularization, otherwise catastrophic reperfusion injury may ensue. The surgeon should then consider the various methods of restoring mesenteric circulation that depend upon cause.

Superior mesenteric artery embolus

Emboli almost invariably lodge beyond the first jejunal branches and the proximal jejunum is usually normal at laparotomy. There is also visible peristalsis in the vessels of the first arcade and a palpable pulse in the root of the mesentery. Since intestine of dubious viability may show good recovery, resection of the bowel is *not* the initial treatment and an embolectomy is required. On reperfusing the mesentery, the initial 500 ml of venous blood should be washed out of the circulation to reduce the consequences of reperfusion following revascularization.

The superior mesenteric artery can be approached inferior to the transverse mesocolon at the root of the mesentery. A longitudinal arteriotomy allows extraction of the embolus and the artery can be patched with vein (there should be no inert material in the presence of ischaemic gut). After removal of the embolus a number 2 Fogarty is inserted distally, taking care to avoid damage to the fragile intima.

Embolectomy is contraindicated when the embolus lodges more distally since the collateral circulation is usually sufficient to limit the ischaemia. Under these circumstances bowel resection alone has a high survival rate.

Thrombosis of the superior mesenteric artery

Any obviously necrotic bowel needs to be resected at the initial operation. If the bowel shows any indication that it may be viable, then more aggressive measures should be undertaken. The earliest reports of mesenteric artery thrombosis suggested thromboendarterectomy of the vessel. The origin of the superior mesenteric artery, however, is posterior to the pancreas and relatively inaccessible, rendering transaortic endarterectomy a technically formidable procedure, particularly in unfit patients. This procedure is no longer considered appropriate when the gut ischaemia is due to a thrombosis of the superior mesenteric artery.

If revacularization of the superior mesenteric artery is considered appropriate, retrograde aortomesenteric bypass is currently the procedure of choice in acute mesenteric artery thrombosis. As there may well be resection of necrotic bowel, an autologous vein rather than a prosthetic graft should be used. The main trunk of the artery may be exposed inferior to the transverse mesocolon as for an embolectomy and the adjacent aorta exposed. A very short graft should then be inserted between the aorta and the superior mesenteric artery. Unless the graft is very short it is prone to kink when the bowel is replaced into the abdomen. For this reason a direct side-to-side anastomosis between the superior mesenteric artery and aorta is considered preferable.

It must be remembered that these revascularization procedures are being performed in critically ill patients, so that the antegrade revascularizations suggested for chronic mesenteric ischaemia (see below) are usually inappropriate, although they offer superior long-term results.

Following revascularization any further necrotic bowel must be resected. Frequently there is remaining doubt about the resection margins and a second look laparotomy 24 h later should be planned.

Mesenteric venous thrombosis

Resection is almost inevitable since the condition is usually diagnosed at laparotomy performed for peritonitis of unknown aetiology. Due to the fact that there is a high incidence of recurrent ischaemia, some have suggested the resection margins should include 15 cm of macroscopically normal bowel. Anticoagulation should be commenced immediately as failure to instigate this can cause a high recurrence rate and mortality.

Venous thrombectomy can be successful on occasions when thrombosis in the portal or superior mesenteric veins is noted at operation. Primary mesenteric venous thrombosis causes more insidious and extensive intestinal ischaemia than arterial occlusion. Consequently, the operability and mortality rates are more favourable than for arterial occlusion. However, when mesenteric venous thrombosis occurs secondary to portal hypertension, visceral infection or systemic hypercoaguable states, the prognosis is similar to that of mesenteric artery thrombosis.

Determination of bowel viability

The traditional intraoperative observations of bowel viability are based on colour, contractility, visible pulsation and bleeding from the edges of the resection margin. If, however, bowel ischaemia is due to non-occlusive mesenteric ischaemia, the serosa may appear normal with a necrotic mucosa.

Although clinical judgement is moderately reliable, surgeons should always err on the side of caution. There are more objective tests of bowel viability available, but only Doppler ultrasound is widely used. The fluorescein dye technique and laser Doppler are advocated by a few.

If bowel viability remains in doubt after primary resection, many surgeons advocate a second-look operation performed 24–48 h later to allow a clearer assessment of the demarcation between viable and non-viable bowel. It is important to realize that the decision to perform the second-look procedure is made at the first operation and not in the post-operative period. At the initial operation, frankly necrotic bowel should be excised and a second-look procedure is indicated when there is doubt about remaining intestine. The threshold for re-exploration should be low as there is evidence that the decision not to reoperate may be incorrect in up to 20% of patients. Overall, a second-look laparotomy is required in approximately 40% of patients.

Chronic mesenteric ischaemia

Aetiology and diagnosis

Chronic mesenteric ischaemia is a rare but well recognized clinical entity. The usual presenting feature is postprandial cramping abdominal pain which has been described as 'intestinal angina'. The cause of the pain is thought to be shunting of blood to the stomach from the rest of the intestine on food intake. Another feature of chronic mesenteric ischaemia is weight loss associated with hunger.

This may be a difficult diagnosis to make and in many cases is reached as a last resort following many normal investigations in the expectation of discovering a gastrointestinal neoplasm.

A significant number of atherosclerotic patients have mild stenoses of the three major arteries supplying the small and large bowel. Furthermore, many patients have severe ostial stenoses which remain asymptomatic. A test to decide which of these is significant has yet to be introduced. Duplex scanning detects stenoses of the visceral arteries but this investigation is very operator dependent and is not straightforward.

The diagnosis is confirmed on aortography which must include lateral views to assess the origin of the coeliac, superior mesenteric and inferior mesenteric arteries. Angiography also provides information on the state of the aorta and the iliac arteries as inflow sites for planned bypass surgery (Fig. 25.1).

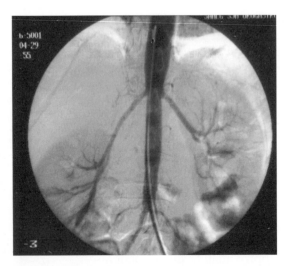

Fig. 25.1. Arterioposterior arteriogram of a patient with chronic mesenteric ischaemia. The aorta and renal arteries are visualized but no branches of the coeliac axis, superior mesenteric or inferior mesenteric are revealed. A lateral view is also essential.

Management

The aims of treatment are:

- to alleviate symptoms by improving mesenteric blood flow;
- (as in carotid endarterectomy) a prophylactic procedure to prevent the possibly dire consequences of arterial occlusion.

Treatment options include:

- angioplasty;
- endarterectomy;
- reimplantation;
- surgical bypass procedures.

Angioplasty

There are a number of reports of angioplasty in the literature. It is not, however, accepted widely as the first-choice procedure. Occlusion has serious consequences immediately and the distribution of the lesions at the ostia of the main vessels renders them more suitable for surgery rather than balloon angioplasty. Stents have not yet made an impact.

Surgery

The issues that have been considered:

- whether an endarterectomy or a formal bypass procedure should be performed?

- if a bypass procedure is performed, what is the optimum graft material?
- should a graft be placed infrarenally (retrograde) or from the supra-coeliac aorta (antegrade)?
- if more than one of the mesenteric vessels is affected, should they all be revascularized or is one sufficient?

Access for endarterectomy of the visceral origins is most easily performed by medial rotation of the viscera. In this way excellent exposure of the coeliac artery origin and superior mesenteric artery are afforded. A left lateral aortotomy is performed and the visceral area of the aorta endarterectomized (Fig. 25.2). This is surprisingly successful. There is anxiety about the distal limit of the endarterectomy and intraoperative Doppler is mandatory if this technique is used.

If bypass is the procedure of choice, certain factors need to be considered. To perform the proximal graft anastomosis on a severely diseased aorta is courting disaster and in some patients grafting from the iliac arteries can be considered. Retrograde revascularization has the disadvantage that any graft may kink once the bowel is returned to the abdominal cavity. To compensate for this, surgeons have suggested that the length of the graft should be very short, or sufficiently long that it may be placed in a retroperitoneal loop from the abdominal aorta along the anterior aspect of the left kidney and lower border of the pancreas to the proximal superior mesenteric artery.

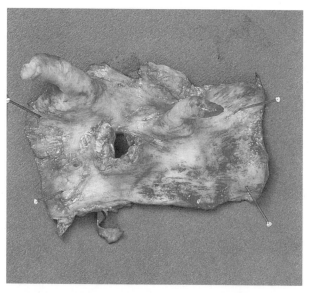

Fig. 25.2. **Endarterectomy specimen from a patient with chronic visceral ischaemia showing the four orifices that have been endarterectomized.**

There is no doubt that supracoeliac clamping is demanding for the surgeon and patient. However, using this method, grafts can be placed antegrade. The supracoeliac aorta is approached from the front through the lesser sac. The crura need to be cut and then swept off the aorta to allow exposure. This approach would appear to be more physiological and there is less risk of graft occlusion by kinking in this situation. Furthermore, this area of the aorta is relatively disease free.

Other methods include transecting the superior mesenteric artery from its origin and reimplanting the non-diseased artery distally onto the native aortic wall. This can be a technically demanding anastomosis and obviously requires the aorta to be relatively disease free. Revascularization of two visceral arteries is optimal although there have been published reports supporting superior mesenteric artery revascularization alone. The graft patency is significantly better where two vessels rather than one are revascularized. This can be achieved by using the proximal end of a vein graft as a plasty of the coeliac artery orifice and tunnelling the graft behind the pancreas to the superior mesenteric artery. Alternatively, a small-calibre Dacron trouser graft can be anastomosed to the supracoeliac aorta and the limbs anastomosed to the coeliac and superior mesenteric artery distally.

Summary

- Mesenteric ischaemia remains a deadly condition with high morbidity and mortality.
- Early diagnosis and intervention is required if outcome is to improve.
- Chronic mesenteric ischaemia is invariably under diagnosed in the UK.
- Weight loss is usually apparent in patients with chronic intestinal ischaemia.
- Mesenteric ischaemia does not occur unless at least two vessels are diseased.

Areas of controversy

- Role of angioplasty in the treatment of stenotic or occlusive lesions of the mesenteric arteries.
- Endarterectomy versus bypass as the treatment of choice.
- Which treatment is best for bypass: vein or synthetic material?

Further reading

- Lewis P, Wolfe JHN. Acute mesenteric ischaemia. In: *Emergency Vascular Surgery*. Greenhalgh RM, Hollier L (eds) London: WB Saunders, 1992, pp 205–216.
- Marston A, Bulkley GB, Fiddian-Green RG, Haglund UH (eds) *Splanchnic Ischaemia and Multiple Organ Failure*. London: Edward Arnold, 1989.

26
Revisional Surgery

A Ross Naylor

Introduction

Over the last 40 years there has been a huge proliferation in the number and extent of arterial reconstructions as surgeons become more experienced and innovative. However, most vascular surgeons would probably concede that some of the most complex problems they currently deal with are those that specifically relate to previous vascular reconstructions, including:

- seroma/lymphocele formation;
- graft aneurysm;
- anastomotic stenosis;
- graft stenosis;
- false aneurysm formation;
- deep graft infection;
- graft thrombosis;
- graft haemorrhage.

Redo surgery of any type is difficult, but revisional vascular surgery can be particularly challenging.

Aetiology

Seroma/lymphocele

A seroma or lymphocele is one of the commonest problems following vascular reconstruction and particularly following repeated explorations through the same wound. Disruption of the lymphatics, usually in the groin, leads to an accumulation of sterile lymph in the deep tissues. It occurs fairly quickly after surgery and can take many weeks to resolve.

Stenosis/thrombosis

Intragraft stenoses are not usually a problem in prosthetic grafts, but are very important in vein grafts. The below-knee or femorodistal vein graft

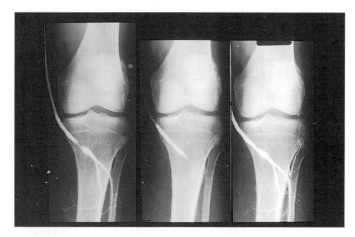

Fig. 26.1. Graft stenosis at lower end on *in situ* vein femoropopliteal bypass
successfully treated by balloon angioplasty.

is prone to localized stenoses in about 30% of patients. The incidence is
maximal in the first year after graft insertion and tends to affect the
lower third of an *in situ* vein graft and the upper third of a reversed vein
graft (Fig. 26.1).

The underlying aetiology is neointimal hyperplasia but it has not, as
yet, been possible to demonstrate conclusively why these should happen.
There is, however, evidence that the graft stenoses do not coincide with
valves or the location of vein graft branches. Anastomotic stenoses are a
particular problem with prosthetic grafts where there is thought to be a
compliance mismatch between the graft and the native artery. This leads
to a proliferation of neointima, particularly at the heel of the graft, which
is frequently responsible for late graft failure (Table 26.1).

The patency of long-term grafts depends on their location, graft type
and the capacity of a vascular unit to optimize patency through regular

Table 26.1. Causes of graft failure.

Early (<30 days)	Incorrect operation
	Poor operative technique
	Inadequate run-off
	Small calibre or diseased vein
	Prosthetic graft thrombogenicity
Intermediate (<1 year)	Neointimal hyperplasia
	Vein graft stenosis
Late (>1 year)	Progression of atheroma
	Deterioration of prosthetic graft

surveillance programmes. For example, the cumulative patency of aorto-bifemoral bypass grafts is about 90% at 5 years. However, the 1-year patency for above-knee femoropopliteal bypasses falls to about 80%, while distal grafts to the below-knee popliteal artery or tibial arteries have an actuarial patency rate of between 25% and 50%, depending on whether vein or prosthetic material was used. However, provided patients with vein grafts are entered into a surveillance programme, the 3-year patency can be maintained at about 70%.

Thrombosis of a prosthetic graft can follow progression of a stenosis at the graft–native artery interface due to intimal hyperplasia or it may be secondary to progressive run-off artery disease below the anastomosis. In patients with a graft or run-off stenosis, the final trigger for acute thrombosis may be a systemic insult such as cardiac failure or dehydration. Vein graft thrombosis most commonly follows progression of unrecognized graft or anastomotic stenoses.

Aneurysms

A *graft aneurysm* is a very rare complication with the newer prosthetic grafts but was associated with the earlier umbilical vein grafts and thinner weave Dacron grafts.

Aneurysms may develop in venous conduits for a number of reasons, including wall weakening after angioplasty of a vein graft stenosis or true aneurysm formation which is occasionally seen in patients who have had vein grafts to bypass popliteal artery aneurysms.

False aneurysms can occur at any anastomosis and may also be due to excessive weakening of the native arterial wall following endarterectomy. Proximal false aneurysms complicate 0.5% of aortic reconstructions (Fig. 26.2) for occlusive disease, while femoral false aneurysms complicate up to 3.5% of groin anastomoses. Carotid false aneurysms are found following 0.7% of procedures.

False aneurysms were initially associated with the use of silk as an anastomotic suture in the 1960s, although this is now never the case. False aneurysms should be considered to be an important predictor of potential infection with low virulence organisms, such as *staphylococcus epidermis*.

Irrespective of the aetiology, there is a progressive weakening at the anastomosis followed by a small leak of blood into a fibrous tissue cavity containing thrombus. As the cavity expands, the anastomosis can eventually become completely disrupted with the graft lying free within the false aneurysm.

Infection

Deep graft infection is the most feared complication after vascular reconstructions, particularly where prosthetic grafts are involved. Aortic graft

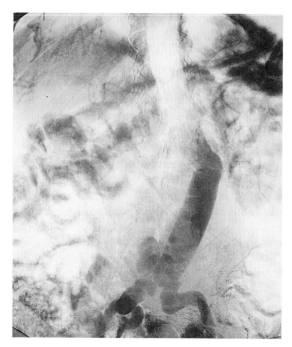

Fig. 26.2. **False aneurysm at lower end of a tube graft used to repair an abdominal aortic aneurysm.**

infections affect 1% of patients with occlusive disease and about 2% of patients with aneurysm disease. Any graft involving a groin wound is associated with a higher risk of infection, possibly up to 3.5%. Groin operations are particularly associated with deep infection because of their location within moist, potentially unclean skin creases.

The commonest micro-organism responsible for deep graft infection is *Staphylococcus aureus*, but over the last decade there has been an increasing frequency of Gram-negative and other organisms, including Proteus, *Escherichia coli* and *Streptococcus faecalis*. The most feared organism is methicillin-resistant *Staphylococcus aureus* (MRSA) which is becoming a major problem in vascular units throughout the UK.

Haemorrhage

Profuse graft haemorrhage is an important presenting feature in deep graft infection. However, in the early postoperative period it may simply be due to defective suturing techniques.

Clinical features

Seroma/lymphocele

Seromas and lymphoceles usually present within the first 6 weeks of surgery as a painless swelling, usually in the groin. Occasionally, the wound will not have completely healed, and there may be a small residual sinus draining clear, yellowish fluid to the distress of the patient with a risk of secondary infection.

Stenosis/thrombosis

Anastomotic and graft stenoses usually develop asymptomatically and may only be detected using Doppler or exercise ankle brachial pressure indices. Family doctors should, however, be warned that any patient with a pre-existing graft who develops new or worsening claudication should be considered to have anastomotic or run-off stenoses until proven otherwise. These patients should be investigated rapidly as once a graft has occluded, it may be particularly difficult to clear.

Aneurysms

Graft aneurysms present as a pulsatile swelling in the line of the graft or acutely with distal thromboembolism.

Graft thrombosis can present with any combination of features typical of acute limb ischaemia including pulselessness, pallor, perishing cold, pain, paraesthesia and paralysis. The clinical features and presentation of acute limb ischaemia are dealt with in Chapter 14.

False aneurysms can present any time from the early postoperative period until years after the initial operation. Irrespective of the timing of presentation, one must always be aware of the potential for infection, even though culture of the sac contents may be sterile to standard cultures.

False aneurysms present with a slowly or rapidly expanding pulsatile mass at a site of anastomosis. The most ominous variety includes those with associated redness and overlying skin necrosis which is a marker of imminent rupture and life-threatening haemorrhage. Alternatively, a false aneurysm is not an infrequent complication of femoral anastomoses in aortic grafts and may be very small and slowly progressive. As such, they may present with nothing more than a prominent pulsation in a groin and do not have the same prognosis as the more rapidly expanding forms.

Infection

Wound infections present with varying degrees of superficial and deep components. Erythema, induration and purulent discharge are well recognized features of wound infection and one must always be aware of the potential for deep involvement and life-threatening haemorrhage.

Deep graft infection presents with a combination of insidious features including: .

- pyrexia of unknown origin;
- night sweats;
- rigors;
- diffuse pains;
- septic emboli;
- graft thrombosis;
- graft haemorrhage;
- induration or even frank abscess formation.

A rare but important complication of aortic procedures is the aorto-enteric fistula where there is a direct communication between one of the aortic anastomoses and the lumen of the gastrointestinal tract, usually the duodenum or jejunum. This can present with life-threatening haemorrhage, usually preceded by a herald bleed. Accordingly, any patient with gastrointestinal bleeding and an aortic graft must be assumed to have an aortoenteric fistula until proven otherwise.

Diagnosis

The diagnosis of most vascular complications requires a high index of suspicion and, occasionally, lateral thinking.

Swellings along the line of the graft or at anastomoses should be examined by duplex ultrasound which will demonstrate whether the swelling is a *false aneurysm* or a *seroma/lymphocele/fluid collection.* If there is a late fluid collection or a persisting seroma which is resistant to treatment, ultrasound can guide aspiration of a small amount of fluid under aseptic conditions in order to allow culture of organisms and selection of appropriate antibiotics. However, one must be aware that the absence of a positive culture on fluid aspiration does not necessarily exclude infection and the microbiologists should be warned so that prolonged cultures can be performed.

False aneurysms of the aortic anastomoses are more difficult to evaluate using ultrasound, but if there is a suspicion of this on examination, the patient should undergo CT scanning and/or angiography (Fig. 26.2). The latter has potential therapeutic importance (see below).

Recurrent and/or graft stenoses cannot be detected readily by clinical examination. Because they are well known to be associated with vein grafts, most centres have a surveillance programme which uses duplex parameters to evaluate the degree of stenosis based on either the peak systolic velocity or the velocity ratio across the stenosis. Those with no access to duplex surveillance can use resting and post-exercise ankle brachial pressure indices and select those with significant falls (>0.15) to proceed to angiography with a view to angioplasty.

Diagnosis of *deep graft infection* can be particularly difficult. The key factor is suspicion. First-line investigations include full blood count and either plasma viscosity or erythrocyte sedimentation rates to look for leucocytosis, etc. An ultrasound scan will provide information on the presence or absence of a false aneurysm and in patients with an aortic graft and upper gastrointestinal haemorrhage, an endoscopy may exclude alternative sources of bleeding such as oesophageal or gastric tumours or ulcers well away from the retroperitoneal bed.

In patients with severe ongoing *haemorrhage*, however, there is little time for investigation and the patient may need to go to theatre straight away. One useful diagnostic and potentially therapeutic development is a percutaneous angiogram through the groin which may demonstrate the bleeding false aneurysm at the proximal aortic anastomosis. This can then be immediately controlled by insertion of an aortic balloon occlusion catheter, thereby allowing stabilization of a rapidly declining haemodynamic status.

Low-grade insidious presentations of infection warrant thorough investigation in order to be entirely sure of the extent and nature of the problem. Aortic grafts are fairly inaccessible and require examination with CT to look for air–fluid interfaces or gas bubbles within the perigraft tissues and/or the presence of a false aneurysm (Fig. 26.3). A CT scan can also permit guided needle aspiration of periaortic fluid for culture which can be invaluable in planning antibiotic therapy.

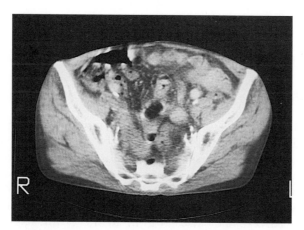

Fig. 26.3. CT scan showing gas bubbles indicative of infection around the right limb of an aortobifemoral bypass graft.

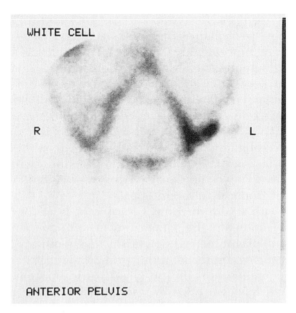

WHITE CELL

R   L

ANTERIOR PELVIS

Fig. 26.4. Indium-labelled white cell scan demonstrating increased uptake in the left groin due to infection of an aortobifemoral bypass graft.

An indium- or technetium-labelled white cell scan can be very useful in evaluating graft infection, particularly in an elderly or frail patient in whom one would not otherwise wish to undertake major revisional surgery unless it was absolutely necessary. A positive white cell scan might, in this situation, mitigate towards a more aggressive approach where conservative measures might otherwise have been continued (Fig. 26.4).

Management

Wound infection

A superficial wound infection can be treated in the standard manner with antibiotics if there is adjacent cellulitis or discharging material. If, however, the infective process extends into the deeper tissues or involves necrosis of the wound edges, then a more aggressive plan of intervention is required. Simple options include excision of wound edges and primary suture, but this is often impossible to achieve. Where there is excessive necrosis or an exposed graft in the groin, it is essential to achieve coverage using a sartorius muscle flap. Gentamicin irrigation beads or impregnated collagen sponge should also be used.

Seroma/lymphocele

In the vast majority of cases, the lymphatic collection will resolve with time. There is no indication for antibiotic therapy unless there is evidence of pyrexia, tenderness, purulence or overlying cellulitis. Repeated aspirations may give transient relief of symptoms but the wound usually fills up with fluid fairly rapidly thereafter and aspiration may predispose to secondary infection.

The most troublesome problem is continued late discharge of lymphatic fluid through the wound. This requires considerable attention to nursing and dressing in conjunction with reassurances to the patient that ultimately the wound will heal. If, however, there are any signs or features of secondary infection, appropriate antibiotics must be started early.

Graft aneurysm

In the unlikely event that a patient presents with a primary aneurysm of the original graft, it is probably wise to excise this segment and replace it with a new piece of prosthetic material or vein. Alternatively, the entire graft can be replaced with more modern prosthetic material or vein as appropriate. Vein graft aneurysms can be monitored until they reach a diameter of 2 cm and then they should probably be surgically corrected. The majority can be treated by resection and end-to-end anastomosis as there is usually a degree of functional elongation as the aneurysm expands. Alternatively, a short segment of interposition vein is perfectly acceptable. A segment of the aneurysm wall should be sent for culture in order to exclude a low-grade infection.

Graft and outflow stenoses

Most vascular units now have a graft surveillance programme where vein grafts are monitored at 1, 3, 6 and 12 months and then 6-monthly or annually thereafter. The highest risk of stenosis formation is within the first 2 years and some centres advocate stopping the surveillance programme after that time period. In Leicester we survey the grafts indefinitely as we have had a number of failures beyond 2 years due to late undiagnosed stenoses.

Each unit must select its own criteria for intervention. In Leicester we use a peak systolic velocity ratio of ≥3 across the stenosis. Stenoses with a velocity ratio <3 should be monitored closely in the surveillance clinic.

There is no consensus as to the best way of treating a vein graft stenosis but the majority are amenable to percutaneous transluminal angioplasty (Fig. 26.1). An alternative option is to perform a patch angioplasty over the site of a recurrent stenosis or to replace a segment of the graft with

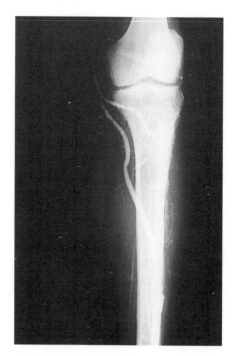

Fig. 26.5. Jump graft from lower end of femoropopliteal graft to tibial level.
The existing graft was failing due to progression of disease at the popliteal
trifurcation.

an interposition vein graft or jump graft to the native distal arteries. A
distal jump graft can be anastomosed to a piece of previously undissected
artery and then tunnelled as appropriate to join up with the original vein
graft (Fig. 26.5). If there is no long saphenous vein available in the ipsilateral leg, then cephalic vein from the arm can be used.

On occasions it is not unusual to have recurrent stenoses at the very
distal anastomosis which recur within a relatively short period of time. In
elderly and frail patients, it is probably worthwhile to persevere with
repeated angioplasties but the natural history is such that these patients
are at very high risk, ultimately requiring amputation (see Chapter 17).

The question of surveillance of prosthetic grafts is more controversial.
In Leicester we introduced a policy of prosthetic graft surveillance in
1992, but abandoned it in 1994. Although a number of run-off stenoses
were detected and treated, this greatly increased our interventional
radiology workload and did not alter long-term patency or clinical
outcome. Accordingly, we have now abandoned this practice, but we do
advise GPs to refer patients urgently should they develop worsening
symptoms.

Anastomotic stenoses may not respond well to angioplasty due to excessive neointimal hyperplasia. Revision of a popliteal anastomosis is difficult and a better option is a jump graft to a lower level or complete graft replacement (Fig. 26.5). A more recent development is removal of the hyperplastic stenosis with a percutaneous atherectomy catheter (Fig. 26.6). A stenosis at the femoral anastomosis of an aortobifemoral bypass should be treated by local revision using a patch of Dacron or vein to widen and extend the anastomosis.

Routine surveillance of angioplasty sites is not justified but duplex surveillance of stents may be. Stents may result in better initial dilatation than angioplasty alone but some patients develop marked neointimal hyperplasia, especially in low flow vessels. Stents that occlude may be difficult to recross and reintervention is easier before occlusion occurs. Like anastomotic stenoses, angioplasty alone may not be effective and atherectomy is one option to consider (Fig. 26.6).

Recurrent symptomatic carotid stenoses following endarterectomy are extremely rare but do occasionally require reoperation. In some patients, this can be an entirely straightforward procedure, while in others there can be a very dense inflammatory reaction around the bifurcation with a risk of cranial nerve injury.

If the recurrent carotid stenosis is late and of an atheromatous nature, then a second endarterectomy and patch can be performed. More commonly, however, there is a pearly-white shiny neointimal hyperplastic stenosis which is often impossible to endarterectomize. In this situation it may be preferable to perform an interposition carotid vein bypass where the vein graft is passed over the distal limb of a Pruitt-Inahara shunt. All carotid vein bypass grafts must then be entered into a surveillance programme.

An alternative to surgery in the situation of a secondary stenosis due to neointimal hyperplasia is percutaneous angioplasty.

False aneurysm

False aneurysms of the carotid artery are extremely rare and complicate 0.7% of endarterectomies. The cause is usually excessive endarterectomy or infection and treatment requires urgent re-exploration with proximal common carotid control, excision of the bifurcation and an interposition vein graft. Great care must be taken to ensure proximal control as mobilization through infected friable tissues can lead to catastrophic haemorrhage. The use of transcranial Doppler ultrasound indicates the urgency or necessity for shunting.

False aneurysms of the proximal aortic anastomosis are generally not detected clinically although on occasions, very large infected false aneurysms may present as an abdominal mass. More likely, they will be

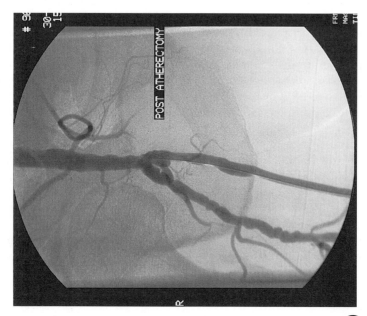

(B)

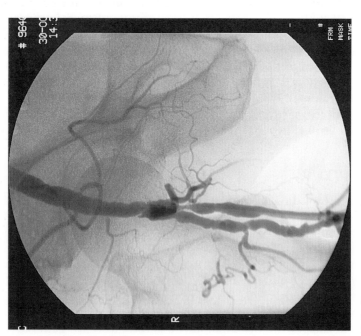

(A)

Fig. 26.6. Recurrent stenosis at proximal end of prosthetic femoropopliteal bypass (A) before and (B) after treatment by atherectomy.

encountered as part of the investigation of a patient with suspected graft infection (see below).

Groin false aneurysms are the commonest type of false aneurysm encountered. The traditional approach is to maintain a watching brief in those with a diameter of <2.5 cm. However, should they start to expand beyond this, or if the rate of expansion is rapid, they should be considered for revisional surgery. The commonest scenario is that of an aortic graft limb passing under the inguinal ligament with partial disruption of the anastomosis onto either the common femoral artery or the profunda femoris artery. Injudicious dissection over the aneurysm may lead to considerable bleeding and therefore it is prudent to mobilize the aortic graft limb via an extraperitoneal flank approach to gain control. Once the vessels have been mobilized, the distal limb of the graft is excised along with the anastomosis and specimens of the false aneurysm sac, graft and anastomosis sent for histological and bacteriological assessment. The latter is essential because a number of false aneurysms are related to low-virulence infections, and a positive culture is very helpful to guiding appropriate antibiotic therapy.

If infection is not suspected, then an interposition graft can be fashioned between the original graft limb and either the conjoint orifices of the superficial femoral and profunda femoris arteries or the profunda femoris artery lumen as an extended profundaplasty. In the absence of autologous vein it is probably wise to use either polytetrafluoroethylene (PTFE) or coated Dacron grafts with rifampicin bonding as both of these should have a greater resistance to secondary infection. If, however, there is a strong suspicion of infection, then placing a redo prosthetic graft in the original bed should be avoided if possible. The interposition graft should be anastomosed to the aortic graft limb via the extraperitoneal incision and then tunnelled through the obturator canal down to the profunda femoris artery which can be exposed via a separate incision on the medial aspect of the thigh. Alternatively, the graft can be extended down to the above-knee popliteal artery.

For these obturator bypasses, it is sensible to use either PTFE or Rifampicin-bonded Dacron grafts as veins may kink on passing through the obturator foramen. The original groin wound should then be debrided thoroughly and can be either irrigated with antibiotics, the original bed closed over gentamicin beads or over a collagen sponge impregnated with gentamicin. The latter has considerable benefits over gentamicin beads as it does not need to be removed and achieves very high tissue concentrations whilst maintaining very low systemic blood levels with no need for plasma monitoring.

Deep graft infection

Infected carotid patch

Fortunately, this is a rare problem but it can be very challenging when it does occur. The management principles involve treatment with antibiotics preoperatively, proximal control of the common carotid artery prior to exploring the carotid bifurcation and excision of the infected patch. Therapeutic options thereafter involve replacement of the prosthetic patch with a saphenous vein patch, resection of the bifurcation with insertion of an interposition vein graft or closure of the distal internal carotid artery. The latter option is the least satisfactory but in some patients it may be the only option because of the potential of ongoing infection with virulent organisms such as MRSA.

Infected aortic grafts

This is one of the most difficult complications to treat and management is largely dictated by the initial presentation of the patient. Any patient with upper gastrointestinal haemorrhage and an aortic graft must be considered to have an aortoenteric fistula until proven otherwise. Sadly, this is often ignored in non-surgical wards and unnecessary time is wasted whilst investigating other possible aetiologies. If the patient is bleeding vigorously, then a life-saving intervention may well be insertion of a balloon catheter over a guidewire via one of the groin vessels. This can be inflated at the site of the false aneurysm or just above it to enable rapid restoration of the circulating blood volume. It also enables a safer dissection around the friable periaortic tissues.

Patients with less urgent bleeding or those with clinical features of stable aortic graft infection have a number of treatment options available to them. Simple conservative management and treatment with systemic antibiotics will not work and some form of invasive therapy is necessary. Irrigation of the perigraft tissue with antibiotics via percutaneously or operatively placed catheters has been demonstrated to be successful in certain patients, but the exact role and long-term outcome remain uncertain. It is, however, a good option in the very frail patient.

For the majority, however, one is faced with the prospect of total graft excision (TGE) and some form of revascularization. A number of factors will guide the surgeon as to the appropriateness of one choice of intervention over another. These include the extent and severity of infection and the type and nature of the graft. For example, if the original proximal aortic anastomosis was end-to-side then the aortic graft can be removed and the defect closed with autologous vein. In addition, the general condition of the patient is a major mitigating factor as is the experience of the surgeon. Low-grade virulent organisms such as

Staphylococcus epidermidis present a different problem from the more aggressive MRSA which can at times be almost impossible to treat.

Thus, the options largely return to TGE with extra-anatomic vascular reconstruction or TGE in association with anatomical vascular reconstruction. Extra-anatomic vascular reconstruction involves:

- TGE preceded by axillobifemoral bypass;
- TGE with synchronous axillofemoral bypass; or
- TGE with delayed axillofemoral bypass.

The latter is now rarely performed as by the time the patient is found to need an extra-anatomic reconstruction, he is not only severely ill from the original operation, but has gross peripheral ischaemia to contend with as well. There is considerable debate as to whether the axillofemoral bypass should precede TGE or immediately follow graft excision. The advantages of the former are that the peripheries have a circulation maintained throughout the procedure but the disadvantage is that there is a risk (perhaps 40%) of secondary axillofemoral infection. Synchronous axillofemoral bypass immediately after graft excision significantly prolongs the procedure but is currently the preferred option in the standard approach to aortic graft infection management. One must accept, however, that extra-anatomical revascularization is a compromise, as it is associated with worse patency rates, reinfection and a 20% risk of aortic stump blow-out from the oversewn aorta.

More recently, there has been a vogue towards restoring 'anatomical' vascular continuity as this is thought to improve long-term patency. One option is to remove the aortic graft and achieve distal revascularization by using superficial femoral vein bypass grafts to the groin vessels. Cryopreserved arterial cadaver allografts are also resistant to infection but prone to late aneurysmal degeneration. Another alternative is the use of rifampicin-bonded, collagen-impregnated Dacron grafts. In this situation, a collagen/gelatin or albumin Dacron-coated graft is bonded with 600 mg of rifampicin for 20 min. Following TGE, the new graft is anastomosed into the *in situ* position following debridement of the graft bed. Early studies suggest that this may have some benefits over the extra-anatomic methods, but no conclusive trials are available to confirm or refute this. Late follow-up studies are vital and preliminary evidence from Leicester suggests they probably are ineffective in the management of MRSA-infected aortic grafts.

Total graft excision is a difficult procedure. The retroperitoneum is usually grossly fibrosed and indurated, particularly if there is a duodenal or enteric fistula. In practice, it is wise to mobilize the aorta at the diaphragm in order to have proximal control should unexpected haemorrhage occur. The traditional exposure of the aorta, i.e. dividing the small bowel mesentery, is difficult and access is greatly facilitated by mobilizing the right colon over towards the left, taking with it the duodenum and head of pancreas. This exposes the inferior vena cava and left renal vein and there is usually an area of undisturbed native aorta immediately below or above the renal arteries where ready access can be achieved. Once full access has been obtained, the aorta can be cross-clamped. It is then possible to open up the graft and define the extent of the fistula without having had to dissect this off during the mobilization phase. A further alternative is to mobilize the left colon, spleen, pancreas and left kidney medially to expose the suprarenal and diaphragmatic aorta. This facilitates access to the suprarenal aorta and minimizes uncontrolled blood loss.

Groin anastomotic infections

The principles of managing these are similar to those for false aneurysms. The main difficulty, however, is knowing just how extensive the infection is. If it is suspected that only the groin anastomosis is infected, then it may be possible to do a partial limb excision of a distal aortic graft limb with an obturator bypass to the profunda femoris artery or above-knee popliteal without traversing old tissue planes. Alternatively, a subscrotal approach from the opposite groin may enable revascularization. The use of autologous conduits such as saphenous vein or superficial femoral vein should reduce the risk of re-infection.

The management of significant groin wound infections following femoropopliteal reconstructions are largely dictated by the condition of the patient, clinical presentation and virulence of the organism. In our experience, MRSA in any graft requires total graft excision as it is incredibly difficult to eradicate. Infections secondary to less virulent organisms such as *Staphylococcus epidermidis* can be treated by partial graft excision and revascularization supplemented by wrapping the secondary graft with gentamicin sponges. If a new graft must be placed within an infected bed, then it may be possible to enlarge the calibre of a vein graft by a spiral saphenous vein graft or a panelled vein graft where the saphenous vein is split down its length and the two segments joined together to create a large calibre conduit. Cryopreserved arterial cadaver allografts are an alternative infection-resistant conduit.

Graft thrombosis

Prosthetic graft occlusions can usually be thrombectomized, preferably as soon as possible after the presenting event. Aortic graft limb thrombosis is usually caused by an outflow stenosis and in addition to thrombectomizing the graft, it is important to insert a patch angioplasty over the distal anastomosis. A rubbery pseudo intima can be a difficult problem to treat and it may require the passage of ring strippers to restore adequate inflow. Ring strippers should, however, be used with caution as they can easily become stuck within the proximal graft, thereby precipitating a more major surgical exploration than was initially envisaged! If it does prove impossible to clear the graft, then alternatives to revascularization include a femorofemoro cross-over graft or an axillofemoral bypass.

Below-knee femoropopliteal prosthetic grafts are often difficult to clear surgically and may benefit from percutaneous thrombolysis. If successful, underlying run-off stenoses may be demonstrated which can then be angioplasted. Failing this, it may be possible to thrombectomize a prosthetic femoropopliteal graft with a balloon embolectomy catheter. However, in the long run, redo femoropopliteal bypass will often be necessary. Femoropopliteal/distal bypass vein grafts are amenable to surgical thrombectomy provided the patient is taken to theatre within a few hours of onset, as otherwise there is rapid organization of the luminal thrombus with adherence to the vein graft wall. Catheter-directed thrombolysis in such patients using recombinant tissue plasminogen activator (rtPA) or streptokinase, with secondary angioplasty of any underlying graft or run-off stenoses, is probably a better option.

A not uncommon problem associated with surgical thrombectomy of both prosthetic and vein grafts is the situation where the graft has been cleared but there is evidence of residual thrombus within tibial vessels. This can often be lysed with 100 000 units of streptokinase or 10 mg tPA dissolved in 100 ml normal saline and infused down the graft over 30 min (Fig. 26.7).

Outcome

Wound infections, though troublesome, tend to resolve with antibiotic therapy and relatively few progress to deep problems. Blackening and skin edge necrosis is an ominous sign and some form of secondary revision is usually necessary, but rarely compromises the long-term limb salvage rate. Similarly, seromas and lymphoceles resolve with time and reassurance, and it is extremely rare for a primary lymphocele to infect the underlying graft.

In the absence of a femoropopliteal vein graft surveillance programme, cumulative 5-year vein graft patency is around 25–30%. This can be improved to about 70% with regular surveillance. However, there is no evidence that surveillance of prosthetic grafts alters clinical outcome and it does not consistently predict those grafts at risk of late occlusion. Surveillance of stents in high-risk positions may be justified.

Deep graft infection is a major problem. Left untreated, virtually every infected aortic graft will ultimately cause loss of life. There are conflicting reports in the literature concerning the outcome of the

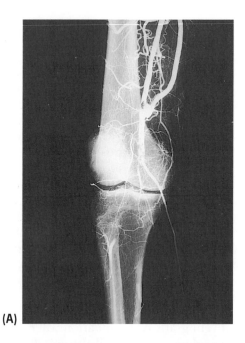

(A)

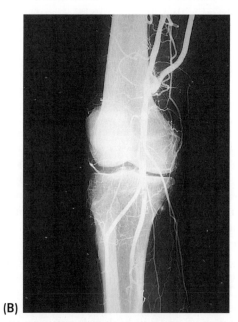

(B)

Fig. 26.7. (A) Angiogram after thrombectomy of prosthetic above-knee femoropopliteal bypass showing persistent thrombus at the level of the knee joint. (B) After thrombolysis with streptokinase there is complete clearance of the run-off.

various treatment options of major aortic graft infection but the combined mortality and amputation rate for total graft excision and axillofemoral bypass is between 40% and 70%. Evidence suggests that there is a reinfection rate of axillofemoral bypasses implanted prior to graft excision of between 25% and 40%. However, this may fall with the use of antibiotic-bonded prostheses. Aortic stump blowout occurs in 10–20% of patients following total graft excision and aortic stump oversewing and is almost invariably fatal. The role of total graft excision and rifampicin-bonded *in situ* graft replacement is under evaluation, but ongoing evidence suggests an overall mortality rate of about 20%. The outcome of peripheral graft infections is slightly better in that the overall mortality is probably lower but the rate of limb loss may be just as high.

In our experience, the presence of MRSA is an ominous predictor of outcome with a very high mortality and morbidity/limb loss rate. As a general rule, it is best to plan a reconstruction using autogenous vein if a preoperative diagnosis of MRSA infection has been made. The main problem is, however, that diagnosis of this organism is not usually made until after the revisional procedure has been performed.

Summary

- Revisional procedures now comprise a large component of a vascular unit's annual workload.
- The aetiology is variable and, as a general rule, revisional surgery is complex and not to be undertaken lightly.
- The most important problems relate to procedures to maintain graft patency and specifically the treatment of graft infection.

Areas of controversy

- Prosthetic or autogenous venous conduit material for above-knee femoro-popliteal bypasses?
- How long should you follow-up a vein graft in a surveillance programme?
- What is the appropriate velocity ratio in a graft surveillance programme for intervention with angioplasty/surgical revision?
- Is it worth attempting thrombolysis of prosthetic grafts when they occlude or should a redo femoropopliteal bypass be performed?
- Is total graft excision with *in situ* replacement with a rifampicin-bonded prosthesis safer in the long-term than total graft excision, aortic stump oversewing and extra-anatomic revascularization?
- What is the optimal treatment for infected prostheses culturing methicillin-resistant *Staphylococcus aureus*?

Further reading

- Campbell B (ed). *Operative Complications in Vascular Surgery; A Practical Approach to Management.* Oxford: Butterworth-Heinemann, 1996.
- Greenhalgh RM, Fowkes FGR (eds). *Trials and Tribulations of Vascular Surgery.* London: WB Saunders, 1996.
- Calligano KI, Veith FJ (eds). *Management of Infected Arterial Grafts.* St Louis: Quality Medical Publishing, 1994.
- Aortofemoral graft infection. *European Journal of Vascular and Endovascular Surgery* 1997;**14**(Supplt).

27
Vascular Malformations

James Jackson

Introduction

One of the major problems encountered when addressing the subject of vascular malformations is the confusion regarding their correct classification. On the basis of cell kinetics two major types of vascular birthmark, which are histologically distinct, have been demarcated:

- *haemangiomas*, which demonstrate endothelial hyperplasia;
- *malformations*, which have normal endothelial turnover.

This biological classification is now the official nomenclature used by the International Workshop of Vascular Anomalies. The term haemangioma should, therefore, be reserved for the acquired vascular tumour of infancy which enlarges by rapid cellular proliferation and always undergoes involution (sometimes incomplete).

Vascular malformations, on the other hand, are inborn errors of vascular morphogenesis and may be subclassified into high- or low-flow types depending upon the presence or absence of arteriovenous shunting, with the low-flow category further subdivided into capillary, venous, lymphatic or mixed lesions according to the type of vessel which is predominantly involved. They are present at birth and are usually evident at that time, although they may occasionally only become obvious many years later due to progressive vascular ectasia. They grow commensurately with the child, although a sudden increase in size is not uncommon during adolescence or pregnancy or as a response to trauma.

Aetiology

The cause of vascular malformations is unknown. It is generally held that anomalous vascular structures arise from arrest or misdirection of the normal development of the vascular tree during one of the three stages of vasculogenesis:

- stage of undifferentiated capillary network;
- retiform stage consisting of large plexiform structures formed by coalescence of the original equipotential capillaries;

- stage of appearance of mature vascular stems after the disappearance of the primitive elements.

It has been suggested that the lack of associated anomalies in practically all patients with sporadic vascular malformations means that these birth-marks are not the result of extraneous factors but occur purely by chance during the extremely complex developmental history of the vascular system.

Most vascular malformations are sporadic but they may rarely occur in a familial form when they are usually multiple. Recent work has identified a locus on chromosome 9p for familial venous malformations in two large kindreds in whom the condition was inherited in an autosomal dominant fashion. It has been suggested that this locus may represent a new (or unmapped) gene involved in vasculogenesis as none of the numerous angiogenesis factors that has been described maps to this region.

Arteriovenous malformations involving the pulmonary circulation may occur in association with hereditary haemorrhagic telangiectasia (HHT) which has an autosomal dominant trait. Genetic linkage for this condition has been established on the long arm of chromosome 9 and the gene at this site has been identified as Endoglin, an endothelial protein involved in the growth and function of blood vessels. Patients with this form of the disease (HHT1) have an approximately 30% chance of developing pulmonary artoriovenous malformations. Genetic linkage of HHT has also been established on chromosome 12 and families with this form of the disease (HHT2) are considerably less likely to develop pulmonary arteriovenous malformations (only 3%) but are at greater risk of arteriovenous malformations on the systemic side of the circulation, notably within the liver.

Pulmonary arteriovenous malformations lie outside the scope of this chapter and are not discussed further.

Clinical features

All malformations are present on the day of birth although they may not be evident at that time. Those with a dermal component are clearly visible, although it is important to remember that the clinically obvious cutaneous mark may represent only a small part of the total lesion. Large, deeply seated malformations may also be visible at an early stage because of associated deformity, such as localized swelling or limb hyper-trophy, although it is sometimes surprising how extensive a lesion can be without being clinically obvious.

The nature of the symptoms caused by a particular malformation depends to some extent upon its site, size and the type of vessel pre-dominantly involved.

Low-flow lesions

Capillary

These malformations, which are often the least impressive in terms of findings on clinical examination, are not uncommonly the cause of severe symptoms, particularly pain, especially when there is involvement of muscle. Examination may be unremarkable other than perhaps some minor soft tissue swelling with or without an overlying dermal stain despite extensive diffuse involvement of deep tissues on MRI. Local hyperhidrosis is common; ulceration and bleeding rarely occur.

Venous

When large, these are often the cause of severe cosmetic deformity and they may change considerably in size when the part of the body which is involved is held dependent. They not infrequently cause considerable pain, which may be due to venous engorgement when held dependent or to spontaneous thrombosis, which is common. An increase in pain often associated with swelling is not uncommonly reported after exercise of the affected part of the body and this is presumably related to an increase in blood flow through the lesion. Such discomfort may last for only a few hours or may persist for several days.

A mild consumptive coagulopathy may be evident on testing but this is rarely of clinical significance.

Overlying varicose eczema and skin ulceration may occur, particularly when there is lower limb involvement, due to unremitting venous hypertension and this is often very difficult to heal once it has developed.

Limb soft tissue and skeletal overgrowth is also a common problem with large lesions, especially when sited around the growth plates of the long bones; lower limb overgrowth causes a limp, and a painful scoliosis may develop if the leg length discrepancy is not recognized and corrected.

Lymphatic

Lymphatic lesions are often large and may be associated with dermal vesicles. They commonly present because of deformity, weeping of lymphatic fluid or secondary infection.

High-flow lesions

High-flow lesions may be asymptomatic, but many patients will complain of pain (which may be severe), local hyperhidrosis, ulceration and bleeding; the last two complications may occur with a malformation involving any superficial site but are a particular problem when the lesion involves a digit, probably due to a combination of local severe venous hypertension and distal tissue ischaemia due to a steal effect through the high-flow shunts. When massive, they may cause high-output cardiac failure, although this is fortunately rare and occurs with only the most extensive of arteriovenous malformations.

Diagnosis

In the majority of patients the diagnosis of a vascular malformation is simple and requires nothing more than a good clinical history and examination. Many patients present during early puberty with a history of an increase in the size of, or the development of symptoms related to, a soft tissue mass which has been present for many years (perhaps noted at the time of birth). Presentation is equally common, however, in patients in their second or third decades, although once again they are often aware that there was a pre-existing abnormality which had caused them little, if any, symptoms in the past.

Findings on clinical examination will vary from no abnormality to a massive lesion affecting a large part of the body. A cutaneous stain may be the full extent of a malformation or the sign of a much larger, deep-seated abnormality. A soft-tissue mass should be carefully examined and its various characteristics recorded, including:

- size;
- consistency;
- presence or absence of tenderness and pulsation;
- whether it can be transilluminated.

Soft, compressible lesions which fill rapidly when compression is released and which swell more when the part of the body which they involve is held dependent are characteristic of venous malformations. Phleboliths are often palpable within these lesions. Firm, non- or poorly-compressible lesions which are pulsatile and over which a bruit may be heard are characteristic of arteriovenous malformations.

A hand-held Doppler probe is one of the most useful instruments to have available in the outpatient clinic as this will allow the demonstration of arteriovenous shunting in some lesions in which pulsation cannot be detected clinically.

Other signs may be present which indicate that a particular lesion is long-standing such as soft-tissue and/or skeletal hypertrophy.

There are occasions, however, when the diagnosis may be less clear cut. In the neonate who has been noted to have a soft tissue swelling at, or soon after, birth it may be very difficult to be sure at initial presentation whether this represents a vascular malformation or an haemangioma. A history of development a few days or perhaps weeks after birth associated with early rapid growth strongly favours the latter diagnosis but such a clear-cut history is not always available. In such cases the true diagnosis will only become apparent on follow-up after a few months.

Post-traumatic arteriovenous fistulae may occasionally mimic a high-flow vascular malformation particularly if long-standing. There will usually be a history of significant trauma and the diagnosis can generally be easily confirmed by selective arteriography.

It is obviously critically important that a malignant soft-tissue neoplasm is not labelled as being a benign arteriovenous malformation and if there is any concern about the nature of the lesion because of an atypical history or clinical examination, then further investigation and in many cases a biopsy are mandatory. Certain lesions may mimic high-flow vascular malformations, including primary lesions such as angiosarcomas and alveolar soft part sarcomas, and metastatic vascular deposits typically originating from renal or thyroid neoplasms (Fig. 27.1). Such metastatic deposits may appear many years after treatment of a primary tumour and this again reiterates the need to obtain a good history at the time of first presentation.

A biopsy, when necessary, may be performed surgically as an open procedure. However, suitable tissue may be obtained in most instances using a percutaneous cutting biopsy needle, although image guidance is recommended when taking a core from the more vascular lesions. Ultrasound, computed tomography (CT) or magnetic resonance imaging (MRI) may usefully demonstrate portions of the 'tumour' to be biopsied which are less vascular than others. Alternatively, the biopsy can be performed during angiography. This is a useful technique, not only because it allows optimal placement of the biopsy needle in the lesion away from the largest vessels but it also allows embolization of the 'tumour' after biopsy as a primary treatment or if bleeding does occur.

Radiological investigations

Because of their rarity it is not uncommon for patients with vascular malformations to have been referred to several different specialists and hospitals before the diagnosis is even suspected and such individuals will often have undergone a variety of different investigations and sometimes even a biopsy. By the time they are referred to a clinician with a good knowledge of these lesions, they are only too relieved to be informed of the benign nature of the malformation and many of them require nothing more than a discussion about their condition and reassurance that the malformation is a 'birthmark' and not 'cancerous'. These individuals will often have a 'lump' which is not associated with any symptoms and they do not require further investigation.

In those patients in whom the diagnosis is in doubt, or who are being considered for treatment, the best investigation(s) will depend to some extent on the type of malformation and on the form of therapy which is being proposed. In practically all cases, however, an MRI scan provides

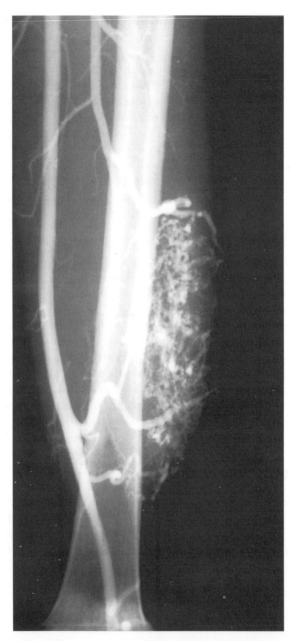

Fig. 27.1. **Highly vascular alveolar soft part sarcoma mimicking an arteriovenous malformation. This early arterial phase from the left femoral arteriogram demonstrates a highly vascular mass within the left thigh with rapid arteriovenous shunting. This angiographic appearance is not unlike that of a high-flow arteriovenous malformation, but the vessels within this mass are more irregular and the limits of the mass are better defined. A subsequent biopsy demonstrated this lesion to be an alveolar soft part sarcoma.** (Kindly supplied by Dr Peter Rowlands, Royal Liverpool University Hospital.)

the most useful information and is often the only radiological investigation which is required.

Plain films

These are rarely necessary but may be useful when assessing associated
bony abnormalities. Marked bony deformities may result from long-
standing compression by an adjacent malformation (particularly venous
lesions). These deformities are often especially notable when they involve
the facial bones as extensive facial asymmetry may result. Full-length
films of the lower extremities are seldom necessary when assessing leg
length discrepancy as an accurate measurement can usually be obtained
by careful clinical examination with the use of blocks of varying height
positioned beneath the shorter leg. If a radiological measurement is
required, however, this is best obtained by performing a CT tomogram.
Calcified phleboliths are commonly seen in venous malformations.

Ultrasound

Colour Doppler ultrasound will clearly differentiate high- from low-flow
lesions and may give an idea of the extent of the abnormality. When the
malformation has a single arteriovenous communication ('truncal'
arteriovenous malformation), the site of this may be clearly delineated
and this may be helpful during treatment. It is also a useful, non-invasive
tool for follow-up examinations, particularly of high-flow lesions.

Certain low-flow malformations may be associated with deep venous
anomalies, including aplasia or hypoplasia, and colour Doppler represents the most accurate method of assessing these vessels. It is extremely
important to appreciate the association between deep and superficial
venous abnormalities; the stripping of superficial varicosities in the presence of deep vein aplasia is likely to make matters worse rather than
better.

Computed tomography

This has been largely replaced by MRI when investigating vascular malformations because of the latter's considerably better soft-tissue delineation. Helical CT with 3D reconstructions may, however, be very useful
either when assessing bony deformity if corrective surgery is being
considered or when an MRI scan is contraindicated.

Magnetic resonance imaging

This is the most useful investigation for both initial assessment and
follow-up. The full extent of high- and low-flow vascular malformations,
including soft tissue and bone involvement, is beautifully delineated
using this modality and images may be performed in any plane which is
helpful to both the surgeon and the radiologist when planning therapy

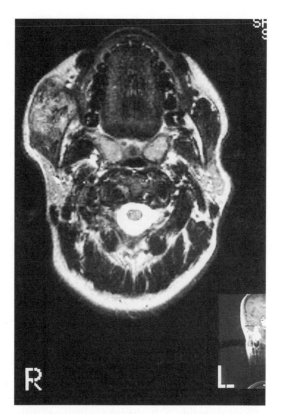

Fig. 27.2. Axial MRI scan demonstrates a mass of mixed signal intensity involving the right cheek and distorting the adjacent masseter muscle.

(Fig. 27.2). A fat suppression sequence will usually provide the best contrast between the malformation and surrounding normal tissue.

Angiography

Imaging of the arterial supply to a malformation is only required for those lesions which have been shown to be of high-flow type on clinical examination and Doppler and are being considered for treatment. Pure low-flow lesions may not show any angiographic abnormality or will be demonstrated as an increased capillary stain without arteriovenous shunting and/or some punctate staining of abnormal veins, and these findings are not useful when planning therapy.

Those low-flow lesions with an abnormal venous component as demonstrated on clinical examination, Doppler and/or MRI may be delineated by direct puncture venography and the deep veins may be separately studied at this time if there is still doubt as to their involvement.

Diagnostic direct puncture venography of these venous malformations is often combined with percutaneous sclerotherapy (*vide infra*).

Arteriography for high-flow lesions is principally performed to assess the type of arteriovenous communications which are present within the malformation which will determine the best approach for treatment by embolization (*vide infra*). This diagnostic angiogram is often combined with therapy. Occasionally, the decision will have been made by this time that surgical excision provides the best chance of long-term palliation or cure and arterial embolization is performed at this first procedure prior to planned surgery which should be performed within 24–48 h.

Management

There have been major advances in our understanding of these lesions and in our ability to treat them by embolization. It should be stressed again, however, that not all patients require treatment. In fact, in a tertiary referral centre for vascular malformations <50% of individuals seen will need any active therapy other than supportive measures, e.g. the prescription of a compression stocking in a patient with lower limb swelling and varicosities related to a venous malformation.

It is equally important to mention that these rare vascular birthmarks should only be treated in major referral centres by those who have a good understanding of the various malformations which occur. A lesion treated incorrectly by surgery or embolization may cause considerable harm and even make the lesion much more difficult to treat later.

For those malformations which are considered suitable for treatment, the different therapeutic options can be divided between:

- surgery with or without preoperative embolization;
- embolization alone.

Surgery

Surgical techniques used in the treatment of vascular malformations can be subdivided into three groups:

- excision;
- compartmentalization by suturing;
- vascular reconstruction.

Excision

Small, superficial arteriovenous malformations may occasionally be cured by surgical excision. Unfortunately, these represent by far the minority of lesions. Most are large and diffuse in nature and involve important normal adjacent structures and are, therefore, exceptionally difficult or impossible to excise.

High-flow lesions which are considered suitable for excision should undergo preoperative arterial embolization in order to reduce blood loss during surgery. Close collaboration between surgeon and radiologist is essential and it is important that both parties recognize that the aim of embolization is only to reduce the vascularity of the malformation and not to reduce the extent of the resection. Satisfactory long-term palliation or indeed cure will only be achieved if the malformation is excised in its entirety.

The surgeon must be fully informed of the extent of the embolization that has been performed. Complete devascularization of a malformation is not always possible by embolization. For example, it is not uncommon for high-flow malformations involving the face to derive some supply from the ophthalmic artery. Embolization of this vessel is not recommended for obvious reasons and if the contribution from this artery is significant, then the surgeon must be forewarned.

Arterial embolization should be performed 24–48 h before the excision as this is the time of maximal devascularization. It can usually be performed with small particles of polyvinyl alcohol. A size of particle is chosen which will produce good peripheral occlusion within the malformation itself without passing through into the venous side. Proximal arterial embolization with large particles, metallic coils or 'glue' should be avoided at all costs for two reasons; firstly, collaterals form almost immediately and satisfactory devascularization will not be achieved; and secondly, this form of embolization will interfere with subsequent arterial access if the malformation recurs.

Sutural compartmentalization

This technique may produce spectacular results in large malformations of low-flow type which are not amenable to surgical excision. A large hand-held needle is used to under-run the malformation in a criss-cross fashion and this induces thrombosis in all of the compartmentalized segments of the lesion because of the obliteration of blood flow. Some skin necrosis between and underneath the sutures is not uncommon but this usually heals in time.

Vascular reconstruction

Because of the increased use of direct puncture techniques for the embolization of even high-flow malformations (*vide infra*), the reconstruction of a suitable vascular access to a lesion for embolization is rarely required. This technique may occasionally be useful, however, when an arterial embolization is deemed to be the best form of treatment and this is denied by previous proximal embolization or by surgical ligation.

Embolization

Low-flow malformations

Venous malformations are best treated by direct puncture sclerotherapy and this should always be performed under imaging control. The technique involves a direct puncture of one of the dilated varicosities forming part of the malformation and venography to delineate its anatomy. Particular note should be made of the amount of contrast medium required to fill the abnormal vascular spaces and the opacification of normal draining veins. Prior to the injection of a liquid sclerosant, it is preferable if the lesion can be decompressed so as to increase the total surface area of the abnormal vein walls which come into immediate contract with the sclerosant. This is not always possible, however, either because the outflow from the lesion is extremely sluggish, or because there is a risk of displacing the needle or cannula from the malformation. The amount of sclerosant should be similar to the quantity of contrast medium which produced filling of the malformation on the diagnostic venogram and this should be injected during compression of normal venous outflow if this is significant. The needle or cannula is then removed and the malformation is immediately compressed.

A variety of embolic agents may be used for venous sclerotherapy, the three most commonly employed being absolute alcohol, 3% sodium tetradechol sulphate (STD) and Ethibloc®. The first of these is extremely painful when injected and, although the prior instillation of a local anaesthetic into the venous sac may relieve the discomfort, the procedure is usually best performed under a short general anaesthetic. STD does not produce the same degree of discomfort and most patients will easily tolerate the procedure with a local anaesthetic alone. Ethibloc® is a vegetable protein, predominantly prolamine or corn amino acids, which is mixed with amidotrizoic acid (for radiopacity), oleum and then with ethanol. It produces an intense inflammatory reaction which may last several weeks and although it is resorbed, this may take many months prior to which it is often discharged through the skin. All three agents produce similar results.

Complete eradication of the lesion is seldom, if ever, achieved but good, long-lasting symptomatic improvement can be expected in terms of a reduction in size, swelling and pain. Recurrent symptoms can be treated by further procedures.

Lymphatic lesions may be treated by percutaneous sclerotherapy and this may be usefully combined with surgery in certain individuals. Some of the best results have been reported with Ethibloc® (*vide supra*). After puncture and drainage of the lymphatic malformation, contrast medium is injected to delineate the anatomy and to assess the volume of the abnormal cavity. The lesion is again drained and sufficient Ethibloc® or other sclerosant (absolute alcohol, 3% STD, tetracycline) is injected to coat the walls of the sac, and compression is then applied. This may produce a satisfactory result in itself but best results are probably obtained if the malformation is subsequently excised.

High-flow vascular malformations

Embolization provides the mainstay of treatment in most high-flow vascular malformations but, whilst excellent palliation may be afforded using this technique, a cure is unlikely. Relatively new technology in the form of co-axial catheters, and the use of liquid embolic agents such as absolute alcohol and 'glue' (N-butyl-2-cyanoacrylate), has allowed embolization via an arterial approach with good clinical and radiological improvement of lesions which were previously considered untreatable.

There are still some lesions, however, which are either extremely hazardous or impossible to treat via an arterial approach because of one or more of the following reasons:

- there may be multiple small feeding arteries supplying the lesion;
- important normal arterial branches may arise in very close proximity to a malformation;
- extreme arterial tortuosity may preclude successful catheterization;
- previous therapy (embolization or surgery) may have occluded arterial access to the central portion of the malformation.

In such circumstances, direct puncture or transvenous embolization techniques may be helpful. One of these two techniques may in fact be the best method of embolization in some high-flow lesions even in the absence of one of the relative contraindications to an arterial embolization listed above (Fig. 27.3).

A knowledge of the different anatomical configurations of high-flow malformations is essential in order to understand how best to approach any particular lesion to obtain the best results from treatment by embolization. Whichever route is employed, embolization must be performed as near as possible to, or across, the arteriovenous communications themselves. Unduly proximal embolization of feeding arteries is to be deplored since, as is the case with surgical ligation, recurrence is invariable and subsequent access to the lesion for more definitive treatment will be severely compromised.

Complications

The complications which are most commonly reported during embolization of vascular malformations are the inadvertent embolization of vessels other than those supplying the lesion, and the passage of emboli through into the venous circulation. Provided that the embolization is performed with meticulous care, these complications should be very uncommon.

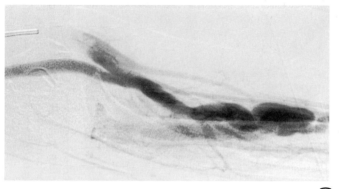

(A)

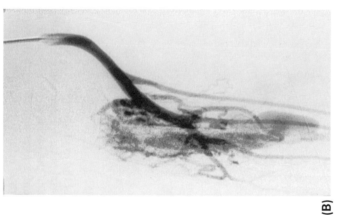

(B)

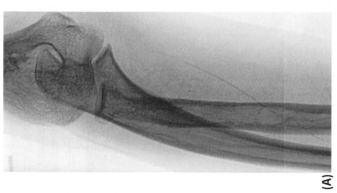

(C)

Fig. 27.3. Right radial head arteriovenous malformation treated by embolization using a retrograde venous approach. (A) Control film of the right elbow demonstrates expansion of the medullary cavity of the proximal radial shaft with enlargement of the vascular foramen. (B) Early arterial phase from right brachial arteriogram demonstrates a high-flow arteriovenous malformation involving the radial head which has numerous arterial feeding vessels. (C) Later phase from same study demonstrates a large emissary vein from the radial shaft draining into a dilated forearm vein.

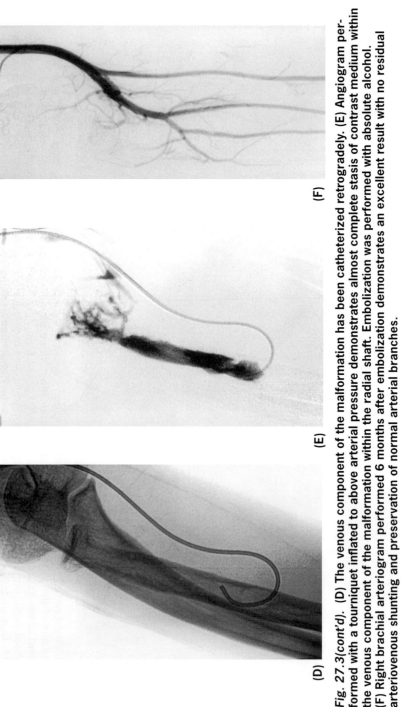

(D)

(E)

(F)

Fig. 27.3(cont'd). (D) The venous component of the malformation has been catheterized retrogradely. (E) Angiogram performed with a tourniquet inflated to above arterial pressure demonstrates almost complete stasis of contrast medium within the venous component of the malformation within the radial shaft. Embolization was performed with absolute alcohol. (F) Right brachial arteriogram performed 6 months after embolization demonstrates an excellent result with no residual arteriovenous shunting and preservation of normal arterial branches.

A 'post-embolization syndrome' which consists of a variable combination of pain at the site of the embolized arteriovenous malformation,
pyrexia, leucocytosis and a general feeling of malaise, is common after
the procedure, particularly if the malformation is large. The condition
generally lasts for only 24–48 h but may persist for a week or more before
it disappears. Symptomatic treatment is usually all that is required.

The more serious complication of infection at the site of embolization
is exceedingly rare but could produce the same symptoms as the 'post-
embolization syndrome' and the possibility of this complication should
always be considered. Blood cultures should be taken in any case
featuring pyrexia and leucocytosis.

Summary

- Vascular malformations are uncommon.
- Cause often unknown but some evidence for genetic associations.
- They are classified as low and high low lesions.
- Treatment options are lesion specific.

Areas of controversy

- Role of embolization prior to surgery.
- Need for treatment of asymptomatic vascular malformations.

Further reading

- Mulliken JB. Classification of vascular birthmarks. In: Mulliken JB, Young AE (eds) *Vascular Birthmarks. Hemangiomas and Malformations.* Philadelphia: WB Saunders, 1988, pp 24–37.
- Young AE. Pathogenesis of vascular malformations. In: Mulliken JB, Young AE (eds) *Vascular Birthmarks. Hemangiomas and Malformations.* Philadelphia: WB Saunders, 1988, pp 107–113.
- Allison DJ. Interventional radiology. In: Grainger RG, Allison DJ (eds) *Diagnostic Radiology. An Anglo-American Textbook of Imaging,* 2nd edn. Edinburgh: Churchill Livingstone, 1992, pp 2329–2390.

28
Vascular Access

Derek Manas

Introduction

Recent advances in surgical technique, the development of poly-tetrafluroethylene (PTFE) synthetic grafts and the introduction of per-cutaneous central vein catheter kits have allowed high-risk, elderly and diabetic patients to benefit from both dialysis and kidney transplantation. Nevertheless, the task of ensuring patency and function of any vascular access procedure remains a significant challenge.

In the mid to late 1950s, establishing patients on haemodialysis required repeated cannulation of distal arteries and veins at each 'sitting'. In 1960, Quinton *et al* introduced an external silastic shunt as a means of repeated vascular access. Although this was a significant advance, the shunt was associated with multiple complications. In 1966, Brescia *et al* introduced the arteriovenous fistula (AVF), an endogenous shunt utilizing the cephalic vein and radial artery. Although there are now many variations of the technique, this 'endogenous fistula' is still regarded as the 'gold standard' method of establishing haemodialysis access.

Selection of mode of access

Modes of access available

Currently, the standard approaches include:

- arteriovenous fistula (AVF) (Fig. 28.1).
- 'bridge' graft (PTFE) (Fig. 28.2).
- central venous line.

Although few studies have compared these approaches in a prospective, randomized fashion, most access surgeons would agree that the native AVF, typically constructed as a side-to-side cephalic vein to radial artery anastomosis, remains the procedure of choice because of its superior long-term patency and low frequency of early and late complications.

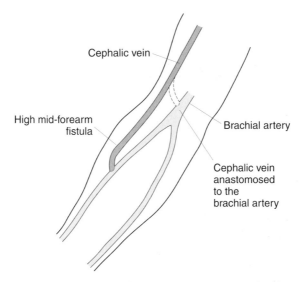

Fig. 28.1. **High mid-forearm arteriovenous fistula.**

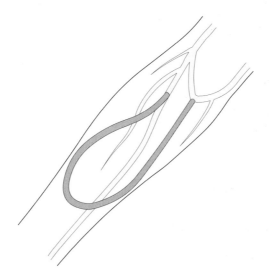

Fig. 28.2. **'Bridge' graft for arteriovenous access.**

The preoperative evaluation

Permanent cuffed venous catheters are associated with an unacceptably high rate of large vein stenosis, thrombosis and subsequent AVF dysfunction, especially long-term subclavian lines. Therefore, all patients requiring chronic haemodialysis should be evaluated for a surgically created shunt.

The preoperative assessment involves a physical examination and/or colour Doppler of the native vessels. As a result, suitable blood vessels that have not been damaged by infection or thrombosis can be identified.

With a venous tourniquet in place, the entire course of the cephalic vein should be examined for patency from the wrist to the shoulder. Gentle percussion of the distended vein at the wrist should transmit a wave that can be felt or heard using a hand-held Doppler at the ante-cubital vein and beyond. This simple test can be performed in the consulting room and used to screen out patients who require further preoperative investigation such as a colour Doppler ultrasound or venography.

If the cephalic vein is patent, the site of the access can be planned. The anastomosis to the radial artery should be as distal as possible. The anatomical 'snuff-box' fistula between the tendons of the extensor polli-cis longus and brevis is the most distal of the endogenous AVFs and gives the longest length of cephalic vein. Published results for snuff-box fistulae show a mean actuarial patency of 76% at 1 year and 73% at 2 years, which compares favourably with the 75% 2-year overall cumulative patency rates with Brescia–Cimino fistulae (Fig. 28.3).

When planning the access, one should ensure that a sufficient length of adequately sized vein is available after arterialization to allow two needles to be inserted sufficiently far apart to avoid recirculation of dialysed blood. The availability of a suitable vein remains the limiting factor and in up to 30% of patients, suitable native vessels will not be available and a prosthetic PTFE 'bridge' fistula will be necessary.

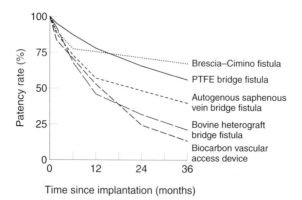

Fig. 28.3. Cumulative patency rates for different access procedures as a function of time.

Fistulae that use small or inadequate veins, although technically feasible as shown by a patent anastomosis, are difficult to cannulate, fail to provide efficient dialysis and usually occlude soon after placement due to difficult and traumatic cannulations. The use of small veins in the hope that the increased blood flow will dilate them enough to give adequate dialysis is a mistake. In the event of early failure due to poor vein quality or size, one should proceed proximally to the cubital fossa.

Brachiocephalic fistulae have excellent short- and medium-term patency rates, presumably because the anastomosis is technically easier to perform, with the upper arm veins being generally larger than those of the forearm. Nevertheless, brachiocephalic and brachiobasilic fistulae, although technically feasible, may only arterialize a short segment of superficial vein that cannot be used for repeated long-term needling. In the case of a brachiobasilic fistula, the resultant arterialized vein may be far too medial for practical and comfortable needling. In such circumstances, the basilic vein can be superficialized and transposed medially. In addition, the proximal cubital fossa AVF may predispose the elderly, atherosclerotic or diabetic patients to a distal 'steal' syndrome because of its tendency to enlarge over time. Care should be taken to keep the arteriovenous anastomosis within the recommended 5–7 mm length.

Although the cephalic vein of the non-dominant arm is the vein of choice, the quality of the cephalic vein is the limiting factor in determining both early and long-term outcome. Therefore, if the venous anatomy of the dominant arm better conforms to the required specifications, that side should be used rather than stubbornly trying to enforce the 'non-dominant' rule.

Access techniques

Chronic venous access catheters

Two basic types of catheters are available:

- those for 'short-term' (<1 week) temporary use;
- those for 'long-term' (weeks or months) or more permanent use.

Catheters for 'short-term' use are indicated for acute dialysis, plasmaphoresis or haemofiltration and carry a relatively low risk of early complications (<5%). Those for long-term use are indicated because of failure to recover rapidly from an acute event or in established end-stage renal disease (ESRD). Often patients in acute renal failure are metabolically and haemodynamically unstable, making them poor candidates for any surgical procedure. More permanent catheters (teflon, polyurethane and silastic) have been developed for patients who have exhausted all access sites or who have severe cardiac failure.

Subclavian vein catheterization is still used, especially for temporary access. A growing body of evidence appears to suggest that these catheters are associated with a 50% incidence of large vein stenosis and thrombosis. As consequence, catheterization of the subclavian vein for 'short-term' dialysis should be avoided and the placement of long-term double-lumen cuffed venous catheters should be restricted to the internal jugular veins unless there are exceptional circumstances. The long-term complications of subclavian vein thrombosis and stenosis can impair venous drainage of subsequent fistulae in the upper limb.

The actuarial survival rate of chronic venous catheters is difficult to assess. Some centres report 1- and 2-year survival rates of 50% and 41%, respectively.

Arteriovenous fistulae

Once selected, the chosen limb should be 'protected' from venesection and intravenous cannula insertion prior to fistula formation.

Constructing an AVF under general anaesthesia or a regional nerve block may be associated with unnecessary morbidity and unwanted hypotension. Moreover, local anaesthetic infiltration is simple, has equivalent results and allows for more flexibility when dealing with the elderly patient with chronic renal failure.

Radiocephalic fistulae

The artery and vein are exposed through a longitudinal or transverse incision at the wrist. The radial nerve is carefully preserved. Whichever technique (end-to-side or side-to-side) is selected, it is important to remember that approximately 30% of the blood flow through any fistula comes from the distal artery and a side-to-side anastomosis can produce increased venous pressure down stream, with painful venous congestion of the ipsilateral thumb. Therefore, if a side-to-side AVF is performed at the wrist, the distal limb of the vein should be ligated at the end of the procedure.

Venous resistance to flow or pain on flushing are features indicative of undiagnosed venous obstruction or inflammation and render the vein unsuitable.

Patients should be adequately hydrated prior to surgery to reduce the risks of early thrombosis associated with hypotension. Vasospasm from handling the vessel, particularly the artery, can be reduced by the local use of papaverine.

Small calibre vessels increase the probability of technical failure (30%). This problem can be minimized by the use of optical magnification and continuous non-absorbable fine sutures (7–0 prolene or CV7 Goretex); some surgeons adopt the microvascular approach of 8–0 interrupted sutures. Vascular clips (VCS) are now available and preliminary data suggest they allow a shorter operation time and give improved success rates.

If the flow is inadequate after completion of the anastomosis, a number of factors may be responsible:

- poor technique;
- poor run-off;
- vasospasm;
- inadequate mobilization of the vessels.

A common error is to assume a pulse distal to the anastomosis is indicative of a successful fistula. Pulsatile flow indicates a patent anastomosis but the absence of a thrill usually indicates a proximal obstruction or low flow and in the absence of reversible factors such as hypotension or vasospasm is a poor prognostic sign. Tissue lying across the vein should be divided to reduce the inevitable compressive effect.

After surgery the limb is kept warm and the blood pressure maintained to avoid hypotension. If the flow ceases, then the patient should only be returned to the operating room if the surgeon feels that the problem is remediable. A difficult anastomosis with tiny vessels is unlikely to be remedied. The failure should be accepted as due to inappropriate selection. Patency rates at 1 year can be expected to be of the order of 65%.

Brachiocephalic fistulae

The second choice after a radiocephalic fistula is a brachiocephalic fistula constructed in the antecubital fossa. It gives patency rates that are generally better than those for radial fistulae but arterial steal is the chief complication. These anastomoses are either performed side-to-side or end-to-side (vein-to-artery). The length of the anastomosis should be restricted to minimize the risk of 'steal' (<6 mm). All other technical factors are similar to those discussed for radial fistulae.

'Bridge' grafts for vascular access

A bridge graft uses a graft to join the artery and vein. This has the advantage that many more sites are available but has the disadvantage of lower patency (Fig. 28.2). Arm grafts are preferable to lower limb grafts because of the higher infection rate with the latter, which may result in amputation or death. The following materials can be used:

- autogenous saphenous vein grafts;
- semi-synthetic bovine carotid and human umbilical vein grafts;
- synthetic PTFE grafts.

Complications

Chronic central venous lines

These have the following complications:

- *Haemopneumothorax* (2%).
- *Haemomediastinum and cardiac tamponade* (guidewire puncture of the right atrium or of the superior vena cava).
- *Catheter occlusion* (25% of long-term catheters). The most expeditious way of managing occlusion is to reinsert another catheter. A method of unclotting catheters is to use thrombolytic agents as a slow continuous infusion over hours (streptokinase, urokinase or thromboplastin activator).
- *Subclavian vein thrombosis and stenosis* (20%). These are directly related to the duration of catheter placement. Most are not clinically recognizable until after placement of an AVF. Venous angioplasty is successful if the stenosis is detected prior to complete occlusion. Unfortunately, recurrence following angioplasty is common (1-year patency of 45% and 12% at 2 years). Vascular endoprostheses have been used for patients in whom stenoses recur <2 months after angioplasty. The Wallstent, a stainless steel multifilament tube device, is the most commonly used.
- *Infection* is the leading cause of morbidity and the second leading cause of death in haemodialysis patients. Central venous catheters become colonized in 20% of patients and bacteraemia develops in 10%. The risk of line sepsis can be minimized by the use of topical antiseptic wraps and antibiotic prophylaxis at the time of line insertion.

Arteriovenous fistulae and 'bridge' grafts

These have the following complications:

- *Acute thrombosis* is the commonest early complication of any access procedure and is usually a result of technical error or hypotension.
- *Early Infection* (within the first 72 h) is most commonly due to a Gram-positive (staphylococcal) organisms, is often superficial and can be prevented by routine use of prophylactic antibiotics.
- *Venous stenosis* which develops in the proximal third of the arterialized vein is an ominous and difficult problem to treat. With regular surveillance these lesions can be identified angiographically prior to complete occlusion and treated by percutaneous transluminal angioplasty (PTA).
- *Venous aneurysms* commonly occur with radiocephalic fistulae. They usually require no treatment provided the skin overlying the fistula is

intact. These aneurysms usually remain stable for many years and, provided the dialysis staff needle the fistula intelligently, never cause major problems.

- *Ischaemia* secondary to steal is a rare complication of radiocephalic fistulae, but a common complication of brachiocephalic fistulae, especially in diabetics, and is related to a progressive increase in fistula size, with reversal of flow in the distal radial artery.
- *Venous hypertension* is caused by proximal venous obstruction. The affected limb becomes engorged, painful, hyperpigmented and ulcerated. Phlebography can confirm the diagnosis and treatment includes percutaneous radiographic stenting (Palmaz or Wallstent) with or without thrombolytic therapy, surgical bypass or fistula ligation.
- *Late infection* of PTFE grafts usually results from contamination due to direct inoculation at the time of needling. Most graft infections are again staphylococcal in nature, the majority occur in the first 6 months post placement and can be prevented with the use of appropriate anti-staphylococcal antibiotic cover. Established infections need aggressive treatment. Localized graft infection may be amenable to local excision and bypass but systemic sepsis requires complete removal.
- *Late thrombosis* occurring after 3 months is most often related to neo-intimal hyperplasia and narrowing of the anastomosis or disruption of the neointima at needling sites with exposure of the thrombogenic surface. Management includes PTA and/or thrombolytic therapy. Endovascular stenting in more peripheral veins and across anastomoses are now becoming commonplace but the long-term outcome of these procedures is still awaited. Prospective screening may allow early intervention and prolong the useful life of the access graft (Table 28.1).

Table 28.1. **Assessment of haemodialysis access.**

Flow	Electromagnetic flow probe
	Duplex ultrasound
	Recirculation of dialysed blood (urea)
	Indicator dilution methods
Structure	Angiography and intra-access pressure measurements
	Duplex ultrasound
	Venous dialyser pressure

Summary

- The cephalic vein-to-radial artery arteriovenous fistula is the first choice method of vascular access.
- Permanent cuffed venous catheters have a high complication rate.
- Vein is the best conduit but should be of adequate size.
- Arteriovenous fistulae fail because of poor technique, poor run-off and vasospasm.
- Bridge grafts have lower patency rates.

Areas of controversy

- Timing of access.
- What is the best angioaccess in the elderly (>70 years)?
- Under what circumstances should PTFE 'bridge' grafts be used as primary access?
- Which PTFE graft is best: Diastat *vs* ePTFE?
- Long-term outcome of peripheral and central endovascular stenting.

Further reading

- Dow R. Surveillance of angioaccess shunt function. In: Ernst CB, Stanley JC (eds) *Current Therapy in Vascular Surgery*. BC Deciker, 1991, pp 932–934.
- Marx AB, Landmann J, Harder FH. Surgery for vascular access. *Current Problems in Surgery* 1990;**27**:1.
- Haimov M. Direct arteriovenous anastomosis for angioaccess. In: Ernst CB, Stanley JC (ed) *Current Therapy in Vascular Surgery*. BC Decker, 1991, pp 922–926.
- Haimov M, Baez A, Neff M. Complications of arteriovenous fistulae for haemodialysis. *Archives of Surgery* 1975:**110**:708–712.
- Schanzer H, Schwartz M, Harrington E *et al.* Treatment of ischaemia due to 'steal' by arteriovenous fistulae with distal artery ligation and revascularization. *Journal of Vascular Surgery* 1988;**7**:770–773.

29

The Future of Vascular Surgery: Areas of Controversy and Research

Roger M Greenhalgh

Introduction

Vascular surgery has developed almost entirely over the last 50 years. Michael DeBakey had the concept and developed the roller pump for cardiopulmonary bypass when he was a medical student. He moved to Houston, Texas and introduced Dacron in the early 1950s for the replacement of many of the great vessels. He also stressed the surgical importance of the profunda femoris.

In the late 1940s, Dos Santos in Lisbon developed endarterectomy and this was further developed by EJ Wylie in San Francisco and Cockett in London. The first publication on carotid surgery in 1954 was from Felix Eastcott, but it was Jesse Thompson who set the standards in carotid surgery and showed what could be achieved.

Robert Linton demonstrated the importance of the calf perforating veins. Kinmonth at St Thomas' and Gerry Taylor at St Bartholomew's in London produced the first lymphogram and virtually all of the knowledge on lymphoedema.

Almost all the pioneering work has taken place in university centres. At first, many of the pioneers were single-handed, but they soon found that this was not a suitable option and aggregation of services has taken place slowly over the years.

Organization of vascular services

There are many problems for the single-handed vascular surgeon, not least that it is difficult to get time off. A single-handed vascular surgeon seldom has a trainee who has a dedicated interest in a future in vascular surgery. It has not been practicable to concentrate all the investigative requirements and necessary staffing around a single vascular surgeon.

The latest concept as outlined in a provisional document on vascular services prepared for the Vascular Surgical Society of Great Britain and Ireland by the Vascular Advisory Committee recommends, as a first choice, that regional centres should be created to serve populations of approximately 600 000. The old concept of the District General Hospital (DGH) was developed in the 1960s to serve a population of some 250 000. It follows that in future vascular surgery may not be offered at every DGH. If this is to be the case, then a number of options are possible for the aggregation of vascular services or co-operation between vascular teams. The final picture will largely depend upon the geographical needs.

There is a clear need for the establishment of an emergency vascular rota with a consultant, dedicated vascular surgeon to be on-call, say 1 night a week, or 1 in 5, and 1 weekend in 5. Ideally, under each consultant there would be a dedicated vascular trainee. Many regional vascular centres have such trainees, but only in a university hospital are there likely to be junior surgeons in training perform research and under such circumstances, they can earn extra money and take emergencies in 1 in 5, just like the consultants. It is becoming increasingly important that a consultant radiologist and his juniors are also available to the same extent as the surgeons (see below).

A regional vascular service serving a population of approximately 600 000 can only be achieved if there is an aggregation of vascular services. At such a centre there will need to be the highest quality of diagnostic facilities and, ideally, a one-stop vascular diagnostic centre where vascular technologists can work alongside vascular surgeons. The technologists have recently created their own professional body and work largely with colour Doppler to achieve non-invasive diagnosis in most vascular conditions. They are largely available by day only, but in the future it may become essential to have an on-call rota for them also, or if not, for vascular or radiological trainees to learn the technique of colour Doppler scanning in their training.

Vascular nursing is another discipline which has developed in recent years. Perhaps the specialist vascular nurse emerged when the skills of the four-layer bandage technique were taken into the community for the healing of venous ulcers. This service is largely in the hands of specially trained nurses who achieve a network across the community in association with general practitioners and primary care centres, and linked with regional centres. These links with the community can be developed further through the vascular nurse system and with the development of the Primary Care Group concept.

It is helpful if the regional centre is based at a university centre as this enables clinical trials to be performed to settle some of the controversies in vascular surgery. It is generally felt that a randomized controlled trial is likely to answer specific questions, but at present there seem to be more 'tribulations' in vascular surgery where it is thought the answer is known but the evidence is extremely weak. There is a slow move towards vascular surgery with an evidence base. Novel endovascular technologies are being introduced rapidly and each will require extremely careful evaluation and most will need to be subjected to a randomized controlled trial.

Emergency services account for the majority of admissions in vascular surgery and it is absolutely vital to have expert imaging out of hours. The vascular radiologist is at least as vital as the vascular surgeon, hence the call for an equivalent rota for vascular radiology. Frequently today, acute thrombotic episodes can be managed more effectively by lytic therapy than blind interventional surgery aiming to fish out a clot. The partnership of radiologists and surgeons in the emergency situation inevitably leads to a better grasp of the diagnosis of a truly acute ischaemia and an acute on chronic one. Radiologists and surgeons can combine to decide if the critical lesion is best managed by balloon angioplasty, stenting or surgery. The radiology–surgery partnership is never so necessary as for the endovascular repair by stent graft of an abdominal aortic aneurysm.

Around the vascular surgeon and radiologist has developed the vascular biologist within university centres. There has been a tremendous increase in the knowledge of the causation of vascular disease, particularly that of aortic aneurysm, vein graft stenosis and perhaps the whole restenosis process. In this decade, the Marfan gene was found on chromosome 15 and on chromosome 16 to be a cluster of genes has been found to be responsible for matrix metalloproteinases and their inhibitors. It has also been demonstrated that the aneurysmal disease process is always associated with greater inflammation. It is inevitable that medical trials will shortly be reporting on outcomes of the control of inflammation or genetic-manipulation in the expansion rate of an aortic aneurysm. It is known that patients who smoke have a faster expansion rate than those who do not, and so there is potential for influencing the expansion rate of aortic aneurysms by altering environmental factors.

For the low-flow situation and small arteries, the vein bypass has been shown to be the best material and is used widely for coronary artery bypass and distal bypass in the limb. Unfortunately, vein graft stenoses occur and there are now increasing data to show why this occurs and medical intervention to limit vein graft stenoses should be available shortly.

Vascular surgery over the 50 years has developed largely around university centres in large part because vascular surgery has moved so fast. It is perhaps developing faster now than ever before and vascular surgery can be expected to advance at least as fast over the next few decades. If regional centres aggregate around universities, then it is absolutely vital that surgeons and radiologists share sessions and hold outpatient clinics at nearby DGHs. Only in this way, using the so called 'hub and spoke' system, can a whole population be served optimally. There has to be a continuum of referral from the primary health care professions, the community, the DGH and the specialist centre. General practitioners are becoming more sophisticated and they are likely to refer patients the extra yard to a specialist vascular unit than to the nearest hospital if the vascular services there are scanty.

Future trends in vascular research

Arterial disease

Since the reporting of the North American and European carotid trials for symptomatic disease, the profession has recognized the benefit of carotid surgery for symptoms of transient ischaemic attack (TIA) and mini stroke. Whether carotid surgery is effective for established stroke, progressing stroke or crescendo TIA is much less certain. Progressing stroke is a fairly unusual presentation and implies a deterioration of neurological deficit over at least a 24-h period. Reports of urgent interventions for progressing stroke have been good, but for crescendo TIA the outcome is far less reliable.

Originally, it was suggested that surgery should be delayed for at least 3 months after an established stroke, in order not to cause bleeding into an infarction. There is now a much less rigid application of this rule and there have not been reports of the precipitation of intracranial bleeds by doing operations too soon after an established stroke.

The results of carotid surgery for symptomatic disease, particularly TIA and amaurosis fugax, are improving with careful cerebral monitoring, transcranial Doppler, EEG and other modalities, and stroke rates are falling in expert centres.

Radiologists are looking to implant wall stents to trap the embolizing atheroma after balloon angioplasty in the carotid bifurcation, but it is not certain whether this is effective. The recent CAVATAS trial implies an approximately 10% stroke rate for both surgery and carotid stenting. Radiologists suggest this shows that stenting is as good as surgery, but many surgeons suggest that a 10% stroke rate is much too high by 1998 standards in a specialist centre. It is difficult to know what the outcome of this will be and even if short-term results with a carotid wall stent are good, then long-term outcome must be followed by random controlled trial before decisions are made on optimum treatment. Until that time, carotid endarterectomy is without doubt the gold standard.

The justification for carotid surgery for asymptomatic carotid disease is, by contrast, certainly not proven. The outcome of the asymptomatic carotid surgical trial is awaited with enthusiasm. This is based in London, but includes many centres in the UK and Europe. Surgeons and radiologists have recruited patients for whom there is some doubt whether an operation should be performed at all. In practical terms, this means patients with very severe asymptomatic carotid stenoses, almost always >80% and often >90%. Some regard the outcome of the Asymptomatic Carotid Artery Study (ACAS) based in the USA as a justification for carotid endarterectomy for asymptomatic disease. It would be fair to say that the enthusiasm for this viewpoint is stronger in the USA than in Europe.

Management of abdominal aortic aneurysm

The UK small aneurysm trial has recently been reported and there is no benefit for surgery within the first 3 months after randomization against surveillance to 5.5 cm or to tenderness of aneurysm or growth of >1 cm/year. Most vascular centres in the world are interested in the Endovascular Repair of Aortic Aneurysm and the so-called EVAR Trials, which are to commence in the UK in 1999. EVAR1 will compare open repair with EVAR in fit patients and EVAR2 will compare best medical against best medical + EVAR in patients deemed unfit for open repair by being classified as American Society of Anesthesia (ASA) Grade IV. There is considerable healthy scepticism about the durability of EVAR systems, particularly among radiologists.

Thoracoabdominal aneurysms have also been corrected by stent graft systems. This is particularly facilitated if there is a neck just above the renals and one just below the renals. Under these circumstances, the thoracic aneurysm can be corrected separately from an abdominal aneurysm. Where it is impossible to apply an EVAR system below the renals, at open repair a thoracic aneurysm endovascular system can be deployed under X-ray control and then the abdominal repair performed by open surgery. Initial results over the short term seem to be satisfactory and it is suspected that the paraplegia rate will be lower than with the conventional open surgical method. This is by no means certain and is very controversial.

Intermittent claudication

The management of intermittent claudication is determined at the one-stop diagnostic clinic where the extent of the disease is mapped by duplex scan. Many surgeons are prepared to operate on aortic aneurysm and carotid arteries to avoid stroke in smokers. In other words, they will advise patients to stop smoking but will operate without question to save life. When it comes to saving legs, most surgeons perform limb salvage procedures and also give advice to stop smoking, but for intermittent claudication, the urgency to intervene is not the same. Many surgeons demand a 3-month period of no smoking before intervening. This author's view is that it is reasonable to expect a patient to enter a type of contract with the surgeon and radiologist and that before any intervention they should stop smoking in order to reduce the risks of restenosis or bypass failure.

The results for aortoiliac procedures in terms of durability are much better than for femoropopliteal procedures and there is greater enthusiasm for angioplasty in the aortoiliac segment even in the smoker. These days the aortic bifurcation graft is rarely used, whereas 10 or more years ago, it was perhaps the commonest operation performed. Radiologists can almost always correct at least one of the iliac systems by balloon angioplasty, allowing for a femorofemoral cross-over bypass graft.

These days femoral angiography is not usually required as an investigation of intermittent claudication because duplex scanning has become so good in the hands of a trained vascular technologist. The femoropopliteal segment is of interest in the claudicant only when the aortoiliac system is corrected and the patient has stopped smoking. If the lesion is long, the only option is a bypass. Supragensiculate bypass with a prosthetic has been shown to be as good as with vein, but vein bypass is better when it is necessary to cross the knee. *In situ* and reverse vein is equally good.

For the short femoropopliteal lesion of 8 cm or less, there is always the question of whether angioplasty should be performed, or whether the patient should be told to exercise and stop smoking. Trials in Edinburgh and Oxford have pointed to the possibility of exercise being as good as angioplasty after a 2-year period. It seems that a stent gives no improvement in the femoropopliteal segment. The question is whether a supervised exercise programme is better than simple advice and if this is much better after a 2- or 3-year period than balloon angioplasty. The outcome of trials looking at this question are eagerly awaited and the area remains controversial at present.

If a vein is used for bypass, duplex surveillance is routine. The development of vein graft stenoses are plotted and further interventions are recommended. At present, there is no evidence that vein graft surveillance benefits the patient compared with simple clinical follow-up. Certainly, vein graft surveillance and the performance of many additional procedures is expensive and cannot be assumed to be to the patient's benefit. A randomized controlled trial testing surveillance is under way and this should clarify this area of controversy.

The endovascular revolution is hitting the management of aneurysm and carotid stenosis, as well as the aortoiliac and femoropopliteal arterial segments but there are other applications, e.g. the control of a traumatic arteriovenous fistula by a wall stent applied to the inside of an artery in a hostile groin. It is fair to say that just about every arterial procedure can be treated or will be treatable by an endovascular method. The question is whether these novel techniques will improve outcome, and will only be answered by randomized controlled trials.

Venous surgery

The commonest vascular operation is for varicose veins but it is still not known whether non-invasive and, in particular, duplex marking of varicose veins leads to improved varicose vein surgery with more durable results. Trials are underway to address this.

For the management of venous ulcer, the four-layer bandage technique is used. This revolutionized the management of venous ulcers by nurses in the community, but the place of surgery in the management of venous ulcers is still not known. It is suspected that four-layer compression heals ulcers just as fast whether corrective surgery is performed or not, and that once a venous ulcer has healed, the recurrence rate of venous ulceration will be greater if the underlying venous problem is left uncontrolled. Trials are under way to examine this area.

Fortunately, approximately 50% of patients have simple primary varicose veins and these are easily correctable by simple surgery. A further 35% of venous ulcer patients have primary varicose veins and some other deep venous problem. By operating on the simple veins only in these patients, the improvement in venous function could be beneficial in maintaining the healing of venous ulceration. Colour Doppler scanning and the one-stop vascular diagnosis clinics are very useful in the arterial system, but they have also virtually replaced the diagnostic venogram. Deep vein thromboses can be diagnosed accurately with duplex, particularly in the larger veins above the popliteal. In addition, the whole of the venous pathology in venous ulceration can be studied by duplex scan and the outcome of interventional surgery can be monitored by this method also.

Summary

- Vascular surgery is continuing to develop rapidly.
- With radiologists, it appears that most vascular lesions can be treated by the endovascular method.
- Medical cures are on the way with a better understanding of vascular biology.

Further reading

- Greenhalgh RM, Fowkes FGR. *Trials and Tribulations in Vascular Surgery.* London: WB Saunders, 1996.
- Darke SG. Vascular Advisory Committee of the Vascular Surgical Society of Great Britain and Ireland. *The Provision of Vascular Services.* A provisional document presented to the VSS at the AGM, November 1997.

Index